CHILD AND ADOLESCENT
MENTAL HEALTH

CORE HANDBOOKS IN PEDIATRICS

CHILD AND ADOLESCENT MENTAL HEALTH

Editors

David L. Kaye, M.D.

Associate Professor of Clinical Psychiatry
Director of Training in Child and Adolescent Psychiatry
SUNY at Buffalo School of Medicine and Biomedical Sciences
Children's Hospital of Buffalo
Buffalo, New York

Maureen E. Montgomery, M.D.

Clinical Assistant Professor of Pediatrics
SUNY at Buffalo School of Medicine and Biomedical Sciences
Buffalo, New York

Stephen W. Munson, M.D.

Associate Professor (Part-Time) of Psychiatry and Pediatrics
Director, Child and Adolescent Psychiatry Residency Training Program
University of Rochester School of Medicine and Dentistry
Rochester, New York

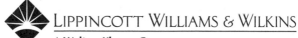

LIPPINCOTT WILLIAMS & WILKINS
A **Wolters Kluwer** Company
Philadelphia • Baltimore • New York • London
Buenos Aires • Hong Kong • Sydney • Tokyo

Acquisitions Editor: Timothy Y. Hiscock
Developmental Editor: Michael Standen
Production Editor: Emily Lerman
Manufacturing Manager: Tim Reynolds
Cover Designer: Jeane Norton
Compositor: Circle Graphics
Printer: R. R. Donnelley, Crawfordsville

Library of Congress Cataloging-in-Publication Data

Child and adolescent mental health / editors, David L. Kaye,
Maureen E. Montgomery, Stephen W. Munson.
   p. ; cm. — (Core handbooks in pediatrics)
  Includes bibliographical references and index.
  ISBN 0-7817-3015-5 (alk. paper)
   1. Child mental health. 2. Teenagers—Mental health. 3. Adolescent
psychology. 4. Child psychiatry. 5. Children—Mental health. 6. Child
mental health services. I. Kaye, David L. II. Montgomery, Maureen E.
(Maureen Elmer), 1948- III. Munson, Stephen W. IV. Series.
   [DNLM: 1. Mental Disorders—Adolescence. 2. Mental Disorders—Child.
3. Adolescent Psychology. 4. Child Psychology. WS 105.5.M3 C536 2003]
RJ499.3 .C457 2003
362.2′083–dc21

                    2002072983

---

10 9 8 7 6 5 4 3 2 1

♣ Contents

Contributing Authors

Helen R. Aronoff, M.D., *Assistant Professor of Clinical Psychiatry, Department of Psychiatry, SUNY at Buffalo School of Medicine; Attending Physician, Department of Psychiatry, Erie County Medical Center, Buffalo, New York*

William J. Barbaresi, M.D., *Assistant Professor, Department of Pediatric and Adolescent Medicine, Mayo Medical School; Chair, Division of Developmental and Behavioral Pediatrics, Mayo Clinic, Rochester, Minnesota*

Michelle S. Barratt, M.D., M.P.H., *Associate Professor, Division of Adolescent Medicine, Department of Pediatrics, University of Texas—Houston Medical School, Houston, Texas*

Dewey J. Bayer, M.A., Ph.D., *Clinical Assistant Professor, Department of Psychiatry, SUNY at Buffalo School of Medicine and Biomedical Sciences, Children's Hospital of Buffalo, Buffalo, New York*

Eugene V. Beresin, M.D., *Associate Professor, Department of Psychiatry, Harvard Medical School; Director of Child and Adolescent Psychiatry Residency Training, Massachusetts General Hospital and McLean Hospital; Department of Psychiatry, Massachusetts General Hospital, Boston, Massachusetts*

Bruce Bleichfeld, Ph.D., *Clinical Assistant Professor, Department of Psychiatry, SUNY at Buffalo School of Medicine and Biomedical Sciences; Erie County Medical Center, Buffalo, New York*

Jeffrey Q. Bostic, M.D., ED.D., *Director of School Psychiatry, Massachusetts General Hospital; Assistant Clinical Professor of Psychiatry, Harvard Medical School, Boston, Massachusetts*

Kathleen Cole-Kelly, M.S., M.S.W., *Professor, Department of Family Medicine, Metrohealth Medical Center, Case Western Reserve University School of Medicine, Cleveland, Ohio*

Gerald E. Daigler, M.D., *Associate Professor of Clinical Pediatrics, Department of Pediatrics, University of New York at Buffalo; Vice Chairman for Graduate Medical Education, Department of Pediatrics, Children's Hospital of Buffalo, Buffalo, New York*

Jeanne M. Dolan, M.D., *Instructor, Department of Psychiatry, Harvard University School of Medicine; Assistant in Psychiatry, Division of Child Psychiatry, The Children's Hospital, Boston, Massachusetts*

Carolyn Piver Dukarm, M.D., *Director, The Center for Eating Disorders, LLC Specialty Center for Women, Sisters of Charity Hospital, Buffalo, New York*

Harwood S. Egan, M.D., Ph.D., *Assistant Professor, Department of Pediatrics, Harvard Medical School; Pediatrician, Department of Pediatrics, Massachusetts General Hospital, Boston, Massachusetts*

Stephanie H. Fretz, M.D., *Private Practice, Buffalo, New York*

William N. Friedrich, Ph.D., A.B.P.P., *Professor, Department of Psychiatry and Psychology, Mayo Medical School; Consultant, Department of Psychiatry and Psychology, Mayo Clinic, Rochester, Minnesota*

Mary Ellen Gellerstedt, M.D., *Associate Professor, Department of Pediatrics, University of Rochester School of Medicine and Dentistry; Director, Behavioral Pediatrics Program, Rochester General Hospital, Rochester, New York*

David L. Kaye, M.D., *Associate Professor of Clinical Psychiatry, Department of Psychiatry, SUNY at Buffalo School of Medicine and Biomedical Sciences; Director of Training in Child and Adolescent Psychiatry, Children's Hospital of Buffalo, Buffalo, New York*

Susan V. McLeer, M.D., *Professor and Chair, Department of Psychiatry, SUNY at Buffalo School of Medicine and Biomedical Sciences, Buffalo, New York*

Deborah A. Merrifield, M.S.W., *Commissioner, Erie County Department of Social Services, Buffalo, New York*

Walter J. Meyer, III, M.D., *Gladys Kempner & R. Lee Kempner Professor of Child Psychiatry, Department of Psychiatry and Behavioral Science, The University of Texas Medical Branch at Galveston; Director, Department of Psychological Services, Shriners Burns Hospital, Shriners Hospital for Children, Galveston, Texas*

Karen J. Miller, M.D., *Associate Professor, Department of Pediatrics, Tufts University School of Medicine; Developmental–Behavioral Pediatrician, Department of Pediatrics, Floating Hospital for Children, Boston, Massachusetts*

Maureen E. Montgomery, M.D., *Clinical Assistant Professor of Pediatrics, SUNY at Buffalo School of Medicine and Biomedical Sciences, Buffalo, New York*

Stephen W. Munson, M.D., *Associate Professor (Part-time), Departments of Psychiatry and Pediatrics, University of Rochester School of Medicine and Dentistry; Director, Child Psychiatry Residency Training Program, University of Rochester Medical Center, Rochester, New York*

Anna, C. Muriel, M.D., M.P.H., *Instructor, Department of Psychiatry, Harvard Medical School; Clinical Assistant, Department of Psychiatry, Massachusetts General Hospital, Boston, Massachusetts*

Caroly S. Pataki, M.D., *Associate Clinical Professor, Department of Psychiatry and Biobehavioral Science, University of California, Los Angeles, School of Medicine; Associate Director of Training, Child Psychiatry Fellowship Program, Division of Child and Adolescent Psychiatry, U.C.L.A. Neuropsychiatric Institute, Los Angeles, California*

Paul D. Pearson, L.L.B., *Fellow, American Academy of Matrimonial Lawyers; Lecturer in Law and Mental Health, Department of Psychiatry, SUNY Buffalo School of Medicine; Attorney/Mediator, Sullivan, Oliverio, & Gioia, Buffalo, New York*

Christopher F. Pollack, Ph.D., *Senior Clinical Instructor, Department of Psychiatry, University of Rochester Medical School, Rochester, New York*

Cynthia W. Santos, M.D., *Associate Professor, Department of Psychiatry and Behavioral Sciences, The University of Texas Medical School at Houston, Houston, Texas*

Cheri J. Shapiro, Ph.D., *Director, Consultation and Evaluation Services, South Carolina Department of Juvenile Justice, Columbia, South Carolina*

Bradley H. Smith, Ph.D., *Assistant Professor, Department of Psychology, The University of South Carolina, Columbia, South Carolina*

Christopher R. Thomas, M.D., *Professor, Department of Psychiatry and Behavioral Sciences, University of Texas Medical Branch; Training Director, Child and Adolescent Psychiatry, Department of Psychiatry and Behavioral Sciences, John Sealy Hospital, Galveston, Texas*

Susan Vinocour, Ph.D., *Associate Professor, Department of Psychiatry, The University of Rochester School of Medicine and Dentistry, Rochester, New York*

♣ Preface

I (D. K.) had completely forgotten the name Hale Shirley, M.D. But there was his book in the same place on my bookshelf. I had not looked at it for years since it was given to me by an old friend whose father had been a pediatrician. In 1948, Dr. Shirley wrote *Psychiatry for the Pediatrician*. As I prepared to write I marveled at how we've once again gone "back to the future." At that time he wrote:

The time, perhaps, is past when the pediatrician needs to be urged to consider the mental as well as the physical health of his patient. Organized pediatrics has increasingly recognized its strategic position in the prevention and treatment of children's behavior and personality disorders. Because of their early and repeated contacts with children and their parents, the pediatrician and general practitioner have an unequaled opportunity to discover situations which may interfere with the normal personality development of the child, to detect early evidences of maladjustment in the child, and to provide opportunity for proper therapeutic measures at an age when treatment can be expected to be most effective. They can also play a vital role in the mental health of their communities by translating to parents, nurses, and teachers the insight, concepts, and attitudes needed in the daily care of children and by giving parents guidance and reassurance in the management of the everyday problems of the everyday child.

Over the past 50 years there has been slow and incremental movement of the two fields towards each other, often punctuated by stutters and stops. In the last ten years this slow progress seems to have improved. In this recent past, within the medical brother- and sisterhood there has been an increasing appreciation for the unity of mind/body/spirit. This has promoted a greater valuation of the doctor-patient relationship by primary care physicians (PCPs) as well as a greater appreciation of the brain by psychiatrists. At the same time that these philosophical orientations within medicine have shifted, the gale winds of managed care have both promoted this collaboration (e.g., by limiting the indications for the "million dollar workup" which fosters a mind-body split; by capitation which fosters prudent use of resources and due consideration of psychiatric and developmental considerations) and also undermined the doctor-patient relationship (e.g., arbitrary and rapid changes in "provider" panels, disregard of the critical need for patient confidentiality, and in many situations promoting a serious conflict of interest for doctors, for example the doctor's financial well being versus the patient's welfare). In spite of these conflicting forces, the reality is that anyone serious about promoting the health care needs of children must address psychiatric and developmental issues.

Child and adolescent psychiatry is a young specialty, developing 25 to 50 years behind pediatrics. The first widely known textbook in the U.S., *Child Psychiatry* (Kanner), was published in

1935. Child psychiatry was not fully recognized as a medical specialty by the American Board of Psychiatry and Neurology until 1957. The major journal in child and adolescent psychiatry, the *Journal of the American Academy of Child and Adolescent Psychiatry,* was established in 1962. Although still quite young, the field has matured; and as it has developed, its fruits have become available to primary care. This is the way of much of medical progress. The evolution of primary care often occurs as a result of a subspecialty problem, which becomes more clearly defined as consensus develops around treatment. At that point, it begins to be incorporated into primary care medicine. For example, some years ago asthma was treated by pulmonologists, but now is routinely handled by PCPs. The same happened with enuresis which was a common problem seen by child and adolescent psychiatrists (CAPs) in the 1960s and 1970s. Now this is a routine pediatric problem that is only seen by a CAP when it is an incidental problem of a child with more severe difficulties. This evolution has now also included attention-deficit/hyperactivity disorder, which is being managed increasingly by PCPs. We think this trend will continue and will accelerate in the future. As pediatricians spend less time on acute illness, they will spend more time on prevention and attention to psychosocial and psychiatric issues. These changes will require that pediatricians and family physicians caring for children be well versed in child and family development, the institutional systems involved in children's lives, and common psychosocial issues and psychiatric conditions. A working knowledge of psychopharmacology will also become essential. We write this book in the hope that it will help to address these issues. While not intended to be exhaustive, it is meant to be current, informed by advances in knowledge, and practical. We hope that, in this way, it will be useful to, and used by, primary care physicians.

David L. Kaye, M.D.
Maureen E. Montgomery, M.D.
Stephen W. Munson, M.D.

Shirley, H. *Psychiatry for the pediatrician.* Commonwealth Fund Press: New York, 1948: vi.
Kanner, L. *Child psychiatry.* Charles Thomas: Springfield, IL, 1935.

🔩 Acknowledgments

Every creative effort has its context. An important context for this book has been the terrorist attacks of September 11, 2001, which has cast its shadow over, as well as inspired, our efforts. One of our chapter authors was directly impacted by these events, and all of us indirectly. These events have served to strengthen our commitments to those personal and professional values we hold dear. This project has involved a lot of work, but was also a joy as we have gotten to know each other better, shared ideas, and enriched ourselves. In doing so, we aspire to add hope and light to the world of children and families.

In completing this book, we first thank our chapter authors, who graciously wrote and rewrote as we evolved the structure and format for the chapters. We are very pleased with their efforts and proud of their final products. We are also grateful to Timothy Y. Hiscock, acquisitions editor at Lippincott Williams & Wilkins, for believing in the concept and the importance of this book. Michael Standen's steady, behind-the-scenes editing should also not go unmentioned. Emily Lerman cheerfully marshalled the book to publication. Emily Ets-Hokin, Ph.D., and Jeff Bostic, M.D., went above and beyond the call with numerous discussions that led to fruitful changes in the book. We also thank the following individuals who read earlier versions of chapters and helped us develop our thoughts: Don Crawford, Ph.D., Henry Cretella, M.D., Michael Cummings, M.D., Kim Dobson, M.D., Eric Glazer, J.D., Dasha Lekic, M.D., Anne Lockwood, Ph.D., David Munson, M.D., David Nathanson, Ph.D., Diana Sanderson, M.D., Patrick Stein, M.D., and Peter Tanguay M.D.

The Yoruba say we sit on the shoulders of those who come before us. And none of this would have occurred without our parents, teachers, and mentors. The inspiration of Muriel and Carl A. Whitaker, M.D., comes through in their belief in families. David V. Keith, M.D., a true artist, has extended these teachings. Gary N. Cohen, M.D., provided fertile ground in the conversations that were the seminal beginnings of this book.

Lastly, we thank and dedicate this book to our families for their persistent encouragement and support: Emily, Madeline and Eliza, Theo, and Paul. They gave up many weekends and evenings, allowing us the time to complete this project. As Eliza said towards the end of the project: "Da—ad, when are you going to be finished *with that book*??" They believed in it as much as, and at times more than, we did. Thank you.

David L. Kaye, M.D.
Maureen E. Montgomery, M.D.
Stephen W. Munson, M.D.

I

Understanding Child and Adolescent Mental Health Problems

1 ♣ Orientation and Organization of this Book

David L. Kaye

One of the chief priorities in the Office of the Surgeon General and Assistant Secretary for Health has been to work to ensure that every child has an optimal chance for a healthy start in life. When we think about a healthy start, we often limit our focus to physical health. But, as clearly articulated in the Surgeon General's Report on Mental Health, mental health is fundamental to overall health and well-being. And that is why we must ensure that our health system responds as readily to the needs of children's mental health as it does to their physical well-being.

> —*David Satcher, M.D., Ph.D.*
> *Surgeon General, U.S.A.*
> *December 2000*

Many children experience mental health problems that interfere with normal development and functioning. The Surgeon General has stated that our nation is facing a public health crisis in this regard. Problems of detection and recognition, access to services, stigma, and discriminatory insurance reimbursement patterns all contribute to this crisis. Primary care physicians (PCPs) are ideally situated to have a significant impact on these issues and improve the health and well-being of children. To address these issues, a PCP needs to be armed with adequate information. We hope this book begins to fill this need.

First, it is important to review the epidemiology of mental health disorders to understand the scope of the problem. Information about epidemiology in child and adolescent psychiatry has grown dramatically in the past 25 years. The optimal method for getting a true picture of prevalence rates is by randomly surveying a population in the community and using standardized approaches to diagnosis (the most widely used of such is the *Diagnostic and Statistical Manual of Mental Disorders* [DSM]). A number of such studies have now been done. Although much work remains, an emerging consensus finds that overall prevalence rates for any DSM-based diagnosis run at **15% to 20%** of children between the ages of 5 and 18 years. Of these children, 33% to 50% are experiencing severe functional impairments (for a detailed review, see Roberts et al. 1998). If one multiplies these percentages by the actual number of children, one comes up with huge numbers of children in the United States with very serious disturbances. Physicians, teachers, and others working with children know this intuitively. The prevalence rates for specific disorders are given in Table 1.1. To put this into perspective, we have also included prevalence rates for selected other pediatric problems.

The next question might be: How many of the children with diagnosable mental health problems receive any kind of help?

Table 1.1.   Prevalence of pediatric disorders

Disorder	Percent
Total DSM disorders	15–20
Anorexia nervosa	0.5–1.0 adolescents
Anxiety disorder (any)	6
AD/HD	2–5
Autistic-spectrum	0.2
Major depression	2 children/5 adolescents
Substance abuse	
Daily alcohol	5 adolescents
Daily marijuana	3
Suicide attempt	5–10 adolescents
Other pediatric disorders	
Cerebral palsy	0.2
Cystic fibrosis	0.03 (whites)
Diabetes mellitus, type I	0.2
Epilepsy	0.3
Traumatic brain injury	0.2

AD/HD, attention-deficit/hyperactivity disorder; DSM, *Diagnostic and Statistical Manual of Mental Disorders.*

Again, although much work remains, the best data we have suggest that **relatively few receive treatment.** In the best study to date, Burns et al. (1995) found in a community survey that less than 20% of the more troubled youth had received any mental health treatment within the past 3 months. Of those who seek treatment, a large percentage leaves treatment prematurely and abruptly. Although many of these children had seen their pediatrician, only 10% addressed the problem with their PCP. The moral is that PCPs are in a unique position to monitor, evaluate or triage, manage a range of problems, and make certain that youth receive appropriate mental health treatment. This has the potential to make an enormous difference in the lives of individual children and families, the pediatric public health, and society as a whole.

The central importance of the family. Throughout this book we convey a particular point of view about children and families and how PCPs can be most effective in promoting their optimal development. At its core, this perspective holds that the **family is at the center** of growth, development, and health for children (and adults as well, we might add). Helping children requires empathy and appreciation for parents and an ability to form a working relationship with them or other responsible adults. It is through active collaboration with families that PCPs are optimally able to help their pediatric patients. PCPs can have a powerful influence through their confirmation of parenting skills and appreciation for what the parents are doing well. This can have an enormously positive effect on parents. Conversely, families who have the sense of being criticized or judged often will withdraw or avoid important issues, limiting the effectiveness of PCPs. Success in forming a helpful alliance requires an appreciation of the **cultural context of the family.**

Organization of this book. This book is organized into two major sections. The first includes chapters on a number of over-arching issues that are critical to helping children. Working with a pediatric population requires understanding the doctor–pediatric patient relationship, as well as the many systems that touch children. We have included chapters on the family, parenting, school, legal system, and social services. Also included is a chapter on the practicalities of organizing a primary care office to address the mental health needs of children and adolescents. The second section of the book addresses the most common clinical problems faced by PCPs. Each chapter has been written by a "team," consisting of a child mental health professional (child and adolescent psychiatrist or psychologist) and a primary care pediatrician to present a blended perspective that is current, informed, practical, and useful. This handbook focuses on the clinical recognition and management of mental health problems in a primary care setting. Although we use the nomenclature found in the current DSM-IV-TR, we have not included its lists of diagnostic criteria. Hence, whereas this is not a diagnostic text or a substitute for DSM-IV-TR (or the version developed for the PCP, the "DSM-PC"), it can be used in conjunction with those references. Each chapter of this section covers a particular clinical problem and follows the same general outline.

I.   **Background.** This provides critical and basic information on understanding the problem.
II. **Office evaluation.** This section delineates the specific questions (for both parents and children or adolescents) useful in evaluating the problem. Standardized questionnaires are included when appropriate.
III. **Triage assessment and treatment planning.** This section provides specific guidelines for triaging the problem (i.e., when should the PCP "watch" the situation, when to "intervene further," and when to "refer"). For this book, a situation to **"watch"** is one in which the parents or child identify a symptom or concern but the situation is likely to improve over time and does not present a danger to the child's physical or mental health. These situations generally require monitoring, education, and support of the child and family, and are commonly addressed by PCPs. Situations to **"intervene further"** are ones in which the PCP has greater concern, and manages the case more actively while retaining primary responsibility for the care of the

child's problem. These cases require closer monitoring, behavior management, advocacy, and perhaps psychotropic medications; consultation with mental health professionals may be sought to assist in management. PCPs can differ in their comfort managing this level of case. By **"referral,"** we specifically mean that the primary responsibility for the case is transferred to a specialist child mental health professional. Problems requiring "referral" are the most serious and very few PCPs will feel competent to manage these situations, although they may be active members of a team treating the child and family.

We offer these as **clinical guideposts for the practitioner on the front lines** while recognizing that these are moving targets. These guidelines will differ, depending on the part of the country, the family, the mental health resources available, and the comfort of the PCP. We also expect that, although these guidelines will change over time, the direction will be that PCPs will take increasing amounts of clinical responsibility for pediatric mental health problems.

A. **Treatment planning.** Following each section on triage (e.g., when to watch), we address in a practical and **multimodal** manner what the PCP can *do* when watching, intervening further, or referring. The sections of the multimodal treatment plan cover the following:

   1. **Psychoeducation** includes suggestions for the psychological approach, the offering of support, patient and family education, and guidance with respect to the specific problem.

   2. **Advocacy** covers recommendations for PCP involvement with schools, social services, and other agencies.

   3. **Psychotherapy** covers approaches that are likely to be most helpful. It is not expected that the PCP will be well versed in, or carry out, these treatments, but rather will be informed on what is likely to be an appropriate approach for a given problem.

   4. The use of psychotropic **medications** provides a brief overview of helpful agents in given circumstances. Recommendations are evidence-based, when possible; if not, they are based on consensus from the literature and clinical experience of the authors and editors.

   5. **Laboratory and other evaluations** provides recommendations for the use of the laboratory and physical examination for the particular problem.

   6. **Monitoring** addresses issues of timing and personnel used for follow-up.

IV. Practical use of medications. A particular issue high-lighted is pediatric psychopharmacology. PCPs are increasingly asked to prescribe these agents for children while receiving modest amounts of education during residency for such treatments. Older physicians are receiving these requests, and at times demands, without benefit of any training unless they have sought this out on their own. For these reasons, we have placed a special emphasis on the role of psychopharmacology. This is not meant to imply that this is the critical component of treatment for all children with mental health problems. Much of the time medications are not central, and even when this is so they should be integrated with other treatments for optimal results. In each chapter is included a summary of information relevant to the psychopharmacologic treatment of that particular condition. At the back of the book are **Medication Appendices** that provide "at-a-glance" summary information about each medication. Following this is a **pediatric psychopharmacology bibliography, including references for parents.**

V. Summary. A brief recapitulation of the most important points concludes each chapter.

VI. Suggested readings. Only a limited number of major, current references (generally review articles) are cited. The interested reader can find more exhaustive bibliographies within these cited references. Also included are Web sites that would be of interest to PCPs, youth, or parents. Relevant self-help groups or books for parents and adolescents are also listed in some chapters.

SUGGESTED READINGS

American Psychiatric Association. *DSM-IV-TR*. Washington, DC: American Psychiatric Press, 2000.

American Psychiatric Association. *DSM-IV-PC*. Washington, DC: American Psychiatric Press, 1997.

Burns BJ, Costello EJ, Angold A, et al. Children's mental health service use across service sectors. *Health Affairs* 1995;14(3):147–159.

Carrillo JE, Green A, Betancourt J. Cross-cultural primary care: a patient-based approach. *Ann Intern Med* 1999;130:829–834.

Roberts R, Attkisson C, Rosenblatt A. Prevalence of psychopathology among children and adolescents. *Am J Psychiatry* 1998;155(6): 715–724.

Web Site

Satcher D. Report of the Surgeon General's conference on children's mental health: a national action agenda. Available at www. surgeongeneral.gov/topics/cmh/childreport.htm. Accessed on 6/20/02.

2 ♣ The Doctor–Patient Relationship in Pediatrics

Eugene V. Beresin

I. **Introduction.** Primary care physicians (PCPs) and allied health professionals play a unique role in the life of a child and family. Besides making important medical diagnoses and providing treatment, the pediatric PCP is one of the few professionals in the life of the child and adolescent who can objectively monitor growth and development. Keeping track of psychosocial development is among the most important functions of outpatient pediatric and family practice because of the high prevalence of psychiatric illness in the population and, perhaps, even more, because of the significant impact of social and environmental forces on youth. Family problems (e.g., marital conflict, divorce, domestic violence, abuse and neglect, substance abuse, unemployment, financial distress, and poor living situations) are only a few of the forces that have an impact on development. Children are also subject to dangerous influences in society (e.g., bullying, sexual harassment and violence among youth, media violence, community unrest, and peer pressure around drugs, sex, and misbehavior). If no adult asks or is in a position for the child to freely disclose how he or she is affected, disturbances in emotions and behavior can erupt when they could have been either prevented or detected and addressed in early stages. To be most effective in this mission, the PCP must develop a relationship that is personal and longitudinal. Continuity of care affords the opportunity to follow change in the child and family over time, and increasingly nurture a doctor–patient relationship that grows in trust, confidence, and depth. Naturally, this is no small task. The PCP must always keep in mind that nothing has to happen, short of an emergency evaluation, in one visit. It is essential to keep in mind that another opportunity will always present for building the relationship piece by piece.

For a doctor in the current professional climate it is not easy to be a confidant for children, adolescents, or parents. Managed care has forced physicians and allied health professionals to see more patients in shorter periods of time. No time seems available to collect psychosocial data. Despite these pressures, physicians can and should be able to make good assessments of psychosocial issues in the lives of their patients. This chapter aims to demonstrate that a strong, caring, and confidential doctor–patient relationship becomes the vehicle for such evaluations and need not sap precious time from busy practices.

II. **Forming a sound doctor–patient relationship**
   A. **Who is the patient?** The practice of pediatrics is unique in that the PCP is doctor for both child and

parent. Whereas most would agree that the child or adolescent is the real patient, many studies of doctor–patient communication have been geared toward the doctor's talking with and to parents. It was thought that the relationship with the parent was essential for "compliance." Better indicated as concordance, "compliance" is indeed dependent on a good relationship with the parent, who administers treatment at home and on whom we rely for important historical data and accurate symptom reporting. However, we now know that a close relationship with the child is also essential. The child is a crucial source of clinical information, needs to learn about the importance of health maintenance early on, and, perhaps most importantly, needs to develop an independent, confidential, and trusting relationship with the PCP, particularly for guidance, support, and treatment in later years. Hence, we face a dual challenge: How do we form independent relationships with both child or adolescent, and caregiver?

B. **Key elements in the clinical interview.** The pediatric interview is the primary means of establishing a relationship that will be productive in gaining information to make reasonable mental health assessments, provide counseling, referral, or both. Discussed below are techniques considered generic to both children and parents, and those specific for children and adolescents, and parents.

1. **General considerations**
   a. The **setting should be quiet, comfortable, and amenable for interviewing** young children and adolescents, as well as families. Toys should be available for young children to play with. The doctor should not sit behind a desk, but be ready to face children at eye level. For school-aged children, this may mean sitting on a low chair at a small desk set up for them, or on the floor. No interruptions should occur, either by phone or others coming into the office. Patients should all feel the meeting is private and confidential.
   b. The **atmosphere should embody both a sense of a time limit as well as timelessness.** Patients do need to know that they only have a certain amount of time for the visit. This helps them try to "get it all in" within the confines of the appointment. They also need to feel that the doctor is providing undivided attention and has no other distractions. In that sense,

"time stops" for everything but the child and parent.

c. The interview should involve **facilitation,** which is achieved by greeting each person cordially and asking how each wishes to be called. It is always important to (a) ask for the **expectations of the child and parent;** (b) allow them to express their concerns by asking open-ended questions permitting them to describe the issues and problems; (c) ask what they hope the doctor can provide and how they have tried to solve the problem; and (d) convey attitudes of acceptance, warmth, and empathy. In addition, the doctor needs to respect the patient's dignity, allow the patient to talk and follow the patient's leads, and not be prematurely reassuring. Each patient needs to be treated a bit differently. It is important to tailor personal interviewing style to the personality of the child or parent, consistent with one's own personality style. For some patients, humor is a wonderful tool. It is particularly useful for young children, who are scared of going to the doctor. Classic examples of this abound in pediatric practice. For example, in an examination of a 4-year-old, asking, "Where is that belly button?" as the doctor peers around a child's back may be helpful. Or, looking in an ear and saying, "I see an elephant in there!" usually gets a giggle. Humor can be used at all developmental levels for children and adolescents. It can be a wonderful way to ease an anxious parent. For example, a joke or two about a comical scene involving an adolescent in a TV show may both ease tension and prepare the parent to discuss tough issues (e.g., sexuality, drugs, or family conflict). On the other hand, some parents may be offended by humor, as if it indicated a lack of true concern for the child or their situation. Learning how to "be a good fit" with each patient is much like the goodness of fit we strive to encourage with each parent–child dyad.

d. **Observe** verbal and nonverbal cues that may indicate problems. Even infants and preschoolers react to parental behavior. Watch for the child's emotional and behavioral responses to parents' reports of issues and problems. Remember that **patients are also observing the doctor.** They are keenly aware of your interest, indifference, preoccupation with other concerns (e.g., a sick newborn in the nursery), disapproval, judgment, and so on. Also be aware of parent–child interactions (i.e., how attached, concerned, appropriate are the behaviors).

e. **Be aware of your own feelings!** Many patients generate strong feelings in physicians, some positive and others negative. Some children will make you angry, frustrated, sad, or anxious. Many parents will torment you, inciting feelings of disgust, hatred, or wishes to get them out of the office quickly or, conversely, to make special arrangements that you would never think of for other parents. It is natural to have feelings about your patients and emotional reactions to them. When these feelings are identified and acknowledged, they are far less likely to impair your decision making or ability to work with difficult kids and parents. If unidentified, the doctor–patient relationship can be threatened and thinking can be blurred.

f. Use **support and education** for both children and parents. The PCP should provide education about normal and abnormal development and both mental health and medical problems to both children and adults. We often forget to inform our child and adolescent patients about the nature, course, and treatment of problems. This phenomenon is well documented in the literature. However, we need to help children in their ongoing strivings for autonomy and to reinforce the attitude of their own responsibility for their mental and physical health.

g. Be aware of the **developmental level and cultural background** of children, adolescents, and parents and **use language and behavior that is consistent, acceptable, and understood by the patient.**

h. For children, adolescents, and parents, **psychosocial screening** in the interview needs to cover five areas: **Friends, Family, School, Play, and Mood** (Chapter 5).

2. **Techniques with children and adolescents**
   a. **Promoting an individual relationship with the child or adolescent.** Young children under age 5 should generally be seen with parents for the entire interview. As children enter the school-age years, the opportunity may present to spend some time alone with them. This can foster the establishment of a personal relationship with the child independent of the parent. Promoting an independent relationship is even more important for adolescents, who are often best seen separately. Time should still be allotted for touching bases with the parents to exchange necessary information and to acknowledge their role as the responsible adults. This also affords an opportunity to observe the parent–child interaction.
   b. **More important than the amount of time spent alone with the child is the communication of respect and inclusion by the PCP in the clinical encounter.** Many children go to see their PCP and rarely get a word in edgewise. It may seem to some young patients that the doctor is really the parent's physician, rather than theirs. The sooner they conceive of the PCP as theirs, the more likely they are to trust the doctor with sensitive and important personal information. Making eye contact with the child, soliciting the child's opinions, and actively inviting the child's questions goes far in promoting a relationship in which the child feels valued and respected.
   c. **Instill lightness** into the experience. Young children need to think of going to the doctor as fun, although they know something painful or uncomfortable may ensue. The presence of toys, stickers, use of puppets when talking to them, and even sitting on the floor and playing a bit are helpful. You can use a puppet to ask questions, or do so while sitting on the floor with puppets. It may be valuable to ask questions such as: "What is your favorite cookie? What is your favorite bedtime book? Do you watch TV? What is the funniest animal you know?" And after breaking the ice, ask, "Do you get scared when the light is turned out? What

is the funniest thing that happened in your family? What is the saddest? Do you or your parents get angry?" As indicated in the flow of questions here, a great technique is to start with rather innocuous, upbeat questions, and move gently to the more difficult ones involving fears, feelings, and relationships. Do not be afraid to ask these questions to very young children. They are often ready and willing to give you their opinion about friends, family, mood, and other psychosocial topics. Just keep the questions in the language they can understand. And remember that questions involving "When did that happen?" or "Why do you say that?" will generally fall flat because young children have a poor concept of time and causality.

d. **Solicit the child's opinions and strengths.** School-aged children really appreciate concern with the many issues in their life. Although they are not ready to discuss abstract concepts, they are increasingly aware of peers, other families, and social rules and can articulate their own emotional reactions to situations. Again, it is best to begin with benign questions, such as "What do you like to do most with your friends? Do you have a best friend? Tell me about him/her. What are you really good at? Do you like sports? What is your favorite one? Have you seen a good movie lately? What was the best part? How do you like your teachers? Who is your favorite? Who is the hardest? Is one really mean and grumpy? How are things at home? What about rules, yuk! Who likes them? Do you have rules or chores? What happens when you get into trouble? Who gets the maddest at home?" Again, humor is highly effective and should be used throughout the interview and physical examination.

e. Using **open-ended questions** is valuable for all children. Let them tell you what they want **before you start asking for specifics.** Open-ended questions should be used to ask questions in each of the five areas noted. Sometimes an open-ended question yields a silence. For example, "How's school?" may not be as good as some of the specific questions noted above. Try an open-ended question first because whatever is on the child's mind may come out and indicate an important area of interest or concern. With no response, go for more specific questions.

f.   **Talking with adolescents requires special attention.** Assessment of adolescents can present a number of additional challenges beyond those involved in assessing younger patients. Parents are often unprepared for the "trials and tribulations" of adolescents, especially their first. They rarely expect the distance needed by teenagers and the inevitable rejection as the adolescent chooses time with friends over family and rarely talks with parents, as was previously the case in childhood. The PCP (or other adults) now has an opportunity to gain information that is generally hidden from parents. Explain this to confused and frustrated parents and let them know that assessment will take place in the office; however, it will be private and confidential.

g.   **Adolescents need to know that the doctor–patient relationship is entirely confidential, unless a danger to self or others** exists. Ground rules need to be established early on, including the role of the PCP as advocate for the teenager. It is useful to move from open-ended questions and upbeat interests to more specific areas that might reveal problems. Remember, adolescents are moving to the stage of abstract reasoning and they are intrigued with questions about identity, justice, morality, and so on. **Asking what they think is a sign of respect.**

Eventually the need arises to inquire about tougher issues, including relationships, sexuality, family conflicts, and other personal issues. Adolescents expect questions about these things, especially drugs and sex. It is sometimes easier to **"take the questions out of the room,"** by asking about such issues in friends' lives. This might make it easier for them to move to issues in their own world. So, you might ask, "Do you know of anyone who has a drug or alcohol problem? How about major family stress in your friends?" These questions could be asked about other topics (e.g., depression, cutting, tattoos, eating disorders, anxiety, or high-risk behavior). **Then you can move to express whether they have any issues with these things.** Another angle is to ask about "stress." Stress is a catchall term for problems and does not carry the stigma of problems with classical labels. It may be easier for an adolescent to discuss depression, anxiety, and family problems under the umbrella of "stress."

Rarely, you could allude to "other kids" you have seen or worked with. You might say, "I see a lot of kids who are confused about what a drug like ecstasy really does. Do you know about this?" The important thing is that they feel valued, respected, and that they are not simply meeting with the doctor to receive another lecture.

h. Most children expect that others in their lives (e.g., parents and teachers) will be talking about them. The PCP should always get **collateral information** about each child and adolescent. It is wise to ask the adolescent for permission to discuss certain issues with others. Usually a series of negotiations with children ensues regarding with whom the PCP is "allowed" to talk. It is always helpful to tell adolescents that information obtained about them will be fed back in future meetings. They need to feel the center of attention and deserving the respect of honest feedback. Sometimes they know they will not like what they hear. The point, however, is to be honest about with whom you are talking and always be up front with a teenager.

C. **Special situations and problems**
  1. **The resistant child and adolescent.** Not all children and adolescents enjoy going to the doctor. Younger children may dread examinations and shots. Some adolescents are resistant to opening up. If they shut down for even routine questions, it is virtually impossible to collect psychosocial information. Here are a few tips for this difficult situation:
    a. **Never insist the adolescent talk.** After reinforcing confidentiality, it is better to view the relationship as a long-term pro-

ject and reschedule visits. Sometimes more frequent short visits are useful.

b. Try to **find some way of empathizing** with the adolescent in developing a relationship. This can be around how difficult things are at home or in school or focus on common interests (e.g., movies, TV shows, or music).

c. Find ways to **advocate for the adolescent,** either with parents or with teachers. Sometimes it is fine to talk with parents (e.g., about increasing privileges, allowing later bedtimes, altering curfew), if appropriate.

d. At times, the adolescent is in real trouble and you simply need to let the teenager know that he or she needs to see you for a big problem and no way is seen around it. On the other hand, perhaps you can suggest that your job may be to help the teen find a way to get out of the particular mess he or she is in.

e. **Be patient!** Teens need time to open up. If they sense you are frustrated or mad at them, they may pull back more.

2. **The difficult parent.** Some parents are truly dreaded by most physicians. Forming a therapeutic alliance is especially troublesome with the following types of parent styles:

a. **Obsessive:** rigid, dogmatic, preoccupied with minute details of treatment, and emotionally constricted.

b. **Hysterical:** overemotional, sensitive, impressionistic, suggestible, overreactive, anxious, and flirtatious.

c. **Denying:** uses denial to cope with stress, inattention to instructions, tends to be noncompliant, and intolerant of emotions.

d. **Dependent:** has unending need for emotional support, may parentify the child, treats doctors as inexhaustible providers, and seems insatiable.

e. **Demanding:** entitled, grandiose, faultfinding, acts as if deserving of special treatment, sensitive to perceived criticism, litigious; are often very important people.

f. **Help-rejecting:** pessimistic, distrusting, nothing is ever good enough, tests others' reliability.

No doubt, we all have had problems with these types of patients. They all require somewhat different approaches. However, a few generalizations may be helpful in building an alliance.

- **Keep the best interests of the child in mind** for the parent and physician. Form your alliance around care of the child.
- **Identify your emotional responses** to each difficult parent and do not let them interfere with your care of the child.
- **Identify and draw on the parents' strengths** (e.g., intelligence, empathy, effective communication skills).
- **Explain the child's problems** in a manner understandable to the parent.
- **Allow the parent to ask questions** about the child's emotional or behavioral problem.
- Be aware that all of these parents have emotional problems themselves and either cannot tolerate the child's mental health problems or feel somehow responsible for it. Be sure to let the parent know that you will get help for everyone.
- Try to use mental health professionals as allies in both understanding the personalities of the parents and how to deal with them, as well as consultants for the mental health needs of child and family.

III. Summary. The relationship with the child or adolescent and parent is the bedrock of all pediatric care. Thinking about and understanding these relationships are critical to establishing and maintaining relationships that nurture and sustain both the family and PCP. Although empathy cannot be taught, many of the technical skills that go into positive relationships can be learned.

SUGGESTED READINGS

Apley J. Listening and talking to patients V: communicating with children. *BMJ* 1980;281:1116–1117.

Beresin EV, Jellinek MS, Herzog DB. The difficult parent: office assessment and management. *Curr Probl Pediatr* 1990;20:620–633.

Green M. The pediatric interview. In: Green M, Haggerty RJ, eds. *Ambulatory pediatrics,* III. Philadelphia: WB Saunders, 1984: 228–240.

Jellinek MS. Interviewing in pediatric outpatient practice. *Curr Probl Pediatr* 1990;20:575–588.

Korsch BM, Aley EF. Pediatric interviewing techniques. *Curr Probl Pediatr* 1973;3:1–42.

Van Dulmen AM. Children's contributions to pediatric outpatient encounters. *Pediatrics* 1998;102:563–568.

3 ♣ Parent Guidance and Consultation

Cheri J. Shapiro and Bradley H. Smith

I. **Importance of parenting.** Few would argue that parents have the most important influence on the lives of their children. Families are the first and most relevant source of socialization and much of what parents do strongly influences children's emotional, social, and cognitive abilities. However, parenting is not simply what parents do to children. Instead, parenting is a complicated multifaceted relationship. The parent has strengths and weaknesses as does the child. Often the match—what has been called the "goodness of fit"—between strengths and weaknesses affects the quality of the relationship. As noted in the introduction to this volume, it is important to recognize that all families have strengths that can lead to solutions to even very difficult problems.

Although all families have strengths, certain strengths are supported by research as being especially important for raising children successfully. Knowing these areas can provide a framework for assessing the parent–child relationship. Four themes in parenting have repeatedly been shown to be characteristics of effective parenting. More specifically, **children with the best outcomes** (i.e., the fewest behavior problems and the best school achievement) tend to be raised by parents who achieve success in the following areas (Steinberg, 1994):

- **Supervision**
- **Structure**
- **Acceptance**
- **Affection**

Additionally, the most effective parents are role models of appropriate behavior and communication.

This chapter describes how to (a) assess families for the areas of competence listed above; (b) guide families who have deficits in these competence areas; and (c) decide about which interventions are appropriate and when. The recommendations can be applicable for most families; however, we provide advice regarding when the family might be referred for intervention that is more intense than what is typically feasible in a primary care setting.

II. **Four characteristics of effective parenting**
   A. **Supervision.** As with most parenting skills, supervision needs to be developmentally appropriate. This means holding and interacting with infants, watching toddlers and young children to be sure they are playing safely, and knowing about an adolescent's activities, including location, peers, and presence of adult supervision.

Supervision refers to knowing the four Ws about the child:

- Where the child is
- When will the child be there
- What the child will be doing
- Who the child will be with

Research has consistently shown that proper supervision is critically important in preventing injuries, reducing aggression and drug abuse, and preventing academic failure and juvenile delinquency.

B. **Structure** refers to providing children with a set of consistently enforced rules and clear expectations that are regularly backed up by positive reinforcement and, when necessary, punishments. This concept is captured in social learning theory as the **"ABCs" of behavior.** "A" stands for antecedents, "B" stands for behavior, and "C" stands for consequences. Behaviors are conceptualized as being influenced by what comes before the behavior (antecedents) and what follows the behavior (consequences). Effective parents communicate clear expectations (i.e., rules) about what type of behavior is expected from their children before the behavior occurs. The rules provide structure and serve as antecedents to help prevent problem behavior in the first place. Structure also refers to the consequences provided for both appropriate and inappropriate behavior. The concepts highlighted here are further detailed later in this chapter.

C. **Acceptance** is the extent to which parents understand their child and are responsive to their child's unique needs. The most **effective parents spend time with their children, recognize appropriate developmental milestones, and understand their child's strengths and weaknesses.** Parent education about normal development is helpful in fostering a sense of acceptance; it can be provided in primary care settings directly or via brief brochures or handouts. In addition to knowledge, an important requirement for acceptance is listening. Even small children who are not really using words need to feel like an adult is listening to them as they struggle to try to speak. Older children and adolescents need to have a chance to express views and opinions appropriately. Parents might not agree with what the child is saying, but they should model good listening skills such as eye contact or restating what their child said. Parents who model these skills are more likely to have their children use those same skills when they are listening to the parent.

D. **Affection.** Last, but not least, is affection. Children need to receive regular, spontaneous, and genuine

affection. Babies grow slowly, lose weight, and sometimes die if they are not shown enough affection. Parents should hug, kiss, praise, and find other ways of
showing honest appreciation of their children. Parents
should also try to catch their children doing well and
let them know the good behavior is noticed and appreciated. Affection comes from the heart and should be
spontaneous and genuine. It can be physical as well
as verbal. Babies and toddlers need a lot of physical
affection in the form of touching, holding, and cuddling. Toddlers and young children need hugs and
regular cuddling (e.g., sitting close while reading a
story). Older children and adolescents benefit from
hugs, good bye and hello greetings, pats on the back,
"high fives," and other physical displays of affection.
Also, as children grow older, verbal expressions of
affection are very powerful. Children who are told
that they are loved have higher self-esteem and are
more confident in their interactions with peers and
more persistent in their schoolwork. Children who
are ignored find other ways to get attention. The best
way to stop bad behavior is to crowd it out with good
behavior. Children who are loved and praised for doing
well are more likely to repeat the positive behavior
than a child for whom the positive behavior is taken
for granted or ignored.

III. **Deciding if there is a problem** depends on having a
conceptual framework for determining if behavior is significantly different from the norm and, therefore, worthy
of further investigation or intervention. The primary care
physician (PCP) is in a unique position to assess the characteristics of effective parenting and detect at a very early
stage problems in the parent–child relationship. **Hints
about parent–child problems may surface during
clinical interactions;** physicians may be alert for the
presence of appropriate supervision, structure, affection,
and acceptance in the office. However, compared with their
typical behavior at home, in many cases children and parents behave differently when visiting a health professional. Therefore, the PCP must **take an active role in
seeking out information about effective parenting.
Direct inquiry of the parents about their parenting
successes and their parenting challenges is essential. Areas of inquiry might include** the child's or adolescent's basic developmental milestones, habits (e.g., sleeping, eating, and routine activities in daily living), and
questions about appropriate role functioning (e.g., school
performance, homework completion, and peer group activity). Parents may not recognize that a problem exists, so
routine screening questions should be phrased in a neutral
manner. Questions can be put on a brief form for parents

to complete while they are waiting for an appointment (see Chapter 5).

IV. **Defining the problem and its ABCs.** When the PCP has decided a problem exists, then information on **problem history, frequency, and severity** must be obtained. Further inquiry is warranted to assess the "ABCs" of behavior, as noted above. **Elements of "B" (behavior) need to be very specifically described.** For example, a vague description of a problem behavior is "my child has a hard time doing her homework". A more specific and useful description is necessary, such as "my child starts her homework OK, but she takes a very long time and we get into arguments about finishing it more quickly." The PCP should **ask enough questions about the behavior to obtain a clear picture of exactly what the problem behaviors are.** A good rule of thumb is the "fly eye view": would a fly on the wall be able to see the behavior being described? If not, further questioning is needed. This is particularly true when the problem behavior has a value-laden description (e.g. "She has a bad attitude"). A more specific description in this case may be "She rolls her eyes at me every time I ask her to do something, then leaves the room without doing what I asked." These highly specific descriptions of problem behaviors help clarify the problem for both the PCP and the parents.

Solutions to the common problem of noncompliance can often be focused on the antecedents of the behavior. For example, clear and specific requests from parents can help many problems with noncompliance. **Rules for effective requests or commands include:**

• Using a **slightly louder but neutral tone of voice**
• Making **eye contact** to deliver the command
• **Requesting briefly and specifically** what needs to happen

For example, shouting from another room for a child to turn off a television and get ready for dinner will likely be met with noncompliance, which may be the behavior the parent is concerned about! Unless asked specifically, the practitioner will never know that the command was shouted from the kitchen, which is down the hall from the room in which the child was watching television. A more effective command would involve the parent going to the room, getting the child's attention by calling his or her name or by standing in front of the television, and then issuing the request.

In addition to appropriate requests, **rules for activities** also serve as antecedents that can be used to prevent problem behavior from occurring. However, such rules need to be very clear and the practitioner should **inquire whether there are clear rules** for the problem situations the parent is describing. A problematic phrase would be "act your age when we go to the store." A more clear and specific request would be "Here are the store rules:

1. Talk in a quiet voice
2. Walk at all times
3. Touch things after I have given you permission"

As this example demonstrates, **it is far better to phrase requests positively (i.e., do this) than negatively (i.e., don't do that).**

Sometimes, behavior can be changed by focusing solely on consequences; however, a "one-two punch" of antecedents and consequences often works best. Having a parent work to establish clear rules about the behavior first, or by having the parent focus on issuing effective requests, is likely needed before moving toward adjusting consequences. The two types of consequences are:

- **Natural consequences for behavior**
- **Rewards or punishments delivered by adults** in response to the behavior

For example, slipping and falling when running in the store is a natural consequence. A treat for following the store rules or a time out for running is something that can be imposed by parents. Understanding consequences following behavior is important. Unfortunately, parents often unintentionally reinforce problematic behavior. For example, parents may reinforce lengthy bouts of whining by saying "no" several times, then finally giving the child what they want. Here, the child learns to whine more to get what is wanted. However, the practitioner needs to ask clear questions to obtain information on such behavior sequences to assess if a problem exits.

Consistent parents enforce their rules in a predictable manner with consequences that can be dependably delivered. When it comes to rules and consequences, the phrase "less is more" is a good guideline. Children (and most parents) cannot easily remember a long, complicated list of rules. Therefore, **parents should write a short list of basic rules (3 to 7, depending on the age of the child),** post the list throughout the household, and concentrate on enforcing these basic rules. Simple, clear rules can also be made for activities outside the home. As noted, good rules tell a child what to do, instead of what not to do. Examples include "be respectful to others," "obey adults," and "be responsible for your belongings."

The idea of **"less is more"** is also appropriate **for consequences,** which are a necessary part of helping parents provide structure for their children. Consistently giving small punishments and rewards is more effective than giving large punishments or rewards. For example, it is more effective to reward homework completion with daily TV watching or another activity that the child enjoys in his or her typical environment (often called natural reinforcers) than to promise a new TV for getting good grades on a report card. Another guideline that is helpful to promote consistent parenting is to **"act right away"**. Children, especially younger children, need immediate feedback. Delaying punishments or rewards can confuse a child. Finally, punishments should be the **"right size"**. For example, grounding may be too strong a punishment for missing one homework assignment, but it is probably an appropriate punishment for not coming home at the appointed time.

V. **Common behavioral interventions**

    A. **Point systems.** Two forms of intervention that warrant specific consideration, given their popularity in the parenting literature, are **point systems** and **time out.** These techniques appear in various forms in most behaviorally oriented parenting literature. **Point systems** refer to ways to document that rules or expectations are being followed or that goals are being met with a token or symbol that represents something the child finds reinforcing. Such systems can also involve the loss of tokens (representing loss of privileges for reinforcers) for negative behaviors. Point systems are designed to help a parent and a child acknowledge on a regular, predetermined basis when a behavior has occurred or not occurred. This regular acknowledgment and reinforcement of goal attainment is critical for developing new skills in children. Using tangible markers of progress, can itself serve as a positive reinforcement for desired behavior. As children get older, the tangible markers of progress (i.e., tokens or symbols) are "traded in" for favored activities or events. **As point systems with younger children commonly take the form of "star charts," we will refer to "star charts" to denote this type of system in this chapter.** One common example to target with such an intervention would be fighting between siblings. The parent would **begin with the establishment of a home rule.** For example, "Treat others with respect" (this rule is the antecedent). Fighting would be a violation of this rule. The parent would also need to know how often the fighting occurs before starting an intervention. The parent would collect information (i.e., baseline data) for several days, which in this case could be a count of the number of fights noted over a period of time (i.e., in a day, a week, and so on). Although a simple tally count of the number of fights is helpful, a more informative method of collecting information would be to ask the parent to keep a simple log tracking the date, time of day of the fights, and what occurred both before (antecedents) and after (consequences) the fighting. This is called **collecting baseline data by**

completing an ABC chart, and can give the practitioner rich information on the context of the fights. Finally, the parent would need to decide what activity would be earned for rule following or decide what privilege the children usually have that can be made contingent on the absence of fighting (**establishing contingencies or consequences**). All of this information would then be put to use to create a star chart to address fights between siblings. For example, the parent creates a chart with intervals ranging from half-hour to several hours, depending on the frequency of fights. For each interval in which the rule is followed (e.g., "treat others with respect") and no fighting occurs, the parent would mark this interval with a **token such as a star, smiley face, sticker, or even a check mark.** If the children are young, the parental smiles or hugs, verbal encouragement, and the earning of the stickers may be rewarding enough to reinforce the rule of treating others with respect (i.e., no fighting). If the children are older, naturally occurring privileges can be earned with the tokens (e.g., time to watch television, ride bicycles, or play with a favored game). If fighting breaks the rule of treating others with respect, the parent would not give the token and the privileges would not be earned.

To summarize, here are a few tips for establishing star charts:

1. **Clearly define the problem behavior** (e.g., tantrums in a 4-year-old). Several behaviors to be targeted can be included in the chart, but tracking more than two or three behaviors can be difficult for the parent.

2. Have the parent **gather baseline information** on each problem behavior over a time period long enough for the problem to occur at least three or four times, to gather some information on the context of the problem behavior. Warn parents that tracking the behavior in this manner will take some work on their part; however, it is necessary to know how often the behavior occurs before you intervene to know if your intervention is effective!

3. Help the parent **create a simple chart covering a time interval** that is appropriate (e.g., if tantrums occur twice a day, the chart should include morning, afternoon, and evening intervals—hourly would be too often in this case and would be too difficult for the parent to maintain).

4. Help the parent **decide how to mark the chart** (e.g., with a smile for time periods without tan-

trums) as well as what the token (in this case a smile) can earn.

5. Help the parent create a **menu of possible re-inforcers** based on how many tokens (smiles) are earned. Having a menu of reinforcers from which the child can choose helps keep the system interesting and engaging for the child. Examples of a menu include 15 minutes of TV, a special treat with a meal, staying up 10 minutes past bedtime, or items suggested by the child.

6. Have the parents **decide when they will begin the system and set up an appointment or phone call to assess progress.** If the system is failing after several attempts, referral to a behaviorally oriented psychologist may be necessary.

B. **Time out.** In addition to star charts, time out is another technique commonly discussed in behavioral parenting literature; it is shorthand for **"time out from positive reinforcement".** What this means is that time out is an ineffective intervention if it allows a child to escape from a situation that they dislike! For example, a child who gets a time out for misbehavior when attending a formal religious ceremony may actually act up more to escape what is perceived as a boring or aversive activity. That is, by earning a time out they can play in the hallway versus sitting still and quiet in a sanctuary. Parents need to **decide beforehand what behaviors would warrant the consequence of time out, and should also designate an area of their home for use during time out.** They will also need to **explain to the child** how they will use it, so the child will understand, before any infraction has occurred, what time out is and the procedures for it. Time out can mean sitting to the side of an activity for a few moments or removal to a separate area of the home. **Rules of thumb for length of time out vary, but should be developmentally appropriate.** Length of time is less important than the child "getting the message" that misbehavior has consequences and that it is better to think before acting. For example, asking a toddler to sit quietly without fidgeting in a time out area for 10 minutes is unreasonable. Expecting a minute or two of quiet might not be. This shorter consequence also more likely results in the child productively focusing on personal behavior versus encouraging the child to focus on the parent's behavior and "unfairness." In short, this promotes the child developing internal self-control. Also, children can be **offered the opportunity for the length of time out to decrease if**

they behave appropriately while in time out. For example, a 9-year-old can be assigned a 15-minute time out, but can earn half that time off for complying with the time out procedure. **Talking to the child** or reasoning with the child while in time out **should not occur.** Brief discussion can occur once the time out has been completed by the parents asking why the time out occurred, and then guiding the child to address the action. For example, if hitting had triggered the time out, **an apology or other form of restitution** may be appropriate. Parents are likely to need direct practice and coaching to implement time out effectively; parents who are having difficulties with this form of intervention may need referral to a behavioral specialist or psychologist.

VI. **When difficulties occur at school.** One issue likely to arise with children and adolescents is the existence of school problems, which are not necessarily accompanied by problems at home. One behavioral intervention designed specifically for school problems is called the **daily report card (DRC).** This intervention is a method of home–school communication and involves having **teachers track very well-defined target behaviors,** positively worded and specifically selected to be achievable, on a daily basis. This is typically done by having teachers rate or count behaviors as described above. If the behavior occurs or the goal is met, the teacher would circle a "Yes" for that behavior for that class. This rating would occur over the course of the day and a **menu of reinforcers** would be **established at home.** The child's access to the menu is determined by how many "yeses" are earned on any given day. The next day the process begins again, so that a child has the opportunity for success each day. A key behavioral concept to understand with DRC is shaping. **Shaping** involves reinforcing successive approximations to the desired behavior. A DRC does not turn a misbehaving child into a "perfect" student in 1 day! The establishment of such an intervention likely requires the assistance of school staff and a behavioral specialist (e.g., a psychologist) to work with the family, the child, and the school to assure proper implementation, maintenance, and eventual fading of the intervention. However, this intervention is common for use with children with disruptive behavior disorders and some basic tips are noted below.

Tips for establishing a DRC involve having a good working parent–school relationship and cooperation from the school (typically the teacher and a school counselor or psychologist; occasionally, assistant principals or principals need to be included in the process). Conflictual parent–school relationships suggest that professional mediation (i.e., referral to a specialist child mental health professional) of the process is needed. Once cooperation is obtained, the teacher would select three to five behaviors to target. As with star charts, baseline information on the problem behaviors is needed before beginning the intervention and, therefore, the teacher needs to track the problem behavior for several days to establish what the DRC target behaviors should be. The DRC format and the menu of home-based reinforcers for goal attainment need to be established. Typically, the child could receive a "yes" for each behavior in each class period. With five periods and four behaviors, the maximal number of yeses that could be earned per day would be 20. The **goal** is for the target behavior to be selected so that the **child is able to earn approximately 80% of possible yeses per day** (16 in this case). Earning far fewer or far more several days in succession suggests that the target behaviors are too challenging or too easy, and need to be adjusted. Parents must also be consistent in reinforcing the DRC each day. Again, as with star charts, a menu of possible reinforcers that the child can earn at home is recommended to prevent the system from becoming too routine. Also, the parents need to **assure that the reinforcers are not available to the child when they were not earned!** When the target behaviors are met consistently, fading the DRC would begin. Fading can occur by decreasing the number of yeses earned per day. For example, by earning yeses for morning and afternoon as opposed to by class. Eventually, the goal is to fade the DRC completely and allow for the natural consequences (e.g., parental approval, better grades, more positive interactions with teachers) to maintain the progress.

VII. **When difficulties occur at home.** When the problem appears primarily to involve the home, practitioners need to appreciate that inquiry about the parent–child relationship and parenting practices is an extremely sensitive undertaking. In fact, discussions about parenting itself happen infrequently enough that significant stigma is still attached to discussion of parenting. This is especially true when mental health issues exist that may be playing a role in the problem for either the parents or the child. Therefore, it is critical for the PCP to begin with the recognition that each and every family has strengths that can become building blocks for future interventions. Interventions should also be designed to promote parental responsibility and self-efficacy. Helping parents to determine what their goals are in interactions with the PCP is one way of implicitly sending the message that parents are responsible and are seen as able to determine any changes that need to be made. The manner in which questions are asked influences the type and amount of information that is gathered and can also influence the parent in terms of whether or not to seek help.

Some problems at home can be addressed by finding ways for parents to improve their appreciation of the child's developmental level and unique characteristics. Thus, **if problems are related to unrealistic expectations, then education about developmentally appropriate goals might be helpful.** Many times tension surrounding problems with supervision, consistency, and acceptance can be helped by **increasing positive time between parents and children.** This concept can be referred to as **building an emotional bank account.** Positive interactions with children are **deposits,** and negative interactions are **withdrawals.** The balance should always be positive! **Deposits** can be made by having the parent catch the child when they are being good and setting aside time for child-directed interactions. Younger children can have special time with a parent through playtime. Whereas, for older children and adolescents, special time involves sharing a favored activity with a parent or having uninterrupted time for enjoying the company of a parent who is not distracted by other things (e.g., siblings or calls from work).

Families that show high or escalating levels of conflict may need prompt and rigorous intervention to prevent child abuse or delinquency beyond simply increasing positive time together. Several studies have shown that **cycles of escalating conflict can be broken with four major steps:**

1. Parents are advised to **reduce the amount of negative talk toward their children.** When a rule is violated, a brief and neutral statement in a calm tone of voice is best.
2. Parents should **avoid harsh or inconsistent discipline.** Because harsh discipline usually makes parents feel bad, it tends to be inconsistent. Also, when using harsh discipline (e.g., yelling or slapping), parents may model inappropriate behavior.
3. Parents should **ignore as much negative behavior as possible.** Parents should intervene only when a rule is broken or safety is compromised.
4. Parents need to **reinforce positive behavior with attention** and, in some cases, tangible rewards.

VIII. **Some parents are not ready to change.** It is critical that PCPs be keenly aware of where the parent is with regard to awareness of a problem or readiness to change problematic behavior. Often PCPs assume that parents know that a problem exists and are ready to change it. Well-meaning and excellent advice can be provided; however, such well-crafted statements or explanations may fall on "deaf ears" if the parents are ignorant of the problem, deny a problem exists, or are unwilling or feel unable to change the problem. If parents seem unwilling or not ready for change, it is time to consider referral to a mental health professional.

IX. **Summary.** In conclusion, one of the few things more humbling and difficult than parenting is giving people advice about parenting. This advice is best given in a form of a menu that is specifically tailored to the needs of a child. When giving advice to a parent, a good thought is how would you react to having a waiter in a restaurant tell you what you should eat? With this in mind, giving parents choices about how to strengthen their supervision, consistency, acceptance, affection, and role modeling can be effective. Multiple studies have shown major improvements in child and adolescent problems as a result of effective intervention. As emphasized by the *Report of the Surgeon General on Child Mental Health,* the PCP is one of the most important gatekeepers for getting help to children in need. Also, the PCP can help provide a "tune-up" for most parenting relationships, which are generally pretty good, but rarely perfect. Indeed, perfection is an impossible goal and finding the right balance between structure and affection is the goal of parent consultation in the primary care setting.

SUGGESTED READINGS

For Practitioners

Dishion T. *The family check-up: a selected intervention for family change. Adolescent transitions program.* This chapter describes the application of the stages of change model to parenting (in press).

Kelly ML. *School-home notes: promoting children's classroom success.* New York: Guilford, 1990. This easy-to-read book is filled with examples and the necessary details for the clinician to use this intervention procedure. This detailed, comprehensive program has a strong empiric base and the application is guided by the direct experiences of a master clinician.

Prochaska JO, Norcross JC, DiClemente CC. In search of how people change: applications to addictive behaviors. *Am Psychol* 1992;47:1102–1114.

Steinberg L, Lamborn SD, Darling N, et al. Over-time changes in adjustment and competence among adolescents from authoritative, authoritarian, indulgent, and neglectful families. *Child Dev* 1994;65:754–770. This research report describes some of the importance of the four characteristics of parenting. Authoritative parents are high on affection, acceptance, structure, and supervision. Children from these families had the best outcomes. The three other types of parenting had deficits in two or more of the critical areas.

For Parents

Boyd-Franklin N, Franklin AJ. *Boys into men: raising our African–American teenage sons.* New York: Penguin Putnam, 2000.

Patterson GR, Forgatch M. *Parents and adolescents living together.* Eugene, OR: Castalia Publishing, 541–343-4433:1987. This book reflects the wisdom of the Director of the Oregon Social Learning Center and one of the leading family therapy researchers of the 20th Century. The practical techniques outlined in the book focus on how to use social learning techniques to foster growth in positive directions. It is full of humorous observations and shows that parenting teens can be serious without being solemn.

Sanders MR. *Every parent: a positive approach to children's behavior,* 1992. This parenting book provides practical concepts to assist parents in developing a positive approach to children's problem behavior. A good reference for parents and practitioners, it is available from Triple P America. Available at http://www.triplep-america.com. Accessed on 6/20/02.

Every Parent's Survival Guide Video. This video, which is part of the internationally successful Triple P-Positive Parenting Program, provides useful vignettes and information for parents and practitioners. The video covers principles of positive parenting, causes of child behavior problems, goal setting and monitoring, strategies for building positive relationships with children, ways to teach new skills and encourage desirable behavior, effective methods for managing misbehavior, and family survival tips to help parents take care of themselves. Available from Triple P America (www.triplep-america.com).

Web Sites

Oregon Social Learning Center, under the direction of Gerald Patterson, is a major research center dedicated to understanding the social and psychological processes related to healthy development and family functioning. They have led the way in understanding the parenting patterns associated with disobedience and conduct problems. Available at http://www.oslc.org. Accessed on 6/20/02.

Parents Anonymous is a national parent-led support, education, and advocacy agency dedicated to strengthening families and preventing maltreatment. This group sponsors local support services in many communities across the nation. Available at http://www. parentsanonymous.org. Accessed on 6/20/02.

Primary Care Triple P. Triple P, the acronym for the Positive Parenting Program, is a multilevel system of programs for parenting and family support aimed at preventing behavioral, emotional, and developmental problems in children by enhancing the knowledge, skills, and confidence of parents. *Primary Care Triple P* is the level of *Triple P* designed specifically to be delivered by physicians and nurses. Training and practitioner resources are available through Triple P America. Available at http://www.triplep-america.com. Accessed on 6/20/02.

Zero to Three is a national nonprofit organization whose aim is to strengthen and support families, practitioners, and communities to promote the healthy development of babies and toddlers. Available at http://www.zerotothree.org. Accessed on 6/20/02.

4 ♣ The Family

Kathleen Cole-Kelly and David L. Kaye

I. **Introduction.** *The family is the patient* is the apt title of a seminal book on the family-oriented approach to working with pediatric patients. The family provides most healthcare for the pediatric patient and the family is the context in which the pediatric patient is growing and developing. Understanding the importance of the family, the family medical (including psychiatric) history, the family structure and functioning, and the influence the family has on the pediatric patient's health and well-being is essential for any pediatric practitioner. Based on the understanding of these factors, the primary care physician (PCP) will adjust his or her care of the pediatric patient. From birth to the teen years, virtually all children come into the pediatric visit with at least one adult. Most adolescents do as well. In short, children and adolescents do not present to their PCP as individuals but as parts of families. Even when a child is out of the home (i.e., foster care) it is helpful to think of the child in the context of the family.

II. **The healthier family.** Having a sense of what is a healthy family enhances the ability of the PCP to appreciate what is good and right in the parenting. Even when the situation is problematic islands of healthy functioning can exist on which the PCP can build. Recognizing these strengths serve not only the parents' but also their children's best interests. On another note: all families have "issues" and problems. None are perfect!! For this reason we use the term "healthier" families. Following is a review of the qualities of the **healthier family.**

A. **Team spirit.** The healthier family has a sense of its whole. The members are proud to belong to their "club." Much of this morale is dependent on the amount of felt freedom to join the others or to act independently. When the consequence for this autonomy is emotional or physical skewering, then the morale of the whole declines. Another factor contributing to this is the emotional and physical warmth in the family. Families in which the parents touch their children warmly (and obviously appropriately) and verbalize their appreciation of their children create healthier climates for children.

B. **Organization.** Healthier families are not democracies! All members do not have the same vote! The metaphor of the army is a useful one (a peacekeeping army ideally!). According to Keith,

> The parents are the commanding officers of the family army. Both are five-star generals. The children are the privates and sergeants in this army, and they gradually

work their way up to junior officer status. Some corollaries are that one five-star general cannot boss another five-star general around. They are peers. Rank has its privilege, and the generals have the right to make unilateral decisions without consulting the soldiers. Rank also has its responsibility and the officers are responsible for the troops' morale.

Another way of saying this is to state that parents and children are of necessity in different generations. They cannot be peers, let alone "best friends." They have different "jobs" with each other and need to respect this reality. Parents need to provide structure, guidance, supervision, limits, and opportunities for their children. Children's "job" is to grow up in as healthy a way as possible, developing their resources and "tools" maximally. Part of their "job" includes school, peers, and extracurricular activities (e.g., sports, hobbies). This works best when a division of labor exists and the roles of each member are clear.

C. **Role flexibility.** While clarity of roles is necessary, it is important to emphasize a need exists for flexibility and change (over time) in the roles or jobs that family members have. Less healthy are situations in which the parent is *never* a peer with the child, the child is *never* allowed to "try on" being an adult, or a sibling is required to be ever responsible. Healthier families promote greater role flexibility while maintaining their basic definitions of father, mother, brother, sister, and so forth. This allows for smoother life transitions (e.g., when children become teens, when grandparents become ill) and also more flexibility to face unexpected difficulties (e.g., divorce, illness, death).

D. **Empathy and emotional honesty** are qualities at the cornerstone of all relationships. Parents who have expectations markedly out of line with those of the culture or the child's developmental needs or abilities create much conflict and symptomatology. Parents with an accurate sense of their particular child's needs and abilities promote the family "team spirit." Expectations that recognize cultural demands also are healthier for children. For example, parents of a 12-year-old child who do not recognize the child's developmental need to be accepted by the peer group by buying the latest Nike footwear create great difficulty when they reject the child's desire for such. Note that parents should not buy all that children desire or that the media encourages, but rather the parents need to understand (i.e., have empathy for) their child's desires. Another example: most parents find (after a few failures!) that long car rides with young children are an invitation for disaster. When parents rigidly insist and expect that they should be able to sit for hours without a break or, more likely, without a "carrot" (i.e., something interesting/fun for them) trouble is likely to find them! Emotional honesty is another matter. Children need to feel they are dealing with something "real" when they interact with their parents, grandparents, and so on. That something "real" is their parent's feelings. When real feelings are avoided or denied, children have greater difficulty, especially in adolescence. For example, the mother in the well-known film "Ordinary People" was unable to show any real feelings about the tragedy that befell the family. Instead, she exhibited a cool composure while golfing at the country club, all the while avoiding or not showing any genuine anguish, remorse, anger, or sadness.

E. **Play and playfulness.** The healthier family has an ability to play and be playful (i.e., have a sense of humor) with each other. This critical quality allows families to cope with the painful circumstances that all people face at some time. Being able to play also allows for a greater range of emotional expression. It is easier to say many difficult things when it is done with a sense of humor. This often takes out the "sting" that creates defensiveness and arguments. Certainly, during severe difficulties (e.g., external disasters, newly diagnosed chronic illness, family disruptions of significance) this sense of play might be suspended but remains within the family's repertoire when hot issues settle down.

F. **Communication and support.** Healthier families are more able to verbalize and discuss feelings. Conflicts are managed without resorting to put-downs, shaming, or physical confrontations. Emotionally charged topics involving one member's sadness, anger, guilt, or humiliation can be "heard" by another member. An emotional expressiveness and responsiveness in the relationships exist. Healthier families are able to support each other emotionally, materially, or both.

G. **Rituals.** The healthier family has a pattern of observing its own unique rituals, which may or may not include religious rituals. Examples of rituals might include dinners together, bedtime stories, Sunday morning pancakes, and kisses before school or work. These contribute to the overall sense of team spirit and history. Families lacking their own rituals are usually in trouble.

III. **Family structure and concepts**

A. **The genogram.** One of the most efficient and effective ways to think "family" from the first pediatric visit is to gather a **three-generational genogram** and place it in the front of the patient chart. The information gathered on the genogram gives the PCP a quick snapshot of the important family members in the patient's life. Quickly, the PCP can find out what family members live with the patient, how many siblings are in the family, significant health issues in other family members, and divorces, remarriages, and deaths of family members. Gathering this information also establishes a positive connection with patients and families for future pediatric care.

With the pressures on today's PCP, how can the genogram be incorporated into clinical practice? Ideally, with any new patient beginning in the practice, the PCP can take a brief 3 to 5 minutes to gather this important information, which will contribute significantly to patient care. This can be augmented with written questionnaires. Questionnaires can include basic demographic information and also pertinent medical and psychiatric histories of family members. **The standard pediatric questionnaire given to new patients should include a checklist for family history of both traditional medical (e.g., cancer, heart disease) and psychiatric conditions (e.g., depression, bipolar disorder, anxiety, substance abuse, suicide, schizophrenia, attention-deficit/hyperactivity disorder, learning disabilities).**

The genogram (Figs. 4.1 and 4.2), which looks like a mobile when drawn, telegraphs the "skeleton" of the family system with children dangling from pairs of married, separated, or divorced adults. This picture of the basic organization of the family conveys a great deal. More detailed information about how the family is organized extends the PCP's knowledge further.

1. **Case example.** *Rosa, age 11, was in for a visit with her PCP. She came with her dad, Mr. L. Rosa has juvenile onset diabetes, which recently had been in poor control. The PCP, glancing at the genogram as she entered the room, remembered that Rosa spends ½ the week with her dad, and ½ the week with her mom. With this in mind, the PCP asked Mr. L. how information about taking care of Rosa's diabetes was getting to her mother. Mr. L. revealed they do not talk much and maybe the PCP or other office staff should give the mom a call.*

   An important piece of information has emerged about how this family is organized. The parents, although sharing the child in joint custody, are not working cooperatively with respect to her chronic illness. Without a sensitive inquiry about the relationship the parents have in working

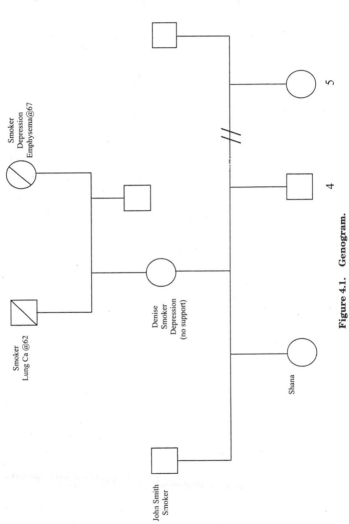

Figure 4.1.   Genogram.

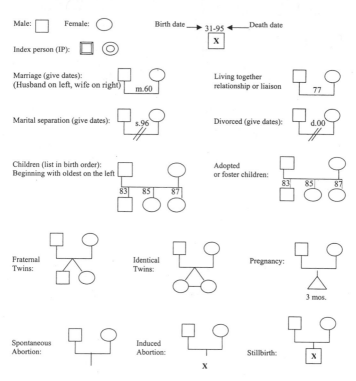

Figure 4.2.   Genogram symbols.

together for consistent management of Rosa's diabetes, unnecessary time would be spent with one parent, making adjustments to diet, insulin, or other interventions. Unnecessary hospitalizations could even occur if all significant family members taking care of Rosa are not equally informed and included in her diabetic care. This example, so familiar to PCPs, is equally relevant when considering mental health problems in children and adolescents.

Each family has a somewhat unique organizational pattern. However, some organizational patterns have been identified as being more conducive to smoother family functioning than others (Chapter 3). An important aspect of family organization is its structure (i.e., clarity of the roles and boundaries). As noted, the healthier family can be thought of as a small army unit with a division of labor and effective, but not rigid, roles. Of course, cultural variations exist and other idiosyncratic exceptions must be appreciated to account for the healthy and normal variation that occurs.

B. **Triangulation.** In addition to the family core concepts already mentioned, a key consideration of family organization merits discussion: **triangulation,** or bringing a third person into a conflict between two others. A child is especially vulnerable to being caught in an unhealthy triangulation when parental conflict cannot be resolved.

1. **Case example.** *Breion brought in his 4-year-old daughter, Aleta, for a cold and cough and sleepless nights. He was worried that she might have an ear infection. After describing the symptoms, her dad commented, "You know, her mother never seems to notice these things early enough. I have told and told her that the minute Aleta gets a cold she should bring her in but she just doesn't seem to act soon enough. I travel so much that I'm not home a lot to do it but I'll tell you, it really seems irresponsible."*

Responding to these situations effectively requires recognizing and understanding them. PCPs usually have little difficulty recognizing their own distress or anxiety when these situations arise. Triangulation occurs as a part of the **natural human tendency to connect with and seek support from others in times of stress.** What creates discomfort for the PCP is the emotional tug of choosing sides, of being loyal to one side over the other. Effective responses take a "yes and," instead of a "yes but" approach. In this situation, the PCP might respond, "I appreciate your input and understand how important it is to you to have agreement with Aleta's mom about how to parent her. I hear your concern and will work with you both to best help Aleta."

Opportunities like this happen often, not only in the PCP's office, but also naturalistically in families. Aleta's mother may promote an intense bonding with her daughter by talking about, for example, how horrible it is that her father travels so much, drinks too much, and criticizes too much. This dynamic puts the daughter in a difficult position that leaves her feeling as if she is betraying her mom if she tries to get close to her dad or vice versa, depending on the circumstances. PCPs need to have a watchful eye for (a) possibilities of being entrapped by parental triangulations that put them in conflict with other family members and (b) triangulation of a child placing them tightly in between parents' struggles, hence hindering their psychological growth and development. These children often present to the PCP with somatic complaints or sleep problems. One note of caution: when concerned that a parent or other adult is abusing a child, the PCP need not worry about triangulation. Instead, it is imperative to attend to the safety issues and follow through with assessing the risk to the child.

C. **Family health beliefs and explanatory models.** Most individuals have personal closely held beliefs or explanatory models for reasons for a nonsignificant illness (you were out without a hat, now look how that's caused you to catch a cold), or with a serious physical or mental illness. Some individuals and families favor physical explanations, whereas others favor psychological ones, but virtually all wish to feel whole and avoid feeling shame or blame for an illness. As noted, parents are highly sensitized to feeling blame for children's problems, physical or mental. It behooves the PCP to bring these beliefs out in the open and thereby steer clear of implying blame to one or both parents.

1. **Case example.** *Dr. Sharma believed that the best way to present the difficult news that the baby born to Andrew and Ann S. had cystic fibrosis was to get as many family members as possible together for this important discussion. Gathered together were the unmarried, young parents of the baby, Ann's mother, and Andrew's father. The PCP posed the question that frequently bore important fruits for discussion and prevented potential resistance to collaborative goals.*

    Dr. Sharma: "I like to ask family members at this time, what they believe caused this condition. I have my own explanations but feel it is important to get out everyone's thoughts so we are all working together."

    Andrew's father: "Well, clearly this has been caused by Ann's genes. We have no asthma in our family; no one even has had bronchitis in our family. I'm just sick to think of this terrible tragedy."

    Had the PCP not inquired about each member's belief, the potential existed for the grandfather to fuel his own and his son's anger at

Ann for her "bad" genetic contribution. This misguided critique would most likely have been played out in painful ways for Ann and the rest of the family had it not been elicited and addressed by the PCP's explanation that cystic fibrosis can ONLY occur when both parents are carriers of the genetic material. This is an extreme example, but it underscores the importance of PCPs exploring family members' beliefs. Culture dictates many beliefs and explanatory models for why people get sick and for the best way to treat the illness. If the PCP fails to elicit these beliefs, a patient or family can be seen as resistant, noncompliant, or difficult, when in fact the problem is a lack of understanding regarding what is driving the patient and family approaches.

D. **Family stress.** Clearly, a close relationship exists between stressful family events and child health. This cycle is closely connected so that events that have an impact on the children, then do so on the adults, which, in turn, affect the children, back to the parents, and so on. This **"multiplier effect"** also includes the grandparents, whose involvement makes the picture more complex.

Often stressful events precipitate physical or psychiatric illness, which can stem from illness in the child or the developmental thrust of the child (i.e., puberty and adolescence), which can then have repercussions for both the child and parents. Stressors can also include marital conflict, separation, or divorce, or illness that affects the children or the parents themselves. It is also important to note that families can become distressed for less obvious reasons (e.g., job loss, financial reversals, and community-wide tragedy or trouble). A particular sequence that the PCP should be alerted to is when a grandparent or other figure important to the parent becomes ill or dies. This reverberates through the family by having an impact on the parents' availability to the children and, hence, affects the children's well-being.

E. **Family support.** One safeguard against family stress is the presence of family support. Social support has been defined as the **emotional, instrumental, and financial help that is obtained from one's family, friends, and other social contacts.** An extensive body of research has demonstrated that social networks and supports can directly improve health, as well as buffer the adverse effects of stress.

Mobilizing a family's strengths and resources can be an excellent counter to the stressful life events all families experience. Eliciting **what has helped the family before and who is available to offer support to the patient or family members** can be useful exploration for the PCP. Knowing the difficulty of coping with single parenthood, stressful marital problems, aging parents, and learning problems in the child, the PCP can empathize with the parent about how hard these challenges are and inquire who else in the social support system (family or otherwise) can offer the parent support.

F. **Family life cycle.** In addition to family organization, the family's life cycle stage can be a useful conceptual consideration for the PCP. Identifying which phase of the life cycle a family is in further helps to orient the PCP to the context of the child.

Family life cycle stages:
1. Leaving home: the unattached adult
2. Couples and pairing
3. Pregnancy and childbirth
4. Families with young children
5. Families with adolescents; grandparents with illness or dying
6. Adulthood and the middle years
7. Graying of the family
8. Death and grieving

Each phase often demands new organizational patterns, altered rules, and new roles to be negotiated. Family therapists have suggested that **problems often emerge** and are plunked on the pediatric table at the nodal point when families are **negotiating a transition** from one phase to the next. With an appreciation of the family issues at each life cycle stage, the PCP can efficiently anticipate what might be causing the pediatric problem being brought "to the table."

IV. **Special family configurations.** Over the past 30 to 40 years, the family has changed dramatically. Trends noted in the United States, but also in most developed and some underdeveloped nations, include the following. More and more children live in configurations other than the traditional two-parent biological family. Although this traditional family still represents the majority, increasing numbers of children live in single-parent households, often headed by never married adults. In recent years, **nearly one third of all births are to unmarried mothers. Divorce rates** increased from 1940 to 1960 (generally, 2 to 2.5/1000 population), rising in the late 1960s, and peaking in the early 1980s (>5/1000), and have **slowly come down modestly over the past 10 to 15 years** (most recently, 4.2/1000). Table 4.1 summarizes selected recent demographics.

Table 4.1. Family and household demographic characteristics, 2000*

Total number of divorces	1.2 million
Divorce rate	4.2/1000
First marriages ending in divorce	40%
Second marriages ending in divorce	50%
Two-parent families with children	26 million
Single-parent families with children	12 million
Total number of children in single-parent families	19 million

* United States Census 2000 data.

A. **Divorce.** Obviously it is much more preferable for children to grow up in harmonious two-parent homes. This is often not the case and the choice for parents is whether to experience the pain of divorce or the pain of staying together with high degrees of conflict. This is equally true for the children, for whom either path has its own set of pain. Researchers on divorce are divided on the impact of divorce on children. Wallerstein and Lewis (1998) suggest that divorce is detrimental to children and has long-lasting negative effects. On the other hand, Hetherington et al. suggest that the picture is highly complex and that the effects on children are less clearcut, with many having difficulty whereas others are actually strengthened. Further, if compared with children who remain in high conflict families who do not divorce, the children of divorce appear to fare better. The two most important **predictors of "healthy" adjustment** to the divorce process are:

1. The **freedom of children from compulsion to be in an alliance** (triangulated) with one parent over the other.
2. A consistent, **loving relationship with each parent.** Regardless of the reason, children who experience their own *divorce* from a parent suffer the most.

If you notice a significant change in behavior or in physical complaints of a child in the beginning or midst of a family divorce, take time with the child to explore what it is like with the changes in the household. It should be noted that **divorce is not an event but a process that occurs over many months and years.** It involves numerous changes for parents and children. For many children, the **peak of stress occurs when the parents actually separate** and one parent moves out. The changes that occur in this initial stage (and continuing for the **next 2 years or so**) are typically the **most tumultuous** for children. The **establishment of regularity and predictability of day-to-day life** is a critical factor in the adjustment of children (most especially younger children) experiencing the divorce of their parents. Sometimes school performance can change, toileting habits of young children can regress, or behavior at home can become erratic. It is important to ask directly how children and parents are faring with the changes. Here are some **tips for guidance of parents** who are in the midst of divorcing:

1. There is a **range of emotional responses** that children show that are normal and expectable. For **younger children,** this includes fear, confusion, crying, and regressive behavior (e.g., sleeping with parents, wetting the bed, baby talk). For **school-aged children,** this often includes anger, defiance, sadness, longing, and regressive behavior. Guilt and self-blame may also be prominent in these children. **Adolescents** often show anger, depression, sadness, and guilt. At times, older children and adolescents do not show much of an emotional response immediately. This should also be considered normal unless it involves extreme and damaging denial or, in some other way, clearly interferes with the child's forward development.

2. The **fantasy of reconciliation** is common and normal. Parents should be prepared for this, accept it, and attempt to be understanding. Little is gained from "confronting" this, although gentle recognition of the reality of the situation can help children accept the unpleasant actuality. When children seem unable to come to terms with this reality, consider referral to a mental health specialist.

3. Some children will express **anger** or other uncomfortable feelings. These feelings should be **acknowledged, accepted, and understood** by parents. Children should not be talked out of their feelings (e.g., "now you shouldn't feel mad, you'll be happier in the long run", "don't be angry, it's no use", "too bad, you just have to deal with it!"). Although it is all right to verbalize these feelings, they should not be acted out. In other words, this acceptance does not extend to destructive or aggressive *behavior*!

4. It is important that the children **not feel that they are to blame** for the divorce. This may require that the parents explain the circumstances

of the breakup. This is especially true in the "civilized" divorce in which no overt conflict has occurred. These are especially difficult for children to come to terms with. In these cases, a general explanation, such as "we had a lot of problems that we just could not work out," is usually sufficient. The explanations are best if the parents acknowledge joint problems that, despite their best efforts and love and concern for their children, could not be resolved. Parents should not go into great detail about why they are divorcing as this draws the child into triangulation and side taking.

5. Parents should **avoid "triangulating"** the children. Despite the intense emotional needs of parents, especially the parent who is "left" and injured, they should resist the temptation to draw any children into taking sides. This generally interferes with a child's forward development and promotes symptomatic behavior. A particularly important corollary of this is to **refrain from:**
   - **"Badmouthing"** the other parent to the children
   - **Continuing overt conflict** in front of the children. Such behavior stunts the child's emotional development, creates deep resentment, and eventually will backfire as the child is damaged. **If the parents can do only one thing to help their children in the face of divorce, it is refraining from badmouthing and continuing overt conflict!** Parents who are unable to refrain from these behaviors should be referred for their own mental health treatment.

6. **Regularity, stability, and predictability** are critical for children's optimal development under any circumstances. This is especially true in the postdivorce situation, in which these qualities can be in short supply. Moves, changes in schools, and loss of financial stability are important and frequent concomitants of divorce. The fewer of these changes the child has to cope with, the better. The **rapid reestablishment of routines** and patterns **at home, school, with peers,** and so on is also paramount. Encourage parents to stick with the predivorce patterns of bedtimes, meal times, homework expectations, chores, and so forth, which helps anchor a child through these rough waters.

7. It is best for children to have **positive relationships with both parents.** Having regular and predictable contact with both parents is

optimal, especially for younger children. In most situations, this requires a written **parenting plan** (Chapter 9) delineating the specific days and times the child will be with each parent. This is generally done as part of the divorce decree. As children become adolescents this issue becomes more complicated as teens become progressively more oriented toward peers and school life. Adolescents also increasingly assert their claims about such matters. This all translates to the need for parents to show greater flexibility as the children get older.

8. Encourage parents to make **extra efforts to be emotionally available** to their children. They should try to stay tuned in to their children's feelings and afford them opportunities to express these feelings in appropriate ways. One way to do this with younger children is **"the 5 minutes,"** in which the parent is instructed to spend 5 minutes with the child on a regular basis (every day is optimal for the youngest children, less often as they move through elementary school). During this time, the parent is "just to listen" to whatever the *child* wants to talk about. "No advice, judgment, good or bad, right or wrong. Just listening and reflecting so the child knows he or she is being heard." Many parents find this a helpful way to stay emotionally in touch with their children. Adolescents are trickier as they need to be able to talk on their own terms, in their own time. Parents can look to create opportunities for their adolescents to talk, recognizing that a "take" can depend on many capricious and unpredictable factors. Ultimately, the adolescent needs to feel that he or she is coming to the discussion voluntarily if it is to be fruitful.

9. It may be helpful to remind parents that these **issues do not go away after the children leave home.** Graduations, marriages, grandchildren, rituals, and holidays continue to be sources of potential conflict that cannot be avoided in the future. It is in everyone's interest to continue to move toward an emotional resolution and settling of feelings, and to do so as soon as possible. The goal is not necessarily for the parents to become "friends," which only occasionally happens, but rather to reach a "peaceful coexistence" in which the emotional tugs on the children are minimized.

B. **Single parents.** A common consideration with single parents is the issue of **social support** for the single parent. Not that having a spouse is any guarantee of having good partner support, but it is inherently a consideration with the single parent. In many cultures and ethnic groups, the maternal grandmother or other relative plays a major role in the raising of children. In these situations, it is incumbent on the physician to **inquire about the other family or others (e.g., friends) who support the patient/family.** Asking, "Who helps you take care of Joey?" is often instructive. The strain of being the sole adult responsible for one or more children can be formidable. PCPs can help the single parent feel understood by acknowledging the strength it takes to persevere in the midst of that strain.

C. **Stepfamilies.** The addition of another adult to the life of the child poses both challenges and opportunities. Much depends on the individuals involved, their "match" with each other, and the adults' abilities to be emotionally available and empathic to the child. However, even in the best of circumstances, adults and children must make many new **adjustments in living together.** This can be the source of much strain. On top of this, all children face the **loyalty binds** presented when living with a new adult (e.g., If I'm nice to him, will dad be hurt or upset?). In more difficult situations children are being tightly pushed or pulled (or both) in ways that interfere with the establishment of a relationship with the stepparent. Or worse, they may be required to live with someone who is abusive or whom they genuinely and legitimately do not like.

D. **Adolescent parents.** Adolescent parenthood is an all too frequent occurrence in the United States. Although the **birth rates for American teens have dropped modestly** in the past decade (from a high of 62/1000 in 1991, to 51/1000 in 1998), nearly **500,000 babies are born annually to teens.** Nearly 80% of these teen mothers are unmarried. In addition to elevated risk of adverse physical effects, these babies are also at substantial psychosocial risk. This age group has multiple needs that require a PCP to scrutinize the family relationships in the pediatric patient's life. Often with the adolescent patient, the **grandparent(s) play a larger role in the child rearing.** Mindful of this, you will need to find out how the adolescent mother and her mother or father are negotiating who is doing what in terms of child care, feeding practices, discipline, and so on. It can be extremely difficult to balance the needs of the infant, which may be better addressed by an older grandparent, with respect for the teenage biological parent. In some situations, the adolescent and parent have agreed that the grandparents, in fact, will function as the parents. Over time, the PCP can help the family members redefine their roles as the teen mother matures and is more able to take on parenting functions.

E. **Gay and lesbian parents** have all the same joys and struggles with children's demands, growth, and development that all parents confront. However, the societal lack of acceptance for gay and lesbian parents can impose a sense of shame that can affect the children as well. Teasing of the children can also be highly problematic. Despite the strong feelings that many have on the politics of this issue, limited data address the actual effects on children. Nevertheless these data, although not definitive, do suggest that the children of gay or lesbian parents **show no greater levels of distress or frequency of psychological problems than children raised by heterosexual parents.** Furthermore **no evidence** suggests that these children are more likely to **become homosexual themselves.** As with other situations, you need to evaluate the child and family on their individual characteristics and qualities.

It may be important to meet with the gay or lesbian parents to find out how and when they are going to talk with their children about their homosexuality. Many resources exist (e.g., Partners Task Force of Gay and Lesbian Couples, www.buddybuddy. com) that can help guide parents and PCPs in addressing these concerns. Multiple factors need to be considered in determining the "right time" to talk with children. One hint may be that the child initiates asking about the adults' relationships. In shaping their responses, the adults then need to consider the child's:
1. Cognitive maturity
2. Emotional readiness
3. Available family support
4. Community and school climate

As in children's questions about adoption, parents often need to address fewer of the "details," and more of the overarching issues that are immediately important to the child (i.e., Are they still safe and secure? Do the adults love and care about them? Will the adults be there to help and support them?). Similarly, large issues such as this one are never addressed at once but rather involve many discussions over a period of years. The discussions change as the child becomes older and different considerations emerge. The most significant contribution you can make to the gay and lesbian couple is to reassure them that you will be available to them, support them, and be open to helping them with any conversations they would like to have with their children. Many communities offer support groups for the children of gay and lesbian families. Mental health professionals should be familiar with available resources.

F. **Grandparents' roles.** The role of grandparents varies tremendously, depending on the parental circumstances (e.g., single parents, blended families, relationships with the parents, geography). Families in which cultural differences exist because of recent immigration, the grandparents may have very different ideas about children's behavior than the children who have become more acculturated to customs in the United States. This can create tension for parents who are trying to bridge the old and new cultures. It is important to ask the parents what role the grandparents play in the child's life and also whether they would like this to be different in any way. In some situations, with single parenting or a parent with a chronic illness, the grandparent may play a more central role in the family and child's life. But these expectations need to be clearly articulated so that boundaries are respected and resentments are avoided. If a grandparent is the one to take the child to the doctor, a mechanism for keeping the parents informed so that their parenting is not bypassed is an important consideration. Making an agreement with parents and grandparents about those roles should be part of a well child visit when issues are to be resolved about which generation is in charge of the child's health and well-being.

G. **Families of children with chronic illness.** Children with chronic illness have a major impact on marriage and the family. Chronic illness can be highly taxing on the parents' resources and exacerbate marital tension and conflict. In turn, this can undermine the parenting of the other children in the family. The family can become so engaged with the care of one child with a chronic illness that the other children receive less than sufficient amounts of time and attention, which has been referred to as the **"hidden patient."** These children often become good at accommodating to "going without" until a stressor precipitates somatic, psychiatric, or behavioral symptoms. Families can also rigidly organize themselves around the chronic illness. These families are at risk of losing healthy rituals that allow the family to function at its best. Helping the family wrestle with **keeping the illness in its place** versus dominating every movement in the family is a valuable intervention for the PCP to make.

Families develop a **division of labor** and involvement in child care. Too often, one parent becomes excessively involved in the care of an ill child, while the other parent is peripheral. This can result in resentments and burn out for the involved parent, and guilt for the other parent and child. Chronically ill children often **worry about being "a burden"** to their families. If parents have unresolved issues in their relationship, focusing on their child's chronic illness can stabilize the tensions in their marriage. This dynamic does not encourage the child to develop independent skills for taking care of him- or herself.

IV. **Summary.** Working with families in pediatric care is inevitable. It also is the avenue to understanding the rich complexity of the lives of patients—their stories, their challenges, their history, and their changes. All pediatric interventions require the good will and concordance of families. Learning effective ways of eliciting, understanding, and intervening with these unique and all-important persons in the pediatric patient's life results in a more effective, as well as satisfying and rewarding practice.

SUGGESTED READINGS

Allmond B, Tanner J, Buckman H. *The family is the patient: using family interviews in children's medical care.* Baltimore: Williams & Wilkins, 1998.

American Psychiatric Association resource document on controversies in child custody: gay and lesbian parenting, transracial adoptions, joint versus sole custody, and custody gender issues. *J Am Acad Psychiatry Law* 1998;26(2):267–276.

Hetherington EM, Kelly J. *For better or for worse: divorce reconsidered.* New York: WW Norton, 2002.

Hetherington EM, Stanley-Hagan M. The adjustment of children with divorced parents: a risk and resiliency perspective. *J Child Psychol Psychiatry* 1999;40(1):129–140.

Keith D, Connell G, Connell L. *Defiance in the family.* Philadelphia: Brunner-Routledge, 2001:5.

Kelly J. Children's adjustment in conflicted marriage and divorce: a decade review of research. *J Am Acad Child Adolesc Psychiatry* 2000;39(8):963–973.

McDaniel S, Campbell T, Seaburn D. *Family-oriented primary care.* New York: Springer-Verlag, 1990.

McDaniel S, Hepworth J, Doherty W. *Medical family therapy: a biopsychosocial approach to families with health problems.* New York: Basic Books, 1992.

McGoldrick M, Gerson R. *Genograms in family assessment.* New York: Jason Aronson, 1978.

Rolland J. *Families, illness and disability: an integrative treatment model.* New York: Basic Books, 1994.

Steinglass P, Horan M. Families and chronic illness. In: Walsh R, Anderson C, eds. *Chronic disorders and the family*. Binghamton, NY: Haworth Press, 1988.

Wallerstein J, Lewis J. The long-term impact of divorce on children: a first report from a 25-year study. *Family and Conciliation Courts Review*. 1998;36(3):368–383.

Wood BL, Klebba K, Miller B. Evolving the biobehavioral family model: the fit of attachment. *Fam Process*. 2000;39(3):319–344.

5 ♣ Management and Assessment of Child Mental Health Problems in the Pediatric Office

Christopher F. Pollack and David L. Kaye

Pediatricians are increasingly being expected to perform in roles that stretch and, in some cases, surpass the boundaries of traditional pediatric training. Although the American Board of Pediatrics (Kelleher, 1995) is increasing ambulatory and behavioral training requirements, which helps to increase awareness of psychosocial problems over the long term, primary care pediatricians in practice struggle to meet today's psychosocial demands.

Health management organizations and other managed care systems increasingly rely on primary care providers (PCPs) to screen, assess, and triage patients for a wide range of both medical and psychological problems. Psychological problems are often difficult to detect or to treat appropriately in a primary care setting (Higgins, 1994). Managed care's additional focus on productivity and profitability has created pressure for pediatric clinicians to limit attention on psychosocial problems, which further increases the difficulty in identifying such problems. However, **early detection and treatment of these problems is the most effective and efficient method of care** (Bennett, 1991). In a review of the literature, Costello (1986) found that **pediatricians generally identify less than one-third the psychopathology found in community-based surveys** in the United States. Another study surveying 300 children, Costello (1989) found that 22% met criteria for a *Diagnostic and Statistical Manual of Mental Disorders,* Third Edition (DSM-III) disorder. However, only 5.7% of children in the population were identified by the pediatrician and a mere 3.8% of the samples were referred for mental health services.

I. **Three models.** Generally, **three models exist for delivering mental health services in the pediatric primary care setting** (Garralda, 2001). Each model has strengths and limitations, but all promote the public health of the pediatric population. They are often combined, so that in any given setting more than one model can be used.

1. **Primary care management model** aims to increase the capacity of primary care personnel for early detection and management of mental health problems.

2. **In-house child mental health specialist model** involves assessment and ongoing treatment by child mental health specialists (typically psychologists or master's level therapists) working in the primary care setting.

3. **Consultation-liaison model** involves a consultation-liaison specialist (typically a child or adolescent psychiatrist or psychologist) working in the primary care setting to provide support for management by PCPs. These specialists can evaluate and make recommendations to the PCP regarding management within the primary care setting. They can also make referrals for ongoing specialist mental health treatment, but would not provide that treatment themselves within the primary care setting.

A. **The primary care management model.** In large part, this book focuses on and promotes this model by augmenting the ability of the PCP to assess and manage mental health problems. This approach is the most important from a public health point of view. Compared with the other models, improved assessment, recognition, management, and referral by the PCP would benefit the greatest number of children and adolescents. However, a variety of factors hamper the PCP's ability to assess mental health issues effectively in the pediatric setting. **Time constraints** placed on the PCP make it difficult to address or investigate adequately mental health concerns. The PCP may only be allotted 10 minutes for a visit, during which he or she is often called on to address a host of concerns. A PCP attempting to conduct a complete inquiry of psychosocial issues with every patient would fall hours behind schedule and face a full and frustrated waiting room. If mental health issues are suspected, the PCP may find it more helpful to schedule a conference to ensure both adequate time and reimbursement for their services. This conference could be scheduled as a **level 5 visit,** with up to an hour designated to assess suspected mental health issues. This method, however, has a significant impact on productivity if used repeatedly. A potentially more cost-effective solution for managing this dilemma would involve the PCP scheduling two **20-minute level 4 visits** on different days to assess mental health concerns. This method does extend the time frame of the assessment, but increases productivity and, therefore, can be used more frequently. **Clear documentation** of the time spent conducting the assessment as well as the procedures and information gathered helps ensure that full reimbursement for this time is received. Additionally, this documentation also provides the PCP with a stronger position if a managed care organization should choose to challenge the billing for these services. (For more detail about documentation and reimbursement issues see Sulkes S: Coding and documentation for reimbursement.)

Telephone contacts with patients also can significantly drain time for the PCP. This drain can be decreased in a number of ways. Many practices find it helpful to have **calling hours,** which are staffed by nurse practitioners or nursing staff. During these hours patients can call to discuss a variety of concerns, including mental health issues. If the issue appears to be involved or the conversation is becoming lengthy, a **nurse practitioner or nurse** can direct the patient to come in for a conference to address their concerns. Pediatricians may also find it helpful to encourage patients to set up conferences to address issues rather than attempting to address these issues over the telephone. Additionally, the use of a mental health professional in partnership with the pediatric practice, as will be discussed below, may facilitate the process of assisting patients and providing good care in a cost-effective manner.

In this model, a premium is also placed on the utilization of other primary care professionals for both assessment and management. It is crucial to **utilize nurse practitioners and physician assistants** to the fullest extent possible. It is incumbent on the PCP to be aware of the legal scope of practice for these professionals to integrate them optimally and creatively into a coherent approach.

B. **The in-house child mental health specialist model** involves the use of specialist mental health professionals within the primary care setting. This model addresses the problem of time management for the PCP and has the benefit of providing ongoing treatment in a setting in which most patients and families feel comfortable (i.e., the PCP office suite). If a mental health professional is to be used, the question arises whether to enlist the assistance of a social worker, psychologist, or psychiatrist. Also, will the mental health professional be an employee, a consultant, or even a partner? Some state laws prohibit practitioners from different professions from being in partnership with one another. However, these laws are changing and in a number of states interesting collaborations are occurring between mental health practitioners and pediatricians. If a clinical social worker, clinical psychologist, or psychiatric educational program is available in the area, it may be possible to arrange for interns or residents to spend time assisting a pediatric office as part of their training.

C. **The consultation-liaison model** involves a contract with a mental health professional for a set number of hours to provide regular consultation regarding mental health assessment and treatment issues. The strength of this model is its appeal to a wide variety of mental health professionals and its provision of access to specialty mental health services to many patients and families. One possibility is to hire a consultant, whose billings would be credited into the practice account. Another possibility is creating a barter system wherein the pediatric office trades support services (e.g., billing and secretarial support, use of physical space for the mental health professional to see patients) in return for consultation and assistance with triaging patients. By using a mental health professional, the PCP can decrease the time spent assessing and referring for mental health issues. For example, the professional or staff member could conduct an initial 40-minute assessment of the patient, with the PCP joining them for an additional 20-minute level 4 visit to complete the assessment. This allows the PCP to conserve valuable time *and* provide rapid assessment of mental health concerns.

1. **Example 1. Limited consultation-liaison: phone triage.** One method would be for the mental health professional to conduct **phone triage.** PCPs, nurse practitioners, and nurses could provide the mental health professional with the background for any concerns regarding various patients (Fig. 5.1). The mental health provider could then contact the patient or the patient's parents to conduct a brief telephone assessment to determine whether the patient would benefit from further assessment.

2. **Example 2. Limited consultation-liaison: crisis intervention.** Another way to use the mental health provider could be in the form of **crisis intervention.** The provider could agree to act as a resource to assess, stabilize, and refer, if necessary, patients who are in crisis. A provider can also be contracted to conduct brief consultation sessions with patients to stabilize them while assessing the need for further treatment.

3. **Example 3. Limited consultation-liaison: continuing medical education.** Another model would involve developing closer relationships with mental health providers in the community. A psychologist could be hired to train and supervise staff in the use of some screening devices as well as to provide consultation regarding the analysis of the data. A mental health professional could be invited to share lunch or breakfast with the PCP, nurse practitioners, or both periodically to provide consultation and

Patient Update/Consultation

Patient Name and
Name of Parent: _____
Patient DOB: _____
Patient Phone #: _____
Date: _____
Referred By: _____

Reason for Referral/Consult:

_____

_____

_____

_____

_____

Disposition: _____ Accepted for Evaluation _____ Accepted for treatment
_____ Brief Consultation _____ Referred Out _____ No action taken

Primary Diagnosis if Applicable:

_____

Plan/Progress/Additional Information:

_____

_____

_____

_____

_____

_____

_____

_____

_____

_____

Figure 5.1.   Sample referral sheet.

education regarding the assessment of psychosocial issues.

4. **Example 4. Bartered consultation-liaison association.** A large PCP office (i.e., 10 pediatricians) entered into an association with a psychologist. Because of state laws, the psychologist was unable to become a legal partner in the practice. Rather than a direct fee for services approach, a barter system was implemented. The psychologist would provide 10 hours per week of consultation, telephone triage, and crisis intervention. Also, the psychologist agreed to provide seminars to the pediatricians and staff on identifying various mental health difficulties, managing strategies for different patients, and current research findings regarding mental health issues. In return, the pediatric group provided an on-site office (a converted examination room in which patients could be evaluated or therapy

conducted) in return for a nominal rental fee. Additionally, the practice provided billing, secretarial, and administrative support for the psychologist.

5. **Example 5. Contracting with managed care.** A number of pediatric practices have made successful proposals to managed care organizations to have mental health services, which have been paid for by the pediatric practice, reimbursed, in part or entirely. One key to making such a proposal successfully is illustrating how such in-house services will decrease both the number of referrals to specialists and, through early intervention, the length of treatment provided by a specialist. As referrals to specialists are less cost-effective to managed care organizations, they may find this type of proposal appealing.

6. **Example 6. Taking advantage of mental health "dead time."** Mental health professionals who specialize in children often have periods during the day when it is difficult for them to fill patient slots because of children being in school. A mental health professional may be willing to conduct brief screening assessments for an hourly fee during those periods. The cost of this system is offset by the decreased time spent assessing mental health issues and the subsequent increase in the PCP's productivity.

7. **Example 7. Utilization of universities.** Another possible system can involve a partnership with a local university or college **graduate program in psychology.** The graduate program could be approached for assistance in scoring screening questionnaires and writing brief summaries for the PCP to review. This would streamline the scoring and analysis of screening measures for the pediatric office and provide the university with data for research and students with practice in scoring and analyzing data. If such an arrangement were entered into, parents would need to provide informed consent for the data to be used for research purposes.

Some communities offer advanced training for child mental health specialists. These include psychiatry programs, psychology graduate programs, or social work programs. Pediatric rotations can be arranged for these trainees in pediatric offices. The pediatric rotation can involve having the trainee work with the pediatric office on developing an assessment program, see patients for short-term treatment, assist with triaging patients to appropriate care, and provide consultation to the PCP. In return, the pediatric office may be asked to support a portion of the intern's salary. However, some programs may not require financial support, as gaining experience may be the primary objective for the intern. Alternatively, a proposal to a managed care organization for such reimbursement to the practice for providing the services, as discussed, may provide the necessary funding. If the intern later becomes a practitioner in the community, the pediatric group will also have developed a working relationship for patient referral in the future.

II. **Screening tools.** From both a clinical and a public health perspective it is cost- and time-effective to use some type of screening measure to detect mental health problems. A decision needs to be made whether to use a **structured diagnostic psychiatric screening interview or a screening questionnaire.** Use of a structured interview would require training staff in conducting the interview and can take between 25 and 45 minutes, or longer. Hence, structured interviews generally are not feasible in the PCP office and are reserved for research purposes. **Screening questionnaires are available both for general developmental and mental health concerns.** Screening for developmental concerns uses parent response questionnaires; mental health screening questionnaires are often available for parents, adolescents, and teachers. It is often helpful to have **mental health screening forms filled out by both parents and teens, obtaining teacher forms only in selected situations.** Screening devices can be completed by parents or the patient **in the waiting room, or mailed to parents prior to their visit.** They offer an extremely powerful tool in the assessment of patient development and mental health, and often are key in opening the door for further exploration and assessment of mental health issues. Depending on the device, scoring of the responses can take between 2 and 10 minutes.

Additional thought needs to be given to how screening will be conducted. Will all patients be given a general or "mass" screening at specific ages? Will patients be screened selectively based on risk factors or the pediatric staff's discretion? Will screenings be included with every physical examination? Obviously, a general screening ensures a greater likelihood of detecting difficulties, but at a significantly greater cost in terms of time and resources. Selective screening may not detect all difficulties, but is the detection rate significantly lower than for general screening? To date, no sufficient amount of research answers this question and these decisions must be left to individual groups of practitioners.

Selected and commonly used general screening tools that may be appropriate in the PCP office will now be briefly described. Screening tools for **specific** clinical problems (i.e., attention-deficit/hyperactivity disorder [AD/HD], depression) are reviewed in those chapters in this book.

A. **Developmental screens**
   1. **Ages and Stages questionnaire**
      Source: Paul H. Brookes Publishers. P.O. 10624, Baltimore, MD 21285. Telephone: 1-800-636-3775.

      Age range: Birth to 5 years.

      Description: Parent questionnaire with 10 to 15 items for each age range. Provides drawings and simple directions to aid parents' description of their children's skills.

      Administration time: 5 to 10 minutes.

      Scoring time: 7 minutes.

      Comments: Gives single pass-fail score; thus best used as a **prescreening** tool.

   2. **Child Development Inventories**
      Source: Behavior Science Systems, P.O. 580274, Minneapolis, MN 55458. Telephone: 612-929-6220.

      Age range: 3 to 72 months.

      Description: Parent questionnaire with three separate inventories for different ages. Each has 60 yes-or-no questions. Screens for language, motor, cognitive, social, preacademic, and self-help skills. A 300-item version is also available for more in-depth assessment.

      Administration time: 5 to 10 minutes.

      Scoring time: 5 to 10 minutes.

      Comments: Excellent standardized screening test.

   3. **Parents' Evaluations of Developmental Status (PEDS)**
      Source: Ellsworth and Vandermeer Press, P.O. 68164, Nashville, TN 37206. Telephone: 615-226-4460. www.pedstest.com.

      Age range: Birth to 8 years.

      Description: Ten-question, evidenced-based triage tool and guidance system for developmental, cognitive, and behavioral concerns.

      Administration time: 5 minutes.

      Scoring time: Few minutes.

      Comments: Excellent standardized screen developed for use in PCP offices and available in English and Spanish. Fifth grade reading level makes this easy to use with parents from a wide variety of socioeconomic backgrounds. Superior tool in most clinical practice situations.

B. Behavioral screens

1. Child Behavior Checklist (CBCL)

Source: http://www.aseba.org/ordering/ordering_start.html.

Age range: 4 to 18 years (separate version for 2 to 4 years).

Description: CBCL/4–18 obtains parents' reports of children's competencies and behavioral or emotional problems. Parents provide information for 20 "competence" items covering their child's activities, social relations, and school performance. Contains 118 items that describe specific behavioral and emotional problems, plus two open-ended items for reporting additional problems. Parents rate their child for how true each item is now or within the past 6 months using the following scale: 0 = not true (as far as you know); 1 = somewhat or sometimes true; 2 = very true or often true.

Administration time: About 30–45 minutes. Can be sent or given to parents to complete at home and return to PCP.

Scoring time: 10 minutes.

Comments: The best normed and most widely used screening measure in mental health settings. An excellent and comprehensive measure with additional forms for teachers and a youth self-report; however, it is often considered too lengthy and time-consuming to score in a pediatric setting (Stancin, 1997). This may still be a good resource if scoring is completed by an outside source or support staff, or if used just as a general mental health "review of systems" without scoring.

2. Eyberg Child Behavior Inventory (ECBI)

Source: Psychological Assessment Resources, P.O. Box 998 Odessa, FL 33556. Telephone: 1-800-331-8378; http://www.parinc.com/

Age range: 2 1/2 to 11 years of age.

Description: A parent report form that consists of 36 short statements of common behavior problems.

Administration time: About 10 minutes, less if parents complete independently.

Scoring time: 5 minutes.

Comments: A good screening device for younger children.

3. **Family Psychosocial Screening**
   Source: Kemper KJ, Kelleher KJ. Family psychosocial screening: instruments and techniques. *Ambulatory Child Health* 1996;4: 325–339.
   Age range: Parent self-report for assessment of family functioning.
   Description: A two-page clinic intake form that identifies psychosocial risk factors associated with developmental problems including (a) four items on parental history of physical abuse as a child; (b) six items on parental substance abuse; and (c) three items on maternal depression.
   Administration time: About 15 minutes, less if parents complete independently.
   Comments: A nice adjunct to the screening devices that focus on the child's behaviors.

4. **Pediatric Symptom Checklist**
   Source: http://www.massgeneral.org/psc/
   Age range: 4 to 16 years.
   Description: Parent report of 35 short statements of problem behaviors, including both externalizing (conduct) and internalizing (e.g., depression, anxiety, adjustment) (Fig. 5.2). **Youth self-report** of 35 similar items (Fig. 5.3). Cutoff scores indicating a potentially clinically significant issue vary according to age. For children between **6 and 16 years of age, a cutoff score of 28** or greater indicates significant impairment. For children between the ages of **2 and 5, a cutoff of 24 or greater is used and the scores on items 6, 7, 14, and 15 are ignored.** The low reading level required allows this to be used with a wide variety of socioeconomic backgrounds.
   Administration time: About 5 minutes; can be filled out in the waiting room.
   Scoring time: Approximately 2 to 3 minutes.
   Comments: A study by Jellinek et al. (1999), involving 395 PCP and 21,000 children, screening was successfully implemented by clinic personnel without the aid of research assistants or other personnel trained specifically for study purposes. This checklist appears to offer the best combination of validity, and ease of scoring and administration for the PCP office.

5. **PortMD system**
   The PortMD system is a more elaborate and systematic alternative to those assessment tools mentioned above. This is a new and innovative

Emotional and physical health go together in children. Because parents are often the first to notice a problem with their child's behavior, emotions or learning, you may help your child get the best care possible by answering these questions. Please indicate which statement best describes your child.

Please mark under the heading that best describes your child:

		NEVER	SOMETIMES	OFTEN
1. Complains of aches and pains	1			
2. Spends more time alone	2			
3. Tires easily, has little energy	3			
4. Fidgety, unable to sit still	4			
5. Has trouble with teacher. (6-16 year old children only)	5			
6. Less interested in school (6-16 year old children only)	6			
7. Acts as if driven by a motor	7			
8. Daydreams too much	8			
9. Distracted easily	9			
10. Is afraid of new situations	10			
11. Feels sad, unhappy	11			
12. Is irritable, angry	12			
13. Feels hopeless	13			
14. Has trouble concentrating	14			
15. Less interested in friends	15			
16. Fights with other children	16			
17. Absent from school..... (6-16 year old children only)	17			
18. School grades dropping. (6-16 year old children only)	18			
19. Is down on him or herself	19			
20. Visits the doctor with doctor finding nothing wrong	20			
21. Has trouble sleeping	21			
22. Worries a lot	22			
23. Wants to be with you more than before	23			
24. Feels he or she is bad	24			
25. Takes unnecessary risks	25			
26. Gets hurt frequently	26			
27. Seems to be having less fun	27			
28. Acts younger than children his or her age	28			
29. Does not listen to rules	29			
30. Does not show feelings	30			
31. Does not understand other people's feelings	31			
32. Teases others	32			
33. Blames others for his or her troubles	33			
34. Takes things that do not belong to him or her	34			
35. Refuses to share	35			

Total score _____

Does your child have any emotional or behavioral problems for which she/he needs help?   ( ) N   ( ) Y
Are there any services that you would like your child to receive for these problems?   ( ) N   ( ) Y

If yes, what services?_____

Figure 5.2.   Pediatric symptom checklist (PSC). (© 1999 Michael Jellinek, M.D.)

online system that includes an initial assessment tool and an ongoing monitoring tool for tracking AD/HD and other selected emotional and behavioral disorders in children and adolescents. This proprietary system was based on DSM-IV diagnostic criteria and developed for the PCP in collaboration with Mark Wolraich, M.D. This promising approach requires the user to have basic computer skills and Internet access. For those able to use the system, it has the advantage of being completed at the convenience of parent and teacher. The instrument takes about 30 minutes for each parent to complete and 20 minutes for the teacher. Data collected are immediately available in the form of easy-to-read

Please mark under the heading that best fits you:

	Never	Sometimes	Often
1. Complain of aches or pains............................	——	——	——
2. Spend more time alone.................................	——	——	——
3. Tire easily, little energy.............................	——	——	——
4. Fidgety, unable to sit still...........................	——	——	——
5. Have trouble with teacher..(6-16 year old children only) ——	——	——	——
6. Less interested in school....(6-16 year old children only) ——	——	——	——
7. Act as if driven by motor.............................	——	——	——
8. Daydream too much......................................	——	——	——
9. Distract easily..	——	——	——
10. Are afraid of new situations.........................	——	——	——
11. Feel sad, unhappy.....................................	——	——	——
12. Are irritable, angry..................................	——	——	——
13. Feel hopeless...	——	——	——
14. Have trouble concentrating............................	——	——	——
15. Less interested in friends............................	——	——	——
16. Fight with other children.............................	——	——	——
17. Absent from school. ..(6-16 year old children only)	——	——	——
18. School grades dropping. ..(6-16 year old children only) ——	——	——	——
19. Down on yourself......................................	——	——	——
20. Visit doctor with doctor finding nothing wrong........	——	——	——
21. Have trouble sleeping.................................	——	——	——
22. Worry a lot...	——	——	——
23. Want to be with parent more than before...............	——	——	——
24. Feel that you are bad.................................	——	——	——
25. Take unnecessary risks................................	——	——	——
26. Get hurt frequently...................................	——	——	——
27. Seem to be having less fun............................	——	——	——
28. Act younger than children your age....................	——	——	——
29. Do not listen to rules................................	——	——	——
30. Do not show feelings..................................	——	——	——
31. Do not understand other people's feelings.............	——	——	——
32. Tease others..	——	——	——
33. Blame others for your troubles........................	——	——	——
34. Take things that do not belong to you.................	——	——	——
35. Refuse to share.......................................	——	——	——

Total Score ____ _____

Figure 5.3.   Pediatric symptom checklist—youth report (Y-PSC).
(© 1999 Michael Jellinek, M.D.)

reports and graphs for the PCP. More information is available at www.help4life.com/index.htm or by calling 866-476-7863.

III. Direct assessment of mental health problems. Once screening is done and a problem identified, the PCP needs to assess directly for mental health problems. In this assessment process, information usually needs to be obtained from:

1. Parents
2. Child or adolescent
3. Teachers

Information from parents is always critical, but especially in children or adolescents with "externalizing" types of problems (e.g., AD/HD, antisocial behaviors, substance abuse). On the other hand, children or adolescents themselves are often better able to report "internalizing" symptoms (e.g., anxiety, depression, sleep problems). It is by putting together the data from all sources of information that the PCP can obtain the clearest and most accurate view of the child's difficulties. These data cover five broad areas: **friends, family, school, play, and mood,** and can be thought of in two domains:

1. History ("subjective")
2. Observations ("objective")

Based on this data collection, the PCP can then generate a thoughtful and appropriate assessment and treatment plan.

A. **History.** This information is usually gathered from talking with the parents and child, along with questionnaires filled out by the child, parents, and teachers. These questionnaires may be general ones (see above) or specific ones used to gather information about particular clinical problems (e.g., AD/HD, depression). These questionnaires are being increasingly used for evaluation and, especially, monitoring of mental health problems. They are **not** used to make a diagnosis, but can be helpful in clarifying areas of concern or giving a "snapshot" of where a child is at a particular point in time. Specific questionnaires are reviewed in the individual chapters covering a given clinical problem. A number of critical areas for historical inquiry are listed below.

Activity level
Aggression and tantrums
Antisocial behaviors
Anxieties, worries, or fears (including avoided activities)
Attention span
Compulsions or rituals
Discipline
Drug use

Expectations for self
Family psychiatric history*
General mood
How frustration and anger are managed (by child and parent)
Obsessions or restricted areas of interest
Parental and family relations
Peer relations
Regression in toileting, speaking, sleeping, and so on
School achievement and behavior
Sexual behavior
Sleeping patterns
Trauma, stress, loss
View of self-likes versus dislikes

B. **Observations.** In addition to direct questioning, much valuable information can be obtained by observing the child's interaction with the parent and observing the child's behavior. Specific areas for observation are listed below.

1. **Parent–child interactions (see also Chapters 3 and 4)**
   - Observe how the parent engages the child. Does the parent seem warm, overly permissive, stern, frustrated, angry, joyful, or sad?
   - What strategies do parents use to gain the child's compliance with requests? Is the parent coaxing, demanding, physically forcing, or calmly stating the request to the child?
   - How does the child respond to these strategies?
   - If the strategy is not working, does the parent change strategies or increase the intensity of the strategy?
   - Does the child use the parent as a secure base?
   - What level of attachment do you see between the parent and child?

2. **Mental status examination**
   - How does the child engage with you? Does the child intrude on you or your office? Avoid you? Friendly? Cooperative? Does the child maintain eye contact?

---

*A note about **family psychiatric history:** This critical part of the history can be efficiently addressed by including it in the initial "patient information form" given to all new patients in a practice. Whereas the typical form includes a checklist that asks about the family history of general conditions (e.g., diabetes, cancer, hypertension), we suggest integrating into this list the following: depression, suicide, anxiety, substance abuse, AD/HD, learning disabilities, schizophrenia, bipolar disorder (or "manic-depression" as many people would call it), and other psychiatric disorders (to capture other problems not identified already).

- Does the child appear alert and aware of surroundings?
- How is the child's dress and grooming? Does the child appear neglected?
- What is the child's mood? Anxious? Fearful? Sad? Angry? Defiant?
- Is the child's speech loud or quiet, flat in tone or full of intonation, slow and moderate, or pressured? How does the child form words? Does the child express his- or herself in an age-appropriate way? Does the child understand appropriately what is being said to him or her?
- What is the child's activity level? Lethargic? Calm? Active? Hyperactive?
- How well does the child maintain concentration?
- Are the child's thought processes, as evidenced by the content of his or her speech, organized and coherent, or disorganized and hard to follow?
- Are there any abnormal movements, unusual vocalizations, or tics?
- Any evidence seen of suicidal or homicidal ideation?

C. **Assessment.** In addition to determining whether psychiatric or psychological symptoms exist, it is crucial to determine the clinical importance of the symptoms. DSM-IVTR diagnoses **require** not only the presence of symptoms, but also significant impairment, distress, and symptom severity.

1. **Impairment** is the degree to which symptoms interfere with the patient's day-to-day life at school, home, with peers, or in the community (e.g., "does _____ get in the way of doing homework, paying attention, success with peers, getting along with parents?").

2. **Distress** includes both the level of distress felt by the patient as well as the level of distress felt by caregivers and others in the child's environment.

3. **Severity of symptoms** is usually closely linked to the first two factors, but on occasion can be independent of them. It also is a major "target" that is tracked to determine if the child is improving.

   Frequency is a crucial aspect. Is it happening once a month, a few times a week, or a few times a day? It is important to get as specific as possible. When parents say "All the time," it may mean only once a week.

Intensity: "He has wild tantrums" can mean anything from saying "No!" and frowning to throwing chairs and punching people.

Duration: How long has this been occurring?

D. **Treatment planning.** Once an assessment has been completed, the PCP is in a position to generate a treatment plan. **Optimal treatment planning** must address multiple areas and, hence, is often referred to as **"multimodal"** by mental health professionals. A corollary of this is that it is **rarely sufficient or appropriate solely to prescribe medication** for children and adolescents with significant mental health problems. A multimodal treatment plan needs to address the following:

1. **Safety** for the child. This is first and foremost, and includes consideration of whether the child is at risk for maltreatment and in need of child protective services. Also included here is whether the child is a danger to self or others and, hence, in need of hospitalization or other protective measures.

2. **Psychoeducation** for the child and parents includes education about the mental health problem, guidance about what to do and expect, and psychological support for the family.

3. The **school** situation. Consideration needs to be given to the child's academic, behavioral, emotional, and social needs in the school setting.

4. Referral for **psychotherapy.** The major types of psychotherapy are cognitive-behavioral treatment, behavior management, supportive therapy, and psychodynamically oriented therapies. These may be carried out in individual, group, or family formats.

5. The possible role of **psychotropic medications.** These agents are often helpful and should be considered in many cases of child mental health problems.

6. The need for **social service supports.** Many children and their families can benefit from programs available through social service agencies (Chapter 8).

7. **Follow-up.** The PCP should be able to determine how frequently a child with a mental health problem requires monitoring by the PCP.

A final note: Looking over the preceding outline, it is a daunting task to obtain all these data, synthesize the compilation, and formulate an assessment and treatment plan. In reality, this is done over a period of time and fundamentally depends on continuity in the relationship. Over time and multiple contacts, the PCP can gradually obtain this information, make parent–child observations, track development, and monitor for symptom development. Orienting oneself to this task from the beginning of contacts with the family and patient makes this task manageable and realistic. When these longitudinal data are not available and continuity is lacking, this task becomes much more difficult within the constraints of the current healthcare environment. Prudent use of nurse practitioners, physician assistants, and, in some cases, support staff can aid in this process. Occasionally, extended visits are necessary and appropriate to make a proper assessment and plan. Under these circumstances, it is helpful to have an in-house mental health specialist or specialist consultant available to the PCP (see earlier sections).

IV. **Referrals.** Once it has been determined that a problem does exist, additional difficulties arise in the referral process. Although many families are comfortable with mental health referrals, some individuals view psychological services as stigmatizing. They may view seeking psychological services as a sign of "weakness," as a failure in parenting, or as a failure on the part of the entire family. Some parents may feel that the PCP is minimizing their concerns or saying that their child's problem is imaginary or "all in their head." The PCP must address all of these issues to improve the likelihood of follow-through with a referral to a mental health professional. Asking directly how the parents feel about the recommendation is often helpful in this regard.

One factor that appears to be beneficial in facilitating follow-through for many families is proximity (Bray, 1995). If PCPs and mental health providers are on the same site, it may be possible to conduct a brief joint session. During this meeting, the PCP can assist the family in forming a therapeutic alliance with the therapist and convey that a close and continued contact will exist between the professionals. Additionally, having the mental health provider at or near the pediatric site can decrease the perceived stigma of seeking mental health services. For parents and children, familiarity with the location also decreases anxiety related to the referral and increases follow-through.

Because of a variety of constraints, it may not be feasible to have a mental health provider on site full- or parttime, or even to have a nearby provider attend a joint visit with the patient. Much can still be done to facilitate compliance with the referral. The PCP is a figure of great authority in the lives of a family and over time becomes a trusted ally. If this ally firmly endorses both the seeking of treatment and expresses confidence in the mental health provider, this significantly decreases family resistance. Of course, this cannot be feigned and it is important for the PCP to **know local mental health referral options and have confidence in those individuals.** It is also crucial for the PCP to **be persistent in following up on recommendations for mental health treatment.** It may be necessary for the PCP to discuss this on multiple occasions with particular families, asking whether they have made an appointment and, if not, why not. Having a nurse or other professional in the office follow up with the family by telephone a few days after a referral has been made can be immensely helpful. For some families, the physician may ask their permission to have the mental health provider call them. If the physician has a close relationship with mental health providers, the providers may be willing to do this to assist in follow-through with the referral. Continued monitoring by the PCP at future appointments (even when not related to the mental health issue) assures optimal outcomes for the child.

For psychological complaints that have a physical component (e.g., many types of anxiety, depression, somatoform disorders, or chronic pain), it is often helpful first to illustrate the **mind–body connection** before bringing up the idea of referral. Have your own examples (e.g., stress decreases immune system functioning, anxiety triggers a distinct physiological response, distraction increases pain tolerance) to use to help parents and children understand this concept. It may be helpful to provide a number of examples of this mind–body connection to "hit" on something the family can embrace. Acknowledge that the patient's body is actually manifesting signs of distress, that these signs are real, and that a psychological perspective may be of use in addressing at least a portion of the patient's difficulty.

Following the referral, **good two-way communication** is vital in providing continuity of care for the patient. Ideally, the PCP would communicate periodically to assure this. However, finding the time to discuss patients over the telephone is often difficult. Additionally, a PCP may refer a patient and then never be given feedback by the mental health provider. This creates frustration and reluctance to refer patients to mental health providers. For general communication, the provider could send a brief summary of the patient (see Fig. 5-1), which also provides a prompt as well as a convenient format to the mental health professional for responding to the PCP. This can streamline the communication process, resulting in improved continuity of care.

V.   **Summary.** Increasingly, PCPs are being asked to evaluate psychosocial issues in children while struggling with how to provide these services effectively and efficiently in the era of managed care. Current research indicates that a significant number of children have psychosocial issues that are not being detected and even fewer treated or referred. A variety of options exist to assist the pediatrician in improving detection rates and in providing these services. Possible methods include partnership with mental health professionals, development of ties with university or college mental health training programs, use of screening devices, and use of a systematic approach to areas of inquiry and observations. Through the use of these methods, the PCP can increase the rate of detection for psychosocial concerns. Following the identification of a significant psychosocial concern, the PCP can gather further information to be able to develop a thoughtful assessment and treatment plan. If referral is indicated, a number of steps are available to the PCP to increase the likelihood of patient follow-through.

SUGGESTED READINGS

Achenbach T, Ruffle T. The child behavior checklist and related forms for assessing behavioral/emotional problems and competencies. *Pediatr Rev* 2000;21(1):265–271.

Bennet FC, Guralnick MJ. Effectiveness of developmental intervention in the first five years of life. *Pediatr Clin North Am* 1991;38:1513–1528.

Bray JH, Rodgers JC. Linking psychologists and family physicians for collaborative practice. *Professional psychology: research and practice* 1995;26:132–138.

Cassidy L, Jellinek M. Approaches to recognition and management of childhood psychiatric disorders in pediatric primary care. *Pediatr Clin North Am* 1998;45(5):1037–1052.

Costello EJ. Primary care pediatrics and child psychopathology: a review of diagnostic, treatment, and referral practices. *Pediatrics* 1986;78:1044–1051.

Costello EJ. Child psychiatric disorders and their correlates: a primary care pediatric sample. *J Am Acad Child Adolesc Psychiatry* 1989;28:851–855.

Garralda E. Child and adolescent psychiatry in general practice. *Aust N Z J Psychiatry* 2001;35:308–314.

Hack S, Jellinek M. Historical clues to the diagnosis of the dysfunctional child and other psychiatric disorders in children. *Pediatr Clin North Am* 1998;45(1):25–48.

Higgins ES. A review of unrecognized mental illness in primary care. *Arch Fam Med* 1994;3:908–917.

Jellinek MS, Murphy JM, Little M, et al. The use of the pediatric symptom checklist to screen for psychosocial problems in pediatric primary care: a national feasibility study. *Arch Pediatr Adolesc Med* 1999;3:254–260.

Kelleher KJ, Wolraich ML. Diagnosing psychosocial problems. *Pediatrics* 1995;95:899–901.

Stancin T, Palermo TM. A review of behavioral screening practices in pediatric settings: do they pass the test? *J Dev Behav Pediatr* 1997; 18:183–194.

Sulkes S. Coding and documentation for reimbursement. In: Coleman W. *Family focused behavioral pediatrics.* Philadelphia: Lippincott Williams & Wilkins, 2001:46–76.

Web Sites

About Our Kids. Extensive information about child mental health issues for parents, children, and professionals. Sponsored by New York University Child Study Center. www.aboutourkids.org/index. html. Accessed on 6/25/02.

American Academy of Child and Adolescent Psychiatry. Excellent resource for information regarding psychiatric disorders, their assessment, and their treatment in pediatric populations. Large series of one-page handouts for parents (*Facts for Families*) on a wide variety of issues. Available at http://www.aacap.org. Accessed on 6/25/02.

American Psychological Association. Interesting articles pertaining to children and current psychological research. Available at http://www. apa.org/psychnet/children.html. Accessed on 6/25/02.

Internet Mental Health. Large Web site with information regarding diagnosis, treatment, and research on various mental health conditions (adult and child focused). Available at http://www.mentalhealth.com. Accessed on 6/25/02.

KidsHealth. Good general Web site for parents with specific information regarding behavior, emotions, and development. Also, the site has specific areas for children and adolescents, with good articles pertaining to mental health issues. Available at http://www. kidshealth.org. Accessed on 6/25/02.

Mental Help Net. Another overview of mental health issues for both patients and professionals. Available at http://www.mentalhelp.net. Accessed on 6/25/02.

Pediatric Development and Behavior. Excellent resource for a variety of developmental and behavioral issues with educational information for physicians, parents, nurse practitioners, and nursing staff. Available at http://www.dbpeds.org. Accessed on 6/25/02.

6 ♣ The Mental Health System

Susan V. McLeer and David L. Kaye

Primary care physicians (PCPs) are often confused by the mental health "system," which has been described by some as an act of creative fiction. As in pediatrics, where one would be hard pressed to find a "system," no mental health "system" is found. Rather, seen are many children with mental health needs, an array of mental health professionals whose roles can be unclear, a confusing array of services of varying efficacy, and an even more confusing variety of payment systems, in both the public and private sector. To access effective treatment too often takes an enormous amount of luck or relentless advocacy. Often, PCPs and parents simply use what is readily accessible, irrespective of whether the treatment offered is effective or appropriate to need. This chapter reviews the following:

- Pediatric mental health needs and access to services
- Financing of mental health services
- Levels of care in the provision of mental health services
- Providers of mental health services
- Psychotherapeutic modalities in mental health treatment

I. **Mental health needs of children and adolescents.** The prevalence of psychiatric disorders among children and youth varies, depending on the study and methodology used to assess diagnostic status. However, most carefully designed studies using random sampling techniques and a broad community base have found that the **prevalence** of **serious emotional disturbances** among community youth ranges from **5% to 8%** (Costello, 1999). If the severity threshold for identification is lowered and the prevalence determined for **any psychiatric diagnosis** with functional impairment the prevalence is approximately **20%** (Costello et al., 1996; Shaffer et al., 1996).

Other index conditions among children and youth not only coexist with other psychiatric disorders, but also frequently contribute to the development of secondary emotional and behavioral problems. The most common of these index conditions are substance use disorders and a variety of neurodevelopmental disorders (e.g., learning disabilities and mental retardation).

A. Substance use disorders are frequent among youth. In a community sample, Kandel et al. (1999) found that **6.2%** of youth met criteria for a substance use disorder. Using a broad-based community sample of adolescents and young adults, ages 15 to 24 years Anthony et al. (1994) found that the rates for substance dependence varied, depending on the nature of the abused substance. The study showed the prevalence of alcohol dependence was 13.6%, cannabis 5.6%, cocaine 2.6%, stimulants 1.6%, and hallucinogens 0.7%. Much substance abuse among children and youth still goes undetected and, hence, untreated. Routine screening for the use and abuse of substances is needed.

B. **Learning disorders** account for significant dysfunction among children and youth and have a secondary impact on both emotions and behaviors. Prevalence estimates from **community samples** are that **15%** of the school-aged population appear to suffer from some form of learning disability (Popper and West, 1999). The 1987 official estimates from the US Centers for Disease Control (CDC) are considerably lower than these community-based studies, with the prevalence estimates being between 5% and 10%. These CDC estimates have been the basis for resource allocation; hence, resources for meeting the needs of learning-disabled youth are significantly less than required. The frequently used guideline of determining gaps between verbal and performance intelligence quotient (IQ) is not an adequate screen for these disorders because several disorders will not be identified through this screening mechanism. Early detection is important to plan for compensatory learning strategies that will maximize educational achievement and minimize secondary emotional or behavioral dysfunction. Under Federal Law PL94-142 schools are required to provide evaluations at no cost to families. However, significant advocacy is oftentimes necessary to ensure that children at high risk with educational problems receive more than an IQ examination and achievement testing to detect subtle, but nonetheless impairing disabilities.

C. Children and youth with other developmental disabilities commonly have difficulties with emotional and behavioral regulation; hence, they frequently have needs that might well be within the purview of the mental health sector. The prevalence of **mental retardation** in the United States is **1% to 3%,** accounting for significant numbers of children and youth who potentially might use mental health services. Among those diagnosed as mentally retarded, 85% will be mildly retarded (IQ between 50/55 to 70); another 10% will be moderately retarded (IQ between 35/40 to 50/55); 3% to 4% will be severely retarded (IQ between 20/25 to 35/40); whereas only 1% to 2% will suffer from profound mental retardation (IQ below 20/25). Need clearly differs, depending on the severity of retardation and level of impairment in adaptive functioning. Children with developmental disabilities in most regions of the country receive services that are supported by different funding streams than those used for mental health services. Because of this, when families and PCPs attempt to access mental health services for these youth, substantial financial barriers to care are encountered. Few settings have been successful in providing a seamless system for mentally retarded children who need mental health and psychiatric care. The determination of payer source has been particularly problematic in accessing reimbursement for hospital aftercare and rehabilitation services.

D. **Service access and availability.** Children and youth with psychiatric disorders or other mental health problems, including mental retardation, learning disabilities, and substance abuse disorders, receive mental health services from many institutions other than programs specifically within the mental health system. Mental health services are, in fact, provided by a multiplicity of programs within both the public and private, not-for-profit and for-profit, sectors of society. Children with mental health problems are more likely to receive services from nonmental health sector programs such as those offered by the child welfare (i.e., social service) system, juvenile justice system, special education programs, developmental disabilities system, alcohol and drug abuse programs, and primary care providers (Garland et al., 2001).

In the first survey of psychiatric disorders among children and youth in a variety of public sector programs, Garland et al. (2001) found that the prevalence of psychiatric disorders was highest, not within mental health sector programs, but rather within special education programs (70.2%). In fact, diagnostic prevalence was found to be only marginally higher in mental health programs (60.8%) when compared with that found in alcohol and drug programs (60.3%). Psychiatric disorder prevalence was 52.1% for children or youth within the juvenile justice system and 41.8% among those receiving child welfare services. In short, children in **all** of these systems have remarkably high rates of psychiatric disorder.

II. **Financing of mental health services for children and youth.** During the 1980s and early 1990s, insurance programs within both the public and private sector provided payment for services based on units of service delivered, "the deliverables." Limits were placed on the length of inpatient treatment, but not on the duration of the ambulatory modes of care, which resulted in overutilization of ambulatory services. This mode of financing care resulted in increased costs and the utilization trends also supported assumptions held by third-party payers who strongly suspected that (a) the costs of psychiatric treatment are uncontrollable and unpredictable; (b) coverage encourages unnecessary and excessive use; (c) mental healthcare is not cost-effective; and (d) providers of mental health services are not accountable to insurers. These factors resulted in a major restructuring of the mechanisms involved in the financing of mental health services. Almost all of the third party systems reduced payments and developed reimbursement systems that lacked parity when compared with coverage for other medical, nonpsychiatric illnesses.

Managed care programs evolved as insurers and employers, both in the private and public sector, sought mechanisms for cost containment. Financial incentives shifted and cost savings were realized through controlling service utilization and rewarding outcome. Mental health benefits provided by health maintenance organizations (HMO) are more limited than those in nonmanaged systems, usually covering a maximum of 20 outpatient visits and 30 days of hospitalization per year. Unbeknownst to most consumers, these maximums are difficult to access because of administrative oversight that stringently limits services. For example, outpatient mental health professionals are often required to submit lengthy reports after a few contacts, after which the payer may authorize a limited number of further appointments. Obtaining authorization for all 20 visits often requires multiple repetitions of this procedure, which often makes it difficult for patients to access the number of visits to which they believe they are "entitled." A similar situation occurs with inpatient utilization, where hospital-based providers must repeatedly argue the case for continued stay beyond a few days, resulting in premature patient discharges. Again, although families believe their policy will cover "30 days" of inpatient hospitalization, it is the "maximum of" clause that rules, leading to few patients actually being able to access those days. Such coverage is far too limited for many children, but especially those with chronic and severe psychiatric disorders. In some instances, the financing of care for children with chronic illness can be shifted from the managed care setting to publicly funded, fee-for-service programs such as Medicaid* and, in rare instances, Medicare without the family sustaining financial ruin.

However, even with mechanisms available for accessing publicly funded coverage for children and youth with chronic conditions, the perception among insurers persists that the financing of mental health services is a "bottomless pit."

---

*Children who have severe and persistent psychiatric disorders are generally eligible for supplemental social security (SSI) (Chapter 8), which automatically makes them eligible for Medicaid.

Consequently, almost all HMO have moved toward a system that allows the offsetting of financial risk through contracting with external vendors rather than providing or overseeing the provision of psychiatric care themselves. Such patterns of delegation of responsibility and risk are referred to as "carve-outs." As an example, Blue Cross–Blue Shield may "carve out" the oversight of their mental health (this generally includes substance abuse also) benefits to Imagine Behavioral Health, a managed behavioral health care company (MBHCC). For a fee, Imagine will oversee and approve utilization—manage the benefits.

Three stages in the evolution of behavioral healthcare "carve-outs," appear nationally. The **first,** as in the example above, is one in which the insurer, self-insured employer, or HMO contracts with a managed behavioral healthcare company to **administer services to all those with psychiatric disorders at a discounted fee-for-service.** The MBHCC seeks to contain costs by maximizing the fee-for-service discount and terminating providers who refer heavily to costly services. This system works when more than sufficient providers are available, a condition that rarely exists for those who are trained and have credentials to provide mental health services to children and adolescents. A **second system** for handling "carve-outs" is through the further down-streaming of financial risk. The insurer or HMO **capitates with the MBHCC** which, in turn, capitates with the behavioral health network of providers. The result of this arrangement is that the middlemen (the administrators) siphon much money out of the system and fewer resources are available for the provision of care. The **third stage** in the evolution of behavioral health "carve-outs" is when the **provider groups or networks assume full risk and contract directly with corporations or government** to provide behavioral health services to a defined population. Data have yet to be collected and analyzed regarding the effectiveness of this last mode of financial organization.

A new trend that is recently emerged is the limiting of "carve-outs" for behavioral health services, with some insurers directly capitating with healthcare networks to provide for all of the healthcare, including mental health, needs of a designated population. This practice passes financial risk on to the healthcare provider network. The networks, in turn, have started "carving-out" behavioral health services through discounted fees for service or capitated arrangements. This model has been used in both private and public systems. However, outcome and financial data have yet to be analyzed.

Whereas managed care has received much criticism, systems dependent on outcome criteria may do much to hasten the application of recent scientific advances to the care of mentally ill children and youth. Managed care systems can supply an incentive for emphasizing quality over quantity, but the trade-off risk is the siphoning off of resources to support administrative structure. At this point it is not clear which of these vectors is prevailing, although it is clear that the percentage of the healthcare dollar that has gone into mental health and substance abuse treatment has decreased dramatically, perhaps by as much as 50%, since the advent of managed care.

What is also clear is that children and youth with serious and persistent mental illness (e.g., schizophrenia, bipolar disorder, recurrent affective disorder, pervasive developmental disorders) can quickly use up the financial resources available through nongovernmental third party payers. Family resources, even among those with significant annual incomes, can be rapidly depleted. Recognizing this, the federal government committed substantial resources to meet many of the needs of families with children who suffer from serious mental illness. In 1992, Congress allocated substantial grants, $60 million, to 25 states and territories for the further development, management, and evaluation of comprehensive community mental health services for children and their families. Administered by the Substance Abuse and Mental Health Services Administration, through its Center for Mental Health Services, the new Child and Adolescent Service System Program was to be based on three principles:

1. The mental health service system was to be driven by the needs and preferences of the child and family from a strength-based versus a deficit-based perspective.
2. Service locus and management were to involve the collaborative effort of multiple agencies grounded in a strong community base.
3. Both the services and service-providing agencies were to be responsive to the cultural context and characteristics of the populations served.

Grantees (the states and territories) were to match federal dollars with local and state money at an increasing level through the 5-year period of funding. The effectiveness of this financial initiative was sufficient that the program was continued with an expanded appropriation in 1997, with more than 6.5 million children having enhanced access to mental health services. Given the devastating impact and chronicity of severe mental illness coupled with the lack of insurance parity in the coverage of psychiatric services, it is essential that public sector support be provided if the youth are to access appropriate and necessary services in the United States.

III. **Systems of care in the delivery of mental health services.** A number of systems provide mental health services for children and adolescents, including the mental health, social services, juvenile justice, mental retardation and developmental disabilities, and school systems. Within the mental health sector, systems of care are organized according to the intensity of services needed, including the following:

A. **Acute and nonacute ambulatory services** (e.g., emergency services or outpatient treatment)
   1. **Acute services** may include not only evaluation, treatment, and referral services in a psychiatric emergency program, but also
      - Mobile outreach services
      - Respite care
      - Home-based interventions

      These programs almost always are supported by public sector money, which includes county, state, and federal funds. All children and families can access such services.
   2. **Outpatient treatment** may be offered in clinic settings, in which case may be found enriched funding from public sector sources for services to children. Such funding makes reimbursement for professional services reasonable for those physicians and nonphysician providers who care for Medicaid-eligible children. However, it is important to appreciate that Medicaid reimbursement for professional services is so low for private psychiatrists that few are able or willing to provide services for this population. Likewise, in states where traditional Medicaid-funded services are managed, private practitioners are infrequently included on the provider panels and, therefore, are ineligible for payment. The PCP must then use public sector clinical programs to access care.
   3. **Enhanced services** (e.g., in-home nursing or behavior management training) are available in many communities to augment outpatient treatment. These services may be accessible through public or private insurance coverage. Another important service is **case management,** which assigns an individual mental health worker (often a bachelor's degree-level social worker) to a severely and persistently disturbed child or adolescent. This worker would then be available to the family 24 hours a day, 7 days a week, to come to the home, provide support and troubleshoot immediate problems, assure treatment needs are met (including arrange transportation under some circumstances), and access additional services as necessary. Case

management is for the most part available only through public resources.

4. **Partial hospitalization programs** are **intensive programs** that generally provide care 5 days per week, for a **few weeks** until an acutely disturbed patient has been stabilized enough to transition to outpatient care. These programs increasingly are garnering support both from the public sector and from a variety of third party payers because the programs are **designed to reduce the need for inpatient hospitalization.** These programs can provide both pharmacologic interventions and a variety of psychosocial interventions, including individual, group, and family treatments. Social skills training with peer groups in a variety of settings, including simulated classroom settings, may be offered.

   Such programs are particularly helpful for children with disruptive behavioral disorders as well as those with severe psychotic illnesses. Partial hospitalization programs seek to provide services that promote early discharge from inpatient settings or reduce the need for inpatient hospitalization. **Costs** for services are usually **30% to 35% of inpatient hospitalization costs.** Consequently, third party payers are becoming increasingly interested in using such programs. This has not always been the case because third party payers have not differentiated between partial hospitalization and day hospitalization programs (see below). The latter have often been subjected to overutilization by providers, resulting in the costs of providing care per client per year escalating significantly beyond what might occur in other clinical settings.

5. **Day hospitalization programs** provide **longer-term care for chronically ill children and youth.** Most often, the children served have chronic disruptive behavioral disorders as well as a variety of coexisting problems (e.g., substance use or abuse, learning disabilities, and severe familial stressors). These programs usually operate 5 days per week with services directed toward improving occupational, educational, socialization, and daily living skills, and medication compliance. Day hospitalization services frequently are **provided in conjunction with a public school system.** The site can be independent of the public school or it may be co-located in a public school setting with

the youngster receiving behavioral health and psychiatric treatment while being mainstreamed into the academic classroom settings. Some programs are privately run and have approved, but private, educational programs integrated with the behavioral health and psychiatric services provided.

All too few treatments available demonstrate efficacy targeting of children with chronic behavioral disorders. Treatment efficacy is further compromised by the existence of comorbid conditions, coupled with significant weaknesses in family supports. Virtually no controlled research has examined outcome for children who receive services in day hospitalization settings as compared with those who receive less intense services. Because of the disruptive nature of a child's disorder, in the absence of day hospitalization service that child might get into further difficulties, perhaps ending up in the juvenile justice system, an outcome which might well have a more significant disruptive effect on his or her developmental trajectory. Hence, the major contribution of day hospitalization may be more that of preventing further and costlier complications arising from the behavioral disorder versus "cure."

Day hospitalization programs almost always have been offered within **public sector settings.** Licensing requirements tend to stipulate relatively low staff-to-client ratios, resulting in lowered daily costs for providing service as compared with other settings. Children, once admitted, typically have **average lengths of stay of 180 to 250 days, with a range of 2 months to 2 years.** Because of the length of stay in these programs, the costs of service per client per year are high. Consequently, managed care and other commercial third party payers have been reluctant to authorize the use of day hospitalization programs. Therefore, access to programs frequently requires that a child be eligible for public sector services (e.g., Medicaid). In some communities, school systems and the mental health public sector jointly fund day treatment programs. Access to these programs in such communities can occur through special education administration (i.e., Committee on Special Education [CSE]) in addition to mental health routes.

Third party payers have reason to confuse day hospitalization programs with partial hospitalization programs because the terminology can change from one state jurisdiction to another. For example, partial hospitalization for children in Pennsylvania is equivalent to day hospitalization in New York State. Conversely, day hospitalization in Pennsylvania more frequently is an admissions diversion program, whereas in New York State these services are provided in partial hospitalization programs. Therefore, it is important for the PCP to determine whether a program targets inpatient admission diversion or long-term treatment for chronic conditions of childhood. One cannot rely on consistent use of the terms defined above across state borders.

B. **Inpatient services.** Inpatient psychiatric units are organized according to length of care considerations.

1. **Acute hospitalization.** Most inpatient services are for acute hospitalization (3 to 15 days). They are used when it is no longer considered safe to treat a patient outside the confines of an inpatient unit. Usually suicide risk or risk of unduly aggressive behavior that is threatening to others is the reason for using acute inpatient services. Once safety is assured, patients are discharged for care to either a partial or day hospitalization program or into a traditional ambulatory setting. With this model of care, definitive treatment occurs outside of the hospital setting.

Acute hospitalization programs are provided both within the public and private sector of care. "Not-for-profit" programs must provide services irrespective of the client's ability to pay and without regard to third party payer source. "For-profit" programs, which do not receive public money, are not obligated to provide services to the uninsured or Medicaid recipients. The private, for-profit programs are oftentimes viewed by families and PCPs as providing "better services" than the "not-for-profits." However, given the substantial amount of public sector resources committed to the provision of mental health services and that academic programs are often coupled with the not-for-profit hospitals, this quality determination may be incorrect. Inpatient services affiliated with medical school programs may experience less of a gap in "technology transfer" (e.g., applying newer research findings in the development of treatment protocols). Hence, treatments offered in such settings may have empirically demonstrated efficacy. Public perceptions, therefore, can contribute to the development of a paradoxical, two-tier system of care. For example, families with considerable financial resources choose to access for-profit private facilities that may not be providing "cutting-edge" services, whereas the poorer families have access only to the not-for-profits, which might well offer a richer array of services with empirically demonstrated efficacy. PCPs really need to familiarize themselves both with the training and experience of the psychiatrists at both the for-profit and the not-for-profit facilities and determine the breadth and depth of services being provided at each facility before making comparative decisions regarding quality. Be aware that visitation by families is allowed, but is more highly restricted than on general medical–surgical units. Commonly, visitation is restricted to a few hours per day (usually the evenings or daytime on weekends) and can be further restricted, depending on the clinical situation. Sleeping over by parents, even for younger patients, is generally not allowed. The PCP can help the parents understand that, because of the brief lengths of stay, their child will not be discharged "all better," but rather stable enough that less intensive treatment can suffice. As in general medicine and pediatrics, this often leads to frustration for both families and physicians who experience patient discharges as premature.

2. **Intermediate stay hospitalization** services are provided for patients who require a more intermediate period of time for stabilization. Length of stays are generally **2 to 6 months,** although the range can extend to 12 to 18 months. Children who are hospitalized in such settings not infrequently have several comorbid conditions, including a primary psychiatric disorder coupled with neurodevelopmental disorders (e.g., a learning disability or mild or moderate mental retardation). It is not unusual for this population of children to have suffered also from a variety of forms of child maltreatment. Families are usually unable to cope with the multidimensional problems that such children have and social support systems are consequently limited. Visitation with families is encouraged as appropriate, although hours are much more restricted than in a general pediatric medical–surgical hospital setting. Services provided in these settings include both biological and psychosocial treatments, educational rehabilitation,

and possibly occupational or vocational counseling, social skills, and daily living skills training programs. Intermediate stay hospitalization is provided both by public and private sector programs. Both for-profit and not-for-profit corporations that have multiple sites throughout the United States provide for private sector programs.

3. **Residential treatment facilities** (RTF) are Joint Commission on Accreditation of Healthcare Organizations (JCAHO)-approved facilities that provide inpatient treatment for children and adolescents who are unable to return to a community setting and require more than intermediate length of stays. Typically, these children and adolescents stay for **1 to 2 years.** RTF are usually freestanding homes, cottages, or small institutions that treat 10 to 50 patients on their "campus." The children live in the RTF, eating and sleeping there. Schooling is also provided on grounds. They receive comprehensive evaluation and treatment, including biological and psychosocial approaches. Individual and group treatment addressing social skills, daily living skills, and self-management are essential. Family therapy and contact with families generally are a integral parts of treatment. Contingent on the clinical situation, visitation with families is encouraged. As children approach discharge, they go home for increasing amounts of time to assess readiness for discharge and to troubleshoot likely problems.

C. **Integrated services between the mental health and child welfare (i.e., social services) sector.** In addition to the specific levels of service noted above, some jurisdictions acknowledge that families with children who have serious psychiatric disorders have other special needs. Hence, the child welfare system and mental health system provide programs that facilitate the maintenance of the child in his or her home through a variety of **"wrap-around services."** Support for these services usually comes from matching programs that utilize federal, state, and county funds. Wrap-around services traditionally include respite care, mobile crisis teams, and home-based services, including the use of mental health professionals in the home who can provide the necessary supervision for suicidal children to avoid inpatient hospitalization. In situations where the home environment is highly unstable or when parents are unable to provide the support and necessary care that children require, the child welfare system will assist in providing alternate living arrangements for the child as well as treatment and educational interventions for the parents. The overarching goal within the child welfare system is family reunification and the services provided are structured in a manner designed to facilitate reunification of the family.

D. **The social service system.** When families are overwhelmed by the psychosocial needs of a child or when families are unable to provide an environment that is free of child maltreatment, the social welfare agencies may support the use of specialized foster care or residential services.

1. **Specialized foster care** provides single-family homes with caretakers who have been trained to care for special needs children (e.g., children with autism or other pervasive developmental disorders, maltreated children with particularly aggressive or sexualized behavioral problems, children with severe and persistent psychiatric disorders). Mental health services, including psychiatric services, must be accessed through community agencies or private practitioners.

2. **Residential facilities** range in size from group homes in the community to larger facilities with a "prep school-like" campus. These facilities have specific programming for education services, a variety of psychosocial treatments and social skills training. Educational and vocational rehabilitation and training services may be provided as well. They generally have limited or no psychiatric services available.

E. **Juvenile justice system.** The number of children and youth in the juvenile justice system who suffer from mental illness is substantial. The prevalence, understandably, for conduct disorder approaches 90% in some facilities. In addition, studies indicate that 19% to 46% of youth are diagnosed with attention-deficit/hyperactivity disorder. Of incarcerated juvenile delinquents, 38% to 50% meet criteria for a major affective disorder. Some youth have undiagnosed psychotic disorders. Studies indicate that most juvenile offenders have suffered from child maltreatment and a significant percentage of those either meet full criteria for posttraumatic stress disorder or exhibit some degree of posttraumatic symptomatology. Learning disabilities are extraordinary in prevalence, with most youth lagging at least 2 years behind their chronologic age in reading skills. Among those youth in the juvenile justice system failing to meet diagnostic criteria for a specific psychiatric disorder, substantial numbers suffer from significant psychiatric symptoms. Suicide has been demonstrated to be a significant risk for youth in juvenile detention facilities. The psychiatric needs of the young people in these facilities have barely been addressed and scarce resources have not been adequately allocated. Some of the national, for-profit corporations that provide contracted physician services have started to address the need for psychiatric services in the juvenile justice system. However, need still vastly out distances service availability and until those youth with mental illness are provided with necessary services, attempts at true rehabilitation are likely to fail or at least be significantly compromised.

F. **The school system** provides both educational and counseling services for children with mental health needs. In fact, this sector may provide the most mental health treatment. To access these services, the child or adolescent must be processed through the CSE. This process and the services available are reviewed in Chapter 7. Recently, a trend has emerged to provide additional mental health services through **school-based health clinics.** These clinics are formed by partnerships with private or public health agencies (i.e., hospitals, clinics) in which child mental health specialists will provide counseling services on school grounds. Evaluation of the need for referral (e.g., for psychiatric services or more intensive programs) and help in linkage to these community-based services is also offered.

G. **Mental retardation and developmental disabilities (MR/DD)** services are often administered through a separate state or local agency. Children with these difficulties commonly have mental health problems, yet mental health services are often meager within the MR/DD system. Most commonly offered is behavior management training for the parents, which may be available in the home. Social and recreational activities are also generally available. Schools and vocational training sites provide further support. Accessing services in the mental health sector can be difficult. Many mental health-based services do not feel they can program adequately for these children. As a result, the children can easily "fall between the cracks" between the systems. These children and adolescents often require psychiatric consultation and treatment, which is available through public mental health clinics or private practitioners.

H. **Alcohol and substance abuse** services are often administered by a state agency separate from mental health. As a result, these services may or may not be offered through general child mental health agencies (i.e., they may be freestanding clinics or facilities). Both private and public programs exist in most communities to address the treatment needs of this population. Chapter 22 describes the range of outpatient and inpatient services generally available.

I.   Barriers to care. It is clear that no one agency appears to take responsibility for coordinating care or assuring that children have access appropriate services according to diagnostic need. This is tragic, given that at no time in our history have we known as much as we do now about which treatments have demonstrated efficacy for specific psychiatric disorders. Compounding the difficulties that families and children experience in accessing appropriate services is the fact that an enormous gap exists between what is known from empiric research findings and the actual practice of mental health professionals and care providers in the community. This means that accessing systems of care provides no assurance that effective treatments will be provided. So many of the exciting developments regarding the efficacious treatment of specific psychiatric disorders never reach the "trenches."

IV.   Providers of mental health services. The numerous professionals, all with differing training backgrounds, who provide mental health services, often confuse PCPs. Because of changing patterns of reimbursement and conceptualizations of mental disorders, "standard" outpatient treatment has changed. Over the past 10 years, child and adolescent psychiatrists (CAP) now conduct psychotherapy less frequently than in the past and, in fact, many see virtually no patients in psychotherapy. Instead, a psychologist, social worker, or master's degree-level therapist typically provides psychotherapy, whereas the psychiatrist administers evaluation and medication management. For a limited number of patients, psychiatrists may conduct psychotherapy, either alone or in conjunction with medication management. In any community may be found a CAP who primarily performs psychotherapy but this is becoming uncommon. The main "players" are:

A.   CAPs are physicians who have completed a minimum of 3 years of residency training in general psychiatry and then 2 years of residency in child and adolescent psychiatry. CAP must pass American Board of Psychiatry and Neurology certification examinations in general psychiatry before sitting for their child and adolescent psychiatry examination. CAP receive training, education, and clinical experience in the neurological and psychiatric evaluation as well as the full range of treatment modalities. Although trained in the psychotherapies, which informs all treatment, most CAP see only a handful of patients for psychotherapeutic treatment only. As noted, the CAP commonly evaluates and oversees medication, whereas another non-MD mental health professional sees the child, family, or both for psychotherapy. This **"split" treatment** allows for the CAP to be involved in treatment for a large number of troubled children and adolescents. This model presents barriers to maintaining adequate communication and can promote "splitting" (i.e., the patient or family sees one as good, the other as bad, such that they are "played off" against each other, which ultimately undermines effective treatment). Little research has been done to evaluate the efficacy of this team approach and it remains controversial among many CAP, who may support an integrated model of treatment whereby the CAP provides all treatment including psychotherapy. Because of this, as well as other factors, some CAP in private practice do not participate with some or all local insurance plans. In some circumstances, insurance companies "close their panels," excluding a CAP from the panel. This can lead to frustration for a PCP who attempts to make a referral of a patient only to find out from the family that the CAP "doesn't accept our insurance." To avoid this, the PCP office will need to be cognizant of the CAP on the major insurers' panels in their area. Until insurance policies become less restrictive and reimbursement improves for cognitive specialists this situation is unlikely to change. The United States has relatively few CAP (~6000) and the demand far outstrips the need. As a result, many areas, especially rural, have no CAP available or only a small number who are overwhelmed by patient care need. It is unlikely that this situation will improve significantly in the near future as the number of residents being trained is only minimally outstripping the number of practitioners retiring or dying. These facts, combined with the magnitude of the public health problem posed by mental disorders, will push PCPs into an increasing role in the evaluation and care of children and adolescents with mental health needs.

B. **Psychologists** have generally completed a doctoral (PhD or PsyD) degree program. The PhD may have been awarded in any of a number of areas within psychology (e.g., clinical, educational, developmental, counseling psychology). To graduate, the candidate must complete class work, clinical externships, a research dissertation, and a clinical internship year. This typically takes a total of 4 to 7 years. The internship year must be completed in an accredited program. This is a clinically intensive year that is akin to a year of residency training. Clinical internships are usually general in their focus (i.e., includes child, adult, and geriatric patients), but child psychology internships do exist. After completion of an internship, psychologists are generally required to have at least 1 additional year of postdoctoral, supervised clinical experience before being eligible for licensure. The licensing procedure varies from state to state and can include examinations in addition to a review of credentials. Licensure in one state is not transferable to another state but rather must be applied for in each state. A national licensing examination (Diplomate in Psychology) is acceptable in all states, but few psychologists take this. Licensure allows the psychologist to operate as an "independent practitioner" and bill insurers for services.* Psychologists receive training in psychological evaluation and testing (including IQ and other cognitive testing) and a full range of psychotherapeutic modalities. They often have extensive training in more research-based treatment modalities (e.g., cognitive behavioral treatment, interpersonal treatment, behavior management). Psychologists primarily provide individual, group, and family psychotherapy. Although they can perform psychological testing, few do this unless they are employed by a school system because insurers infrequently reimburse for this service. Whereas many psychologists develop some knowledge about psychotropic medications, few have any training in this area. Although the American Psychological Association has made it a priority to pursue legislation granting prescription privileges to psychologists, only one state (New Mexico) has yet permitted such a law to pass. Despite this limitation in training and licensure, psychologists often recommend to PCPs that a psychotropic medication be prescribed. Although these recommendations may be helpful, PCPs are advised to make their own determination of the appropriateness of medication and, if so, which medication to use. Psychologists work in both public mental health clinics and also in the private sector, where they comprise the largest group of private mental health practitioners. PCPs should familiarize themselves with the local psychologists who have specialized

---

*Some "psychologists" (e.g., some school psychologists) have had 2 years of graduate school leading to a master's degree in psychology. These individuals generally cannot be licensed as "independent practitioners," but instead may be hired by institutions (e.g., schools, residential programs) to provide specific assessments (e.g., IQ testing) and interventions (e.g., group counseling) in the school or institution setting.

expertise in children and adolescents, as many psychologists do not. As with CAP, psychologists may or may not be providers in a given insurance panel. To minimize frustration, the PCP should keep a list of child psychologists who participate with various local insurance plans. **Neuropsychologists** are psychologists who have completed a doctoral program in psychology and then an internship or postdoctoral fellowship in neuropsychology. These individuals have expertise in advanced psychological testing techniques, in addition to the basic knowledge acquired by other psychologists. Neuropsychologists often work in neurology-related clinical and research settings (e.g., traumatic brain injury, Tourette's syndrome, brain tumors, epilepsy) providing assessments, educational consultation, and psychological treatments tailored for this population.

C. **Social workers** have generally completed a 2-year master's degree program in social work (MSW), although institution-based (e.g., hospital, school, or some clinic settings) social workers may have a bachelor's degree or less. Master's level social workers receive a broad curriculum in social work along with a modest number of practicum courses involving supervised clinical work. If they become social workers performing clinical mental health work (others may work in social services, adoption, foster care, child protective services, and so on), they generally then must work in an agency for a specified number of years (e.g., 5 years) under the direct supervision of a senior social worker, psychologist, or psychiatrist. Most states then allow a social worker to be licensed as a clinical social worker (CSW) or a licensed clinical social worker (LCSW). Many states require further supervised experience to receive special designation (e.g., in New York this is an R number) as an "independent practitioner" eligible to receive third party payments and perform clinical work independently. Social workers' scope of practice generally includes individual, group, and family psychotherapy, but not evaluation. Social workers often work in public mental health agencies (e.g., community mental health centers, Catholic Charities, child and family services) providing the majority of front-line treatment. It is likely that a patient referred to a public mental health clinic will initially be assigned a social worker to do an "intake" evaluation. A senior psychologist or psychiatrist generally reviews the social worker's findings before a final treatment plan is developed. It is generally at this time that a decision will be made whether it is necessary to have a child see a CAP. If the decision is made to provide individual and family therapy, this is often carried out by the social worker (or psychologist if available in the clinic). A CAP may be brought into the case at any time subsequently if deemed appropriate (i.e., to clarify diagnosis, to assess for dangerousness or need for hospitalization, to evaluate for medication). In private practice, clinical social workers can operate an independent office alone or may share space with other mental health practitioners. PCPs should know which social workers in their community have training and expertise in working with children and families. Knowledge about the social workers on specific insurance panels will save aggravation for the physician and family.

D. **Master's level therapists.** Many other graduate programs offer master's degrees in fields related to mental health (e.g., marital and family therapy, rehabilitation counseling, counseling psychology, music therapy, art therapy). States vary tremendously in which degrees they recognize as eligible for licensure (e.g., licensed professional counselor or LPC, and marital, family, and child counselor or MFCC). Licensure is critical because this generally determines whether public mental health clinics can charge insurers for their services or whether they may be an "independent practitioner" accepting third party payments in a private office. Many degrees are not eligible for licensure in a given state. Although individuals with these degrees may work in school or other institutional settings, it is unusual to find them in public mental health clinics even though the quality of their work may be excellent.

E. **Credentialed alcoholism counselor (CAC), alcoholism and substance abuse (CASAC), or chemical dependency counselor (CDC)** is the credential granted to those individuals who generally provide treatment in substance abuse treatment agencies. Individuals are eligible if they have a high school diploma or beyond, and meet specified state requirements. States vary widely in their statutes, but the requirements generally include a combination of coursework, clinical externships, and a specified minimal number of hours of supervised work experience in a licensed substance abuse agency (e.g., in New York State those with a master's degree in a related field need 2,000 hours, those with an associate's degree or high school diploma will need 6,000). Individuals must also pass a national written and oral examination. This credential is not a license and therefore does not confer "independent practitioner" status or the ability to see private patients or bill insurance companies. On the other hand, substance abuse agencies are required to staff their programs with individuals who have this credential. In practice, this credential generally is necessary to work in a substance abuse agency.

F. **Psychiatric nurse practitioners** are being used more frequently, especially in outpatient settings. Private practice CAP can enter into agreement with a child psychiatric nurse practitioner (CPNP) to efficiently take care of larger numbers of patients on medications. Some public sector clinics are taking a similar approach. Scope of practice legislation in many states is changing to allow for an expanded and more independent role for CPNP, which will lead to an increased role in mental health treatment in the future.

V. **Psychotherapeutic modalities in mental health treatment.** Treatment planning for children and adolescents with mental health problems requires a **multimodal approach** (Chapter 5). Psychoeducation, advocacy, medications, and psychotherapeutic approaches are all critical. Most PCPs are familiar with all of these approaches, except for the psychotherapies, which receive little attention in medical school or residency training. For this reason, a brief description of the most commonly used types follows. Although they are each described separately, they do in fact overlap in practice (i.e., most therapists will take a pragmatic approach combining principles from differing approaches depending on the patient, the clinical problem, and the progress of the patient). For the most part, each of the following approaches can be offered in individual, group, or family therapy formats.

A. **Psychodynamic psychotherapy** approaches are based on an in-depth understanding of the inner lives and relationships of children and parents. An emphasis is placed on **understanding** the patterns of current problematic feeling responses and relationships, and their connections to past important versions of the same. Although founded on Freud's original ideas, these approaches have evolved dramatically in the past 30 to 50 years. The current iterations of this therapy are a far cry from the caricatures of the passive psychoanalyst who sees the patient four times per week and strokes his beard while saying "un-huh" a lot. As currently practiced, psychodynamic psychotherapies are conducted usually on a once-per-week basis and continue for a number of months, if not years. Although the therapist is active in the co-creation of the therapeutic relationship, the patient's initiative is nurtured so that the patient generally selects the focus of each session. Psychodynamic approaches can be used in individual, group, and family formats. The goals of this therapy are to catalyze fundamental and permanent changes in the way a patient handles feelings, self-image, and self-esteem, how the patient relates to others, and personal expectations for self and others. In short, this is an ambitious approach and one that requires much from the patient. Specifically, a patient must have the psychological strength and health to contain impulses, observe self, and talk about personal feelings and thoughts. For younger children "play" can be substituted for "talk," so that they must be able to play (use dolls to pretend to hit the adult doll on the head) versus act out their feelings (hit the therapist on the head). For these reasons, pure psychodynamic approaches may not be appropriate for many patients, especially those who have externalizing problems or are the most disturbed. At the same time, this is an approach that has been helpful for many higher functioning individuals and most therapists routinely integrate psychodynamic understanding into any approach they use. Although historically psychiatrists were most likely to embrace this perspective, this is less true presently. Whereas many psychiatrists are well versed in this approach, many others are receiving little training. Psychologists are now the most prominent contributors to the field of psychodynamic psychotherapy. Many social workers and other master's level therapists also incorporate this perspective in their work.

B. **Cognitive behavioral therapy (CBT)** is a time-limited approach that evolved from both the behavioral and psychodynamic traditions. It requires an active and directive therapist who focuses on the here and now (versus the past) and develops in-session exercises and "homework" assignments for patients that target behavioral patterns around symptomatic behavior and the associated automatic thought patterns that underlie it. Symptomatic behavior is seen as stemming from distress emotions (e.g., anxiety, depression) that are mediated by a distorted cognitive appraisal of an event. Treatment focuses on the distorted cognitive (i.e., information) processing. The cognitive component of treatment is done by teaching the patient to observe thought patterns and identify those which are maladaptive. The patient is then encouraged to develop coping strategies to counter the maladaptive patterns. For example, a common maladaptive cognition is "I am a total failure," or all-or-none thinking. The patient is taught to note when such thinking occurs, log its occurrence in a diary, and initiate a preplanned strategy for realistic self-appraisal. Behavioral treatments make use of relaxation training, behavioral rehearsal, sustained exposure, response prevention, and graded task assignment (i.e., breaking down a behavioral problem into small steps). This is a highly structured approach that usually requires sessions once per week for a total of 10 to 20 sessions. It contains an educational component, whereby the therapist acts much like a "coach" to the patient, initiating and directing treatment focus. Outcome research of CBT approaches has demonstrated short-term efficacy when used for a variety of clinical problems (e.g., depression, anxiety, obsessive-compulsive disorders, panic disorder, anger management, substance abuse, social skills). For certain conditions, people, places, and situations can trigger symptom recurrence and therapists have found that "booster" sessions may well be necessary to maintain treatment benefits. Relatively few practicing therapists have extensive training in CBT, although most are familiar with the approach. Psychologists and, to a lesser extent, psychiatrists are most likely to be well versed in this modality. Computerized CBT programs are in the early stages of development and may be used widely in the future.

C. **Behavior management** refers primarily to the "training" of parents in responding effectively to children's behaviors (Chapter 3). This approach is generally directive and educational in focus. Behavior therapists teach parents the "ABCs" of behavior, and help them learn how to make requests (the Antecedent of Behavior) and how to provide rewards and punishments (the Consequences of behavior). They assist the parents in learning how to use time out, and develop "star charts" or commensurate charts for older children. A behavior therapist might meet with the child as well to make the child an active participant in the process, instead of a passive recipient of what the parents decide. Sessions occur from once per week to once per month with from 10 to 20 in total. "Booster" sessions, whereby the family returns months or years later for reinforcement are expected to be necessary. Most psychologists have received extensive training in behavior management. Psychiatrists and other therapists have at least a modicum of training in this approach, whereas some have extensive training and expertise.

D. **Parent guidance** refers to the supportive and advice-giving roles that a therapist can take with parents regarding any aspect of the child's life. This is an aspect of virtually all treatments with children and adolescents and is incorporated by psychiatrists, psychologists, and master's level therapists.

E. **Interpersonal therapy (IPT)** is a new manual-driven and time-limited therapy approach that has been successfully used with depressed adolescents. This treatment focuses on the linkage of symptoms to one of four interpersonal problem areas. It focuses on the here and now and uses a variety of techniques to work through the current life interpersonal difficulty. It requires an active, supportive therapist who meets with the patient once per week for 15 to 20 sessions. Although efficacy has been established for IPT, very few therapists are trained in this approach. As with CBT, this can also lend itself to computerized approaches in the future.

F. **Family therapy** is a generic term that applies to approaches that focus on the relationships between family members in the here and now. Generally it implies the presence of at least two, and usually more, members of a family at each session. The goal is to alter current family interactional patterns and, hence, ameliorate symptoms. Psychodynamic, behavioral, or cognitive-behavioral perspectives have been adapted to a family therapy format. Therapists tend to be active in the sessions, although they will differ in the degree of directiveness. This is generally a short-term treatment approach aimed at immediate symptom relief, although psychodynamically informed family therapy often has broader goals. Virtually all mental health professionals have had training and experience in family therapy methods.

VI. **Summary.** The PCP needs to keep his or her knowledge base current regarding what actually "works" for children with psychiatric illness. The PCP also needs to serve as an advocate to link children and their families to people and systems that can further advocate for the youngsters to improve the likelihood of appropriate and effective treatments being accessed. One mechanism for doing this is to maintain a directory of web sites for a variety of advocate groups, including those who advocate for specific disorders (e.g., Child and Adolescent Bipolar Foundation), as well as those providing for general advocacy and supports for children and families struggling with mental illness. Many of these disease-specific advocacy groups maintain web sites that keep consumers and providers current with particular treatments that have been demonstrated to be effective as well as directions for accessing such treatments. Research advances are also discussed on these web sites. Individual chapters contain addresses for additional problem-specific web sites.

SUGGESTED READINGS

General Advocacy Resources

American Academy of Child and Adolescent Psychiatry. Available at http://www.aacap.org. Accessed on 6/29/02.

American Academy of Pediatrics. Available at www.aap.org. Accessed on 6/29/02.

Bazelon Center For Mental Health Law. Legal Advocacy For The Civil Rights And Human Dignity Of People With Mental Disability. Available at http://www.bazelon.org. Accessed on 6/29/02.

Center for Mental Health Services KEN (Knowledge Exchange Network). KEN Provides information and resources on prevention, treatment, and rehabilitation services for mental illness. Available at http://www.mentalhealth.org/publications. Accessed on 6/29/02.

Child, Adolescent and Family Branch, Center For Mental Health Services. National center supporting research on the diagnosis and treatment of mental illness in children and adolescents. Available at www.mentalhealth.org/child/childhealth.asp. Accessed on 6/29/02.

Connect for Kids. State pages (51) (including the District of Columbia) link visitors to resources at the state and local level. Available at http://www.connectforkids.org/homepage1576/index.htm. Accessed on 6/29/02.

Federation of Families for Children's Mental Health. A national parent-run organization focused on the needs of children and youth with emotional, behavioral, or mental disorders and their families. Information available at http://www.ffcmh.org. Accessed on 6/29/02.

Insure Kids Now. A national campaign to link the nation's 10 million uninsured children—from birth to age 18—to free and low-cost health insurance. Toll-free number: 1-877-543-7669 (1-877-4 Kids Now). Available at http://www.insurekidsnow.gov. Accessed on 6/29/02.

National Mental Health Association. Focuses on improving mental health and preventing mental disorders through advocacy, education, research, and services. Available at http://www.nmha.org. Accessed on 6/29/02.

National Alliance of the Mentally Ill (NAMI). Powerful advocacy group that provides support for families with mentally ill children and youth. Advocates nationally, and through regional branches, for high-quality treatment and the advancement of research on psychiatric disorders. Helpline: 800-950-NAMI. Available at http://www.nami.org. Accessed on 6/29/02.

National Suicide Prevention Hotline. (800) 999-9999

Suicide Awareness/Voices of Education (SAVE). Available at http://www.save.org. Accessed on 6/29/02.

Suicide Information and Education Center (SIEC). Maintains a list of suicide prevention hotlines and services in the United States and Canada. Available at http://www.siec.ca/crisis.html. Accessed on 6/29/02.

References

Aarons GA, Brown SA, Hough RL, et al. Prevalence of adolescent substance use disorders across five sectors of care. *J Am Acad Adolesc Psychiatry* 2001;40:419–426.

Anthony JC, Warner LA, Kessler R. Comparative epidemiology of dependence on tobacco, alcohol, controlled substances and inhalants: basic findings from the National Comorbidity Survey. *Exp Clin Psychopharmacol* 1994;2:244–268.

Centers for Disease Control. Assessment of the number and characteristics of persons affected by learning disabilities. In: *Interagency Committee on Learning Disabilities: Learning Disabilities: A Report to the U.S. Congress.* Washington, DC: US Department of Health and Human Services, 1987:107.

Costello EJ, Angold A, Burns B, et al. The Great Smoky Mountains study of youth: goals, design and prevalence of DSM-III-R disorders. *Arch Gen Psychiatry* 1996;53:1129–1136.

Costello EJ. Commentary on prevalence and impact of parent-reported disabling mental health conditions among US children. *J Am Acad Adolesc Psychiatry* 1999;38:610–613.

Garland AF, Hough RL, McCabe KM, et al. Prevalence of psychiatric disorders in youths across five sectors of care. *J Am Acad Child Adolesc Psychiatry* 2001;40:409–418.

Kandel DB, Johnson JG, Bird HR, et al. Psychiatric comorbidity among adolescents with substance use disorders: findings from the MECA study. *J Am Acad Adolesc Psychiatry* 1999;38:693–699.

Popper C, West SA. Disorders usually first diagnosed in infancy, childhood, or adolescence. In: Hales RE, Yudofsky SC, Talbott JA, eds. *The American Psychiatric Press textbook of psychiatry,* 3rd ed. Washington, DC: American Psychiatric Press, 1999:870.

Rosenblatt JA, Rosenblatt A, Biggs EE. Criminal behavior and emotional disorders: comparing youth served by the mental health and juvenile justice system. *J Behav Health Serv Res* 2000;27:227–237.

Shaffer D, Fisher P, Dulcan MK, et al. The NIMH diagnostic interview schedule for children version 2.3 (DISC 2.3): description, acceptability, prevalence rates, and performance in the MECA study. *J Am Acad Adolesc Psychiatry* 1996;35:865–877.

7 ♣ The School System

Dewey J. Bayer and David L. Kaye

I. **Background.** In the early 1970s it came to the attention of the US Congress that large numbers of school-aged children were unable to receive an education in the public school setting. These estimated millions of children included those with mental retardation, deafness, blindness, autism, and learning disabilities, among other conditions. At that time, if a child required any special educational service it was primarily up to the parent to arrange for such. Some parents were able to afford private schooling. Others who lived in an affluent or progressive area might have had available services in the public school. For most parents, however, their disabled children were either poorly served or were entirely excluded from the school setting. Many children required institutionalization because of a lack of educational resources. All this prompted the federal passage in 1975 of **Public Law 94-142, the Education for All Handicapped Children Act.** This act provided the foundation for the provision of special educational services by legislating that **all children aged 6 to 21, regardless of any "handicapping condition," must be provided with a "free appropriate education"** by the public school system. P.L. 94-142 also set forth the precepts:
1. There would be a number of handicapping conditions that would qualify for services. These included:
   - Deafness or hearing impaired
   - Deaf-blind
   - Mental retardation
   - Multiply handicapped (two or more disabilities)
   - Learning disabled
   - Orthopedic impairment (e.g., cerebral palsy, muscular dystrophy, amputations)
   - Other health impaired (chronic conditions such as epilepsy, sickle cell, heart disease, hemophilia)
   - Serious emotional disturbance
   - Speech or language impaired
   - Visual impairment
   - Note that autism and traumatic brain injured were added to this list by new legislation in 1990. In 1991, attention-deficit/hyperactivity disorder and attention-deficit disorder (AD/HD and ADD) were explicitly included as an "other health impaired" disability (see below).
2. A **committee for special education (CSE)** must be constituted in each school district to oversee the evaluation of each child.
3. Following a multidisciplinary evaluation of a child's abilities, functioning, and needs (i.e., the **"CSE evaluation"**) the school must develop a detailed **individualized education program (IEP).**

4. Every effort must be made to provide services for the child in the **least restrictive environment,** meaning that children should be educated with their peers as much as possible (**mainstreaming,** which generally came to mean in music, art, gym, lunch, and so on).
5. Parents must be given the opportunity for **informed consent** and **due process** with respect to any decisions made by the CSE.
6. **Reevaluation** of the child's progress and placement was required on a yearly basis, with a full review (including retesting the child) every 3 years (**triennial evaluation**).

Beyond this structure it was left to each state to develop the specific mechanics of this process. Each state operationalized (and still does so) the law somewhat differently, so that although the basics are the same throughout the country, nuanced differences exist within each state with which the primary care physician (PCP) may need to be familiar. Since the original act, four major federal revisions have been made:

- 1983 P.L. 98-199 made minor revisions calling for demonstration projects for infants and preschool children, who were included in the original act but for whom services were not mandated. Parents were also given the right to see their child's educational records.
- 1986 P.L. 99-457 extended the rights and protections afforded school-aged children to those 3 to 21 years of age. This prompted the development of **committees for preschool evaluation,** the function and role of which was the same as the CSE for older children, and also established a system of early intervention services for children with special needs from birth to 3 years of age. For these youngest children an **individualized family services plan** would be developed, akin to the IEP for children older than 3.
- 1990 P.L. 101-476 **Individuals with Disabilities Education Act (IDEA)** changed the name of the act to emphasize people first (i.e., "individuals" is the first word vs. "education" in the original act), the need to serve different aged individuals (not just children), and the use of the term "disability" (vs. a "handicap", which implied a more fixed and insurmountable problem). A major addition was to include **autism and traumatic brain injury** on the list of qualifying disabilities. In 1991, an administrative clarification was made to include **AD/HD (and ADD) and Tourette's syndrome** to the list of qualifying disabilities (either as "other health impaired", "learning disabled", or "serious emotional disturbance," depending on the predominant findings). This act also mandated that counseling, assistive technology (e.g., alternative communication

devices) and "transition services" (e.g., vocational, life skills that allow for the transition to adulthood) be included in IEP recommendations.

- 1997 105-17 (**IDEA '97**) mandated greater "inclusion" of disabled students not only in regular classroom teaching but also in state- and district-wide assessment programs; increased parent and student participation in the process of decision making (i.e., not just being given a recommendation by the CSE that they could agree or disagree with); the need for planning of "transition services" for adolescents at age 14; an emphasis on positive behavioral strategies to address misbehavior and a clarification of the disciplinary process especially as it related to seriously emotionally disturbed children. Lastly, retesting for the triennial evaluation could be waived if the IEP team (including the parents and child, if appropriate) felt sufficient information was available otherwise to make a decision.

II. **Obtaining special education services.** The next sections follow the process of obtaining special education services. The PCP can be of significant help to parents and children in this process by:

- **Coaching and supporting** the parents in navigating the school system and special education process
- **Initiating** the process of assessment and identification, when necessary
- **Monitoring** the child's progress after services are begun
- **Advocating** for the child's needs as appropriate

A. **Step I. Identification.** In most districts when a child is having trouble in school, the child has been discussed and initial remedies implemented by the teacher (often in collaboration with the parents), and then by other school personnel (e.g., school psychologist, principal). Each building has a multidisciplinary team consisting of teaching and support staff that comes together on a regular basis to brainstorm solutions for children not experiencing success. It is also possible that special services can be provided under the more accepting and informal mandates of **Section 504 of the Rehabilitation Act** (1974) without the formal process of identifying a child with a disability. The regulation applies to many more children than are covered by PL 94-142. Insofar as school children are concerned, the critical question under Section 504 is whether a student's impairment substantially limits the ability to learn, not whether a "significant discrepancy" exists between ability and academic achievement. Districts vary widely in their use of the statute because funding is not provided by the federal government and is left entirely up to the state and local district. Some districts try to avoid responsibility, others use it freely to initiate special help for children who are doing fairly well academically, although impeded by limitations. A case in point might be a child with impulse control problems (e.g., AD/HD) performing academically near grade level. A district that uses Section 504 could be willing to provide the services of a consulting teacher to adapt the classroom curriculum to better accommodate the child's needs. The possibility of using Section 504 should be explored with the building principal if the efforts of the multidisciplinary team have been insufficient and before referral is made to the CSE.

B. **Step 2. Referral to the CSE.** The responsibility for identifying and locating children with disabilities rests on the school system, but those in the community who know the child, particularly the parents and the physician, may alert the school system that a child may have a handicap. **Requests for evaluation** should be made in **written form** to school personnel, usually the director or chairperson of special education. In some school systems the request should be directed to the building principal or district superintendent. The district, through its CSE, must then immediately initiate a full, **multidisciplinary evaluation.** Under federal rules, the **CSE must include,** at a minimum:

1. An administrator in the school system (e.g., director of pupil services or a building principal). Usually this person is designated the committee chairperson.
2. The child's parent(s)
3. A person knowledgeable about interpreting tests **(usually a school psychologist)**
4. Special education and regular education teachers
5. A social worker

Older adolescents are often included as well in their own CSE meeting. A parent may request additional members (e.g., a medical provider who knows the child well, other advocates) and individual states can mandate other members (e.g., New York mandates a school psychologist). The local school district can include other members on their CSE as well (e.g., some include a pediatrician or child psychiatrist).

Once a referral is made, the CSE decides which evaluations should be included in the assessment of the particular child (e.g. speech or language evaluation, occupational therapy/physical therapy [OT/PT] evaluation, general pediatric, psychiatric). **Individualized psychological and educational testing must be a part of this evaluation.** All these evaluations are paid for by the school district and are **without additional cost to the parents.** The CSE has a "reasonable" time period to complete its evaluation and then must convene to determine the need for special educational services. The chairperson (usually the administrator) assigns personnel to conduct the assessment, monitors time lines dictated by the law, calls meetings, and maintains all records. This is the person the parent or outside professionals should contact with requests, questions, or further information.

C. **Step 3. Meeting the standards.** After evaluations are completed, the CSE convenes to make its determinations. The CSE needs to answer three questions in their assessment:

1. Does the child have a **particular category of disability?**
2. **To what degree** does the disability **affect the child's educational performance?**
3. Because of the disability, does the child **need special education and related services?**

Establishing the presence of a disability often requires documentation from a PCP or other physician, although some categories of disability require other professional evaluations (i.e., speech pathologist's evaluation to document speech or language disorder, psychologist to document presence of mental retardation). Some disabilities (e.g., deaf, orthopedically impaired, visual impairment), by their nature, meet the criteria to receive special services. Others, most notably learning disabled and emotionally disturbed, require that educational performance be impaired. A multipronged assessment should be conducted to determine whether performance is affected. Part of this assessment involves administering culturally sensitive, and standardized educational and psychological tests. A knowledgeable and trained personnel, usually a school psychologist, must administer these tests. **Assessment** is a problem-solving process that includes not only testing but also observation, teacher or parent checklists, interviews, evaluation of curricula, and examination of school records. A good CSE evaluation is an assessment. Because psychological testing is often a central part of assessment, the basic characteristics of the major testing instruments are summarized here (see Section III).

D. **Step 4: The individualized education program (IEP).** If the CSE **with the agreement of the parent** decides that a handicapping condition exists and services are required, it must draw up a personalized plan of treatment for the child, called the "IEP." This plan must involve and be approved of by the parent.

Parents cannot be forced to accept a service plan, and a number of options are available when agreement cannot be reached. Parents should contact the CSE chairperson regarding their concerns, and they can pursue the following:

1. An **educational consultant or advocate** can be brought into the process by the parents to try to help them reach agreement with the school.

2. **Mediation** by a noninvolved party can be requested by the parents to broker an agreement with the school.

3. If disagreement continues, parents can contact an attorney and ask for a **due process hearing.**

4. Lastly, parents can file a complaint with their **state board of education.**

The IEP outlines how the school system will provide a **free and appropriate education** for the given child. This is an extremely important document, meant to guide all the treatments that the child will receive. Because of the operational detail included, the tendency for many IEPs to have a "boilerplate" look to them, and the fact that school districts use slightly different formats for documenting the findings, reading an IEP can be overwhelming at first. Understanding what is included can help to make sense of the document, which parents often feel bewildered by as well. The major areas addressed by the IEP are:

1. The child's **cognitive aptitude and present levels of educational achievement;** usually these scores are found on the first or second page.

2. **Measurable annual goals,** including benchmarks or short-term objectives, expressed in terms of specific behaviors or academic skills (e.g., the child successfully decode four-syllable words taken from a grade-level reader).

3. The **special education services** (including classroom placement, consultant teachers, resource room, and so on.), **supplementary aids** (e.g., a Kurzweil reading machine), and **related services** (e.g., speech therapy, counseling, occupational therapy) to be provided to the child.

4. The **program modifications or supports** for school personnel that will be provided for the child to advance appropriately toward meeting his or her annual goals and to be involved in extracurricular and other non-academic activities (e.g., special bus for trans-

porting child, preferential seating, the use of an individual aid to help child transition from one activity to another).

5. An emphasis on **inclusion** with an explanation of the extent, if any, to which the child will not participate with nondisabled students in the regular class and in extracurricular and nonacademic activities; this includes transportation (i.e., busing).

6. Any **individual testing modifications** to be made in the administration of state and district-wide assessment programs of student achievement, or how the student will be alternatively assessed (e.g., provision of additional time during group examinations at the end of the year).

7. Delineation of the **transition service needs** of the child, beginning at age 14 and updated annually thereafter (e.g., a vocational exploration course).

8. Provision of the needed **transition services** of the child, beginning at age 16 or younger, when appropriate (e.g., a job coach during a work placement).

Many other details are included that are primarily relevant to the teachers and school personnel and will not be reviewed here. The form of the IEP has evolved considerably over the last 25 years, and the current version puts much more emphasis on specifics about goals and treatments, and the involvement of both the child and the parent than did earlier versions. Parents need to monitor whether goals are being reached and can call for change by contacting the CSE chairperson if they are not.

E. **Step 5: Least restrictive environment.** School districts must ensure to the maximal extent appropriate that students with disabilities ages 3 through 21 are both educated with (**"inclusion"**) and participate in nonacademic and extracurricular activities with nondisabled children. Special classes, separate schooling, or other removal of children with disabilities from the regular classroom occurs only when the nature or severity of the educational disability is such that education in the regular class cannot be achieved satisfactorily with the use of supplementary aids and services. For children placed outside of the regular classroom, rules regarding placement require that each student with a disability be educated as close to home as possible, and that each student be educated in the same school he or she would attend if not disabled. At times this is not practically feasible and the child needs to be placed within a school outside the home district. For example, a mentally retarded child who lives in a rural school district may need to be grouped with similar children from other nearby districts in a school outside their local area. Efforts are generally made to avoid this, and any such arrangement must be specified in the IEP. The central role of parents in the IEP planning process makes them important in determining where placement will be. The options to be considered are (in order of increasing level of restrictiveness):

1. **General education ("regular") classroom,** possibly with consulting teacher support (also known as inclusion)

2. **Resource room** (i.e., working in the home school with a special education teacher and a small number of other similar students, outside the regular classroom, for up to 50% of the school day; typically 45 to 60 minutes a day, 3 to 5 days a week). These children are expected to master the same curriculum as those in general education classes.

3. **Self-contained class** (i.e., a full-time special education placement in a regular school building, possibly out of district). The size of these classes varies from state to state but is always smaller than a regular class. Typical options might be for 12 to 15 students with 1 special education teacher, with or without an aide; 6 to 8 students with 1 special education teacher, with or without an aide. Children in these classrooms have a modified curriculum that differs from that in the general education class.

4. **Special school,** also known as an agency placement. Examples might include a school for the blind or deaf, or a mental health day treatment program.

Even where more restrictive placement is required (special class or school), parents can request some level of **"mainstreaming,"** meaning times during the day where the child is involved with nonidentified children, possibly in physical education or library instruction.

With IDEA current emphasis on regular education curriculum and parents' desires not to have their children removed from normally developing peers, inclusion has become a popular placement alternative, even for severely handicapped (autism, orthopedically impaired, mentally retarded) children. Some children thrive on inclusion, whereas others do better with a special placement. In any individual situation the best way to make this determination is to carefully consider what is known about that particular child, his or her strengths and weaknesses, what he or she has responded to in the past, and so forth. It is imperative that all of the data be considered in an open (i.e., without fixed and preconceived beliefs) and mutually respectful discussion. Although the school setting can be intimidating for parents, the PCP can be helpful in coaching the parent to be positive and assertive, rather than adversarial. It is also helpful to remind the parents that **no decision can be finalized without their approval.**

F. **Step 6: The review process,** a formal **yearly review,** allows the IEP team to revisit the terms of the IEP, to determine whether it is adequately meeting the individual needs of the student, and to assess whether the student is making adequate progress toward annual goals. In many school districts, the "annual review" is strategically scheduled toward the end of the school year, allowing the IEP team to review progress at a time when it makes the most sense to do so. Annual reviews held during this time of year allow for more appropriate educational goals or objectives to be written and for placement recommendations to be made before the transition to the next grade. Based on a review of the student's progress during the previous year and input from IEP team members, new IEPs are developed during the annual review meeting that typically go into effect the following school year.

A **more comprehensive review** must take place every 3 years. The requirements for this **triennial evaluation** have changed under the IDEA for 1997. After a thorough review of the information available regarding a student's present level of performance, the IEP committee (this includes the parent) is responsible for making a decision regarding the amount and kind of new assessments needed to address the student's individualized educational program. All involved may agree that no additional testing is necessary at that time. In this case, a new IEP will be developed based on the information already available from teachers, report cards, yearly educational testing, and so forth. On the other hand, the school, parents, or both may deem additional testing and assessment procedures necessary. Informed parental consent must be sought by the school district before any new assessment can take place. The district may proceed with new assessment if it can show that it has taken reasonable measures to obtain this consent and the parents have failed to respond. Conversely, if the parent requests it, a triennial evaluation must include new assessments.

III. Understanding psychological testing.

    A. Intelligence testing. First, a few words about **intelligence quotient (IQ)** testing. Conceptually, **IQ** is defined as the developmental age ÷ chronological age and is supposed to reflect a person's **ability** to learn academic material. **Intelligence** is a much broader concept than what is measured by IQ tests (i.e., IQ tests measure little of creativity, problem-solving, emotional or interpersonal intelligence, and so on). What IQ tests do correlate well with is how able someone is to learn academic (reading, writing, and arithmetic) material. IQ tests do predict how well someone will do in school. Beyond that the data are less clear. Nevertheless, IQ tests have been used in schools for many years and we expect that they will continue to be used for the foreseeable future to help guide educational placement decisions. It is also important to note that **IQ testing alone is not sufficient for the diagnosis of learning disabilities, AD/HD, or** another currently popular concept, **central auditory processing disorder** (CAPD). Diagnosis of a learning disability requires comparison of IQ with educational test scores; AD/HD is a clinical diagnosis (Chapter 12), although IQ tests can provide suggestions of this disorder; and CAPD is a concept that is assessed by specialized language testing.

    All CSE psychological evaluations include testing with a normed cognitive instrument. Tests most often used in the United States are the Wechsler scales and the Stanford-Binet Test. The current **school-age version (6 to 16 years of age)** of the Wechsler test is the **Wechsler Intelligence Scale for Children-III (or WISC-III);** for **preschoolers** (generally limited to use for children 4 to 6 years of age, but can be used in children as young as 3 or as old as 7 years of age), **the Wechsler Preschool Inventory.** Both of them are constructed similarly, have similar (although not identical) subtest scales, but include different items commensurate with the age of the child. The **Stanford Binet IV** is the current version of this test. Earlier versions of this test were thought to be more heavily weighted to verbal abilities and, consequently, it is used less frequently in the United States. The current version is broader based and the test may become more widely used. Because the WISC-III is used most frequently at this time, it will be discussed in greater detail.

    The **WISC-III** consists of items examining verbal and performance (i.e., nonverbal, visuospatial, organizational, visual-perceptual skills) abilities and requires more than an hour to administer. Scores are reported for the **verbal (VIQ) and performance (PIQ) subscales,** as well as a full-scale IQ (FSIQ), which is a composite of VIQ and PIQ scores. The **verbal and performance subscales** are each composed of a **number of subtests** (Table 7.1). The subtests can be read individually or grouped together to generate conclusions about broader factors such as verbal comprehension, perceptual organization, and processing speed. Thus, the evaluator can discuss how basic factual knowledge (information subtest) is significantly lower than short-term memory skill (digit span subtest), with scaled scores of 7 and 13, respectively. These scores along with other information about the child allow for a conclusion about learning needs or disability classification.

B. **Educational testing.** Common **tests of academic skills (or "educational tests")** include the Woodcock-Johnson Achievement Battery (now in the third edition), Wide Range Achievement Test, the Kaufman

---

Table 7.1.   Verbal and performance subscales

Information: factual knowledge, long-term memory, recall. *How many eyes do you have?*

Similarities: abstract reasoning, verbal categories and concepts. *How are shirts and socks alike?*

Arithmetic: attention and concentration, numerical reasoning. *If you have 15 apples and give 7 away, how many are left?*

Vocabulary: language development, word knowledge, verbal fluency. *What is a cup?*

Comprehension: social and practical judgment, common sense. *Why do people wear clothes?*

Digit span: attention, short-term auditory memory. *Memory of digit strings.*

Picture completion: alertness to detail, visual discrimination. *Identify the important part missing from a picture.*

Coding: attention, visual-motor coordination, speed. *Drawing correct symbol under numbers.*

Picture arrangement: planning or organizing, logical thinking, social knowledge. *Put cartoon panels in correct order.*

Block design: spatial analysis (three-dimensional), abstract visual problem-solving. *Reproduce geometric designs using blocks.*

Object assembly: visual analysis and construction of objects (two-dimensional). *Assemble puzzle pieces.*

Symbol search: attention, visual-motor speed, persistence. *Quickly determine whether symbols match target symbols.*

Mazes: fine motor coordination, planning, following directions. *Paper and pencil maze completion.*

Test of Educational Achievement, and the Wechsler Individual Achievement Test, among many others. All of these are broad measures that tap what children **actually have learned** in reading, mathematics, language arts skills (i.e., writing and spelling skills), and other academic areas. They are reported as cluster scores for "total" or "broad" reading, mathematics, and language skills. These, in turn, are composites of subtests that can also be reported (e.g., "letter-word identification," "story recall".) All educational testing is not equivalent. Each battery is different and may measure different skills, leading to different scores. Some tests of "reading" will measure phonetic reading skills, others passage comprehension, and still others story recall or memory. The Woodcock-Johnson III (W-J III), one of the most widely used instruments, includes scores for the following primary cluster areas and individual subtests.

1. **Oral language** consists of **story recall** (recall stories presented using an audio recording) and **understanding directions** (listen to audio-recorded instructions and follow directions by pointing to various objects in a colored picture).

2. **Broad reading** consists of **letter-word identification** (recognizing individual letters or words), **reading fluency** (quickly read short sentences and indicate whether they are true or false), and **passage comprehension** (e.g., read short passages and identify a key missing word).

3. **Broad mathematics** consists of **calculation** (perform basic mathematics operations), **mathemetics fluency** (solve simple addition, subtraction, and multiplication facts quickly), and **applied problems** (solve verbally presented mathematics problems [i.e., "story problems"]).

4. **Broad written language** includes written tests of spelling, fluency of production, and quality of expression.

5. **Academic knowledge** broadly measures the child's knowledge of science, social studies, and cultural facts.

6. **Academic skills** reflects basic achievement skills by aggregating measures of reading decoding, mathematics calculation, and spelling of single-word responses.

7. **Academic fluency** is a combination of **reading fluency, mathematics fluency, and writing fluency.**

When looking at these scores it may also be important to factor in the socioeconomic status

(SES) of the school. All other factors being equal, children from higher SES schools generally will score higher than those learning in schools predominantly made up of lower SES students. A child's scores are reported compared with national norms, although some districts are also able to report locally normed scores.

If the presenting problem also involves behavioral or emotional concerns, either a behavior rating scale (e.g., Child Behavior checklist or a Connors Rating scale) or a projective instrument (a drawing test or story-making test) would be added to these. In these cases, the psychologist must complete a structured analysis of the behavioral problems (Functional Behavioral Assessment) and construct a behavior management plan. Speech and language, occupational therapy, and physical therapy evaluations can also be part of the assessment process.

When the disability is one other than "learning disabled," the condition need only interfere "substantially" with learning for the student to receive services. Disabilities such as autism, hearing impaired, mental retardation, and orthopedic impairment inherently meet such criteria and, hence, qualify for special educational services. The case of learning disability is more complex and usually centers around the discrepancy between aptitude (i.e., IQ scores) and achievement (educational test scores). Policies vary widely from state to state, and application further varies from district to district. Some states require rigidly defined statistical criteria (e.g., 2 SD differences between normed IQ tests and academic achievement tests), but most mirror the federal definition that the differences between aptitude and achievement need only be "significant." This leads to variability between schools and across states. A mixture of normed score comparisons (e.g., verbal comprehension is at the 50th percentile, while decoding skills fall 2 years behind the child's chronologic age) in evaluations and observational data (e.g., "the child spent 50% of the instruction period off-task") are presented in a form that builds toward a conclusion for or against the existence of a disability. If a number of tests are used, if differences among the scores are large enough to generally support the conclusion drawn (a minimum of 1 SD difference), and if the examiner appears to have a good grasp of the child's background and characteristics, then the conclusions should be given more weight than if the report is short, contains few test data, and is based on only one meeting with the child.

C. **Test score overview.** Because most educational and psychological tests use **standard scores (SS)** with a mean of 100 and a SD of 15, a SS of 100 is at the 50% **percentile rank (PR)** level. Psychological tests, such as the WISC-III, report scores for FSIQ, PIQ, and VIQ as a standard score. Overall scores are interpreted as follows:

- Superior above 120
- Above average 110–120 (75% to 90%)
- **Average range 90–110** (25% to 75%)
- Below average 80–90 (10% to 25%)
- Borderline 70–80 (2% to 10%)
- Mental retardation below 70

Table 7.2 outlines the equivalence of alternative ways of reporting test scores.

Educational tests are reported as **standard scores** similar to those used for cognitive tests (means of 10 or 100, SD of 3 or 15) as well as **age equivalent (AE)** scores (i.e., the age that 50% of children achieve an equivalent score), **grade equivalent (GE)** scores (i.e., the grade of the average child earning a particular test score), and as **PR** (the percentage of children of the same age below a child's score). These nationally normed tests compare children with a cross-section of others at the same grade and age levels. An AE score of 6.8 would mean that 50% of children aged 6 years, 8 months would obtain this score. A GE score of 6.3 on a reading test would mean that the child is reading at the level of the average child in the third month of 6th grade. A PR of 22 would mean the child, compared with a nationally representative sample of their same-aged or same-grade

Table 7.2.   **Equivalence of testing scores**

Standard Score	Subtest Score	Percentile Score	Standard Deviation
130	16	98	+2
115	13	84	+1
110	—	75	—
100	10	50	0
90	—	25	—
85	7	16	−1
70	4	2	−2

peers, was able to read as well as or better than 22% (or more poorly than 78%). Psychologists generally place the **most stock in the SS and PR scores,** as AE and GE scores can be less reliable indicators. On the other hand, AE and GE scores often convey more graphically the difficulty a child is having (i.e., a child aged 7 years and 5 months is reading at a 5-year, 3-month level, or at a kindergarten, 4th month level). Some tests are using newer ways of reporting the data. The W-J III reports an "Easy to Diff" score to reflect the age-equivalent range of correct responses, from the easiest to most difficult. It also uses a relative proficiency index (RPI), which reports how well the child would be expected to do relative to age mates. An RPI of 60/90 suggests that the child performs a particular task with 60% proficiency, whereas the average child of the same age would perform at 90%.

D. **Basic interpretation of psychological testing.** Although only psychologists are qualified and trained to make in-depth interpretations of psychological tests, a PCP can become familiar with a basic understanding of these IQ and educational test scores. The following steps may be useful toward this end.

1. **Examine the FS IQ, V IQ, and P IQ.** Discrepancies between the VIQ and PIQ of **greater than 15 points** are thought to be of significance. Most individuals will perform consistently on these two subscales. A significant difference may reflect a learning disability; however, learning differences, motor difficulties, language disorders, and attentional or motivational factors also need to be considered.

2. **Examine the subtest scatter** (i.e., the difference between the subtest scores on each subscale). Although small variations are typical, **differences of 4 or more** on subtests within each domain (verbal or performance) are considered significant.

3. **Integrate areas of relative strength and weakness.** Examine the subtests for consistencies in ability areas. For example, multiple subtests tap attention (i.e., digit span, coding, arithmetic, symbol search); others verbal comprehension (i.e., information, vocabulary, comprehension); still others processing speed (i.e., coding, object assembly).

4. **Review the educational test scores for consistency between themselves and with the child's age.** Scores on broad reading versus mathematics versus writing should be generally

similar and commensurate with the child's age. Large discrepancies on the different domains (i.e., more than 1-year difference between AE scores or more than 1 SD on SS) suggest lack of exposure to an area, inadequate effort, learning differences, or learning disabilities. Large discrepancies between the child's actual scores and those expected based on the child's age may also reflect these factors. Deficits observed in all domains raise the possibility of low average or borderline IQ, or mental retardation.

5. **Compare the IQ scores with the educational test scores.** Children are expected to achieve educational test scores equivalent to their **developmental age.** Children with an average IQ would be expected to achieve at average educational levels for their age (i.e., age equivalent scores in all domains should be commensurate with chronologic age); with below average IQ, AE achievement should be lower than chronologic age; with above average IQ, AE should be above chronologic age.

E. **A sample analysis.** Table 7.3 is a sample report for a child 7½ years of age.

Interpretation

1. **Examine FSIQ, VIQ, and PIQ.** As can be seen, the FSIQ is in the average range. However, a significant 28-point difference is seen between VIQ and PIQ. This suggests a learning difficulty or disability, although other factors could depress the PIQ (e.g., poor vision, fine or gross motor deficits, loss of motivation in the examination).

2. **Subtest scatter.** Verbal subtest scores go from a low of 8 (digit span) to a high of 16 (similarities). This difference is significant and suggests relative strengths in abstraction abilities, and a weakness in sustained attention. The other verbal scores are roughly in the average range. On the performance subtests, scores run from lows of 4 (coding), to 6 (symbol search, picture completion). These performance subtest scores also support a finding of weakness in attention. Visual-perceptual skills also appear to be decreased (picture completion and object assembly are also depressed). The other scores fall within an average range.

3. **Integrate areas of relative strength and weakness.** These test scores suggest overall average cognitive abilities, with strength in the areas of abstract reasoning and weaknesses in attention and visual-perceptual skills.

Table 7.3. The Wechsler Intelligence Scale for Children-III

Verbal Subtests	Score	Performance Subtests	Score
Information	10	Picture completion	6
Similarities	16	Coding	4
Arithmetic	11	Picture arrangement	10
Vocabulary	13	Block design	12
Comprehension	12	Object assembly	7
Digit span	8	Symbol search	6

Verbal IQ = 114
Performance IQ = 86
Full Scale IQ = 101

Woodcock-Johnson III

	AE	Easy to Diff.		RPI	PR	SS
Cluster/Test						
Oral language	6–8	4–6	7–1	69/90	11	82
Broad reading	6–7	6–4	6–10	19/90	8	79
Broad mathematics	7–5	6–9	8–3	89/90	48	99
Mathematic calculation skills	7–5	6–8	8–4	89/90	47	99
Academic skills	6–10	6–7	7–2	44/90	17	86
Academic fluency	6–9	6–0	7–5	73/90	17	86
Individual subtests						
Letter-word identification	6–8	6–6	6–10	8/90	12	82
Reading fluency	6–9	6–5	7–2	83/90	18	86
Story recall	5–7	3–3	9–5	83/90	18	86
Understanding directions	5–9	3–3	9–5	52/90	11	82
Calculation	7–6	4–11	6–7	90/90	49	100
Mathematics fluency	7–3	5–5	9–3	89/90	40	96
Spelling	6–9	6–5	7–1	40/90	19	87
Writing fluency	6–3	5–5	7–2	67/90	17	85
Passage comprehension	6–4	6–1	6–7	12/90	8	79
Applied problems	7–5	6–10	8–1	89/90	48	99

IQ, intelligence quotient; AE, age equivalent; RPI, relative proficiency index; PR, percentile ranks; SS, subtest scatter.

4. **Review educational tests for consistency between them and the child's age.** On the overall **clusters,** the child is achieving in the expected range for broad mathematics and mathematics calculation skills, is slightly delayed in academic skills and oral language, and is significantly delayed (almost 1 year and more than 1 SD) in broad reading. Looking at the **subtest** results, it is evident that the child has areas of being on track (calculation, mathematics fluency, applied problems), of some delay (letter-word identification, reading fluency, spelling), and of major delay (story recall, understanding directions, writing fluency, and passage comprehension). Looking at the SS, we see that the child is functioning at more than 1 SD behind in broad reading and oral language skills, with letter-word identification, understanding directions, and passage comprehension being the primary areas of difficulty. Together, these factors indicate this child is clearly showing signs of significant differences between domains and also in comparison with chronologic age. This is especially pronounced in the areas related to verbal and reading processing and memory, but also writing skills. Mathematics skills appeared to be developing adequately.

5. **Compare the IQ with the educational test scores.** Based only on the FSIQ of 101, we would expect that the child would achieve roughly in the average range across educational tests. As noted, a significant discrepancy is seen between VIQ and PIQ and so it is not surprising that the educational scores were highly uneven as well. This child clearly was not developing skills at the expected levels. An evaluator might conclude that a significant difference (1 SD or more) exists between aptitude and achievement.

   After further discussion of the child's behaviors in the classroom and during testing, the psychologist stated that the child's uneven aptitude skills and relatively low achievement levels supported a conclusion of "learning disabled." The findings and conclusion would then be discussed by the CSE and a decision made about the need for special education. Note that some school districts (and also *Diagnostic and Statistical Manual of Mental Disorders, Fourth Edition Text Revision*) would not see this as qualifying as a "disability," as it is not a 2 SD discrepancy between aptitude and achievement. In this case, the child might be eligible for services through 504 provisions. If no services at all were available through this school district, this situation might well lead to conflict and the need for appeals and due process hearings (see above).

IV. **Summary.** School is a critical part of a child's life. As all parents know, a poor fit between a child and a given school situation can make for a very difficult year, have a serious impact on the child's mental and physical health, and interfere with learning. Although akin to an adult's job or work situation, schools also have the resources and responsibility to address children's emotional and psychosocial developmental needs. This affords the opportunity to have a major impact on children's lives. By understanding the services available in schools and how to access them, PCPs can advocate for and guide parents in obtaining an optimal education for their children.

SUGGESTED READINGS

Sattler J. *Assessment of children: cognitive applications and assessment of children: behavioral and clinical applications.* La Mesa, CA: Jerome Sattler Publishers, 2001. These two texts are the most comprehensive published sources on the psychological assessment of children. PCPs will not generally need (or want) this level of detail.

Wodrich D. *Children's psychological testing: a guide for nonpsychologists.* Baltimore: Paul Brookes, 1998. An accessible guide for the PCP wanting additional information about the subject.

Web Sites

Children and Adults with Attention Deficit/Hyperactivity Disorder (CHADD) is a family advocacy organization with local chapters in most major metropolitan areas. Its Web site has much useful information for parents, teachers, and physicians. Available at www.chadd.org. Accessed on 6/20/02.

Educational Resources Information Center Clearinghouse on Assessment and Evaluation (ERIC) is an outstanding online source of information for all areas of educational assessment, theory, and practice. Links are available to textbooks and articles, frequently asked questions that point to print and online sources, a full "how-to" series on research, measurement, and statistical issues, and short reports that synthesize research and ideas about emerging issues (ERIC Digests). This is a must site for both professionals and parents. Available at www.ericae.net/nav-lib.htm. Accessed on 6/20/02.

Family and Advocates Partnership for Education (FAPE) maintains a Web site for families and other advocates to provide information on special education. Available at www.fape.org. Accessed on 6/20/02.

LDOnline, a Web site developed by WETA, a PBS affiliate, is an excellent source of information on learning disabilities and special education for parents, teachers, and professionals. Available at www.ldonline.org. Accessed on 6/20/02.

The National Information Center for Children and Youth with Disabilities (NICHCY) is the national information and referral center that provides information on disabilities and disability-related issues for families, educators, and other professionals. This site is especially useful for legal information. Available at www.nichcy.org. Accessed on 6/20/02.

Technical Assistance Alliance for Parent Centers is a clearinghouse to provide information to parents with children and youth with disabilities and the professionals who serve them. Funded by the US Department of Education, Office of Special Education Programs, this site provides information by state. Available at www.taalliance. org. Accessed on 6/20/02.

US Office of Special Education and Rehabilitation Services. Guide to the IEP. This is a general guide for parents that outlines the federal guidelines. Available at http://www.ed.gov/offices/OSERS/OSEP/Products/IEP_Guide/. Accessed on 6/20/02.

8 The Social Services System

Deborah A. Merrifield and David L. Kaye

I. **Introduction.** The United States, since the passage of the Social Security Act of 1935, has taken on the responsibility of insuring that basic human needs are met when, for a variety of reasons, a citizen is unable to provide for those needs or the needs of their children. The social service system has developed over 60 years as the combined responsibility of federal, state, and local governments. A social services department in a community can administer a wide variety of government-mandated and -regulated benefits and services falling in the major categories of:
- Child and family support
- Income support
- Healthcare

In any community, the mix of services provided by social service organizations can vary somewhat. The two common variations are the **combined organizations,** providing the array of income support, health, and social support to children and families under one division (e.g., a Department of Social Services) and **the single organization,** wherein one or more of these service sectors has been split off to multiple divisions. For example, in New York City the Administration for Children and Families deals with Child Welfare, whereas the Human Resources Administration deals with public assistance, Medicaid, food stamps, and so on. The primary federal agency regulating these social support programs is the US Department of Health and Human Services, with the principal exception being the Food Stamp program, which is administered by the US Department of Agriculture. The federal agencies set the rules and federal financing scheme for all 50 states. The states, in turn, oversee and regulate the local branch of the government charged with administering these programs. Some states administer their own programs in localities through regional offices, others through a local arm of government, usually a county. Income support, healthcare, and some social services are delivered directly by the local government. Other social services can be provided through contractual relationships between the local government and not-for-profit agencies (e.g., Catholic Charities, Jewish Family Services, Boys and Girls Clubs).

Many communities have formed valuable partnerships among various community systems to improve the effectiveness of the community's response to the issues facing children and families. These blended programs often support **"wrap-around" services,** referring to individualized services provided to the child and family **in their natural settings** (i.e., home, school, community) to prevent the need for institutional placement. These services can support the caretaker (e.g., training in behavior management, problem-solving, or providing respite) or the child (e.g., after-school programs, intensive case managers available 24 hours a day, 7 days a week).

II. **Child and family support programs.** Mandated social service programs to protect children and support families to meet the needs of their children, referred to as **child welfare services,** are generally provided regardless of the family's income. Access to these services is driven by the risk of harm to the child or vulnerable adult. Services can be initiated on a voluntary basis when something has caused a serious decline in a parent's or child's functioning, or when required by Child Protective Services (CPS) (or commensurate agency) in the context of child maltreatment. Child abuse and neglect often occur in the context of such problems as poverty, parental substance abuse, family violence, mental illness, homelessness, and human immunodeficiency virus (HIV) infection. Support services can be directed at any or all of these targeted problems. Many such programs exist in most communities and include mandated social service programs as well as private nonprofit agency programs (e.g., Parents Anonymous, Catholic Charities, neighborhood centers).

The **role of the primary care physician (PCP)** is to identify children at **risk** and to facilitate their families' access to services. Generally, it is best to engage vulnerable families positively and early, referring them for preventive or support services on a voluntary basis. When families are unwilling or unable to engage in services on a voluntary basis, it may be necessary to file a report with the appropriate child protective agency. At times it may not be possible to ascertain what truly happened in a given situation. PCPs should keep in mind that they are **not** forensic investigators and should not attempt to reach a final determination of the facts. **However, when maltreatment is suspected, an agreement by a family to seek voluntary child welfare services cannot take the place of the physician's own report to CPS.**

Child abuse often takes place in families in which domestic violence is also occurring. Parents may have realistic fears that by making a child abuse report or even seeking voluntary support services they will be placed at risk. This issue should be explored by the PCP (i.e., "How do you think the [maltreating] adult will respond to this call? Do you feel safe going home? Are you worried that he or she may become violent or threatening? Has he or she ever done this in the past?"). Appropriate provisions should be made to assure the safety of all family members. This may require referral to a domestic violence shelter or law enforcement agency.

A. **Child protective services.** At the state level, CPS or the commensurate agency has the statutory authority to:
- Investigate allegations of child abuse and neglect
- Secure the safety of the child
- Monitor a plan for remediation of the problems that led to the allegations

A community relies on a local or statewide **child abuse phone access system,** called the "central registry" (or "hotline" in some states) where anyone suspecting harm to children can telephone in their observations. All states have established that certain professionals interacting with children are **"mandated reporters"** and must call this central registry. **Physicians are always among those required to report.** The most recent amendment to the federal laws regarding child maltreatment, the Child Abuse Protection and Treatment Act of 1996, established for the first time national standards in which calls to the central registry **must be investigated** by the local authorities with **"reasonable cause"** to suspect that child abuse or neglect exists. At a minimum, this can be met by any **recent act or failure to act** (i.e., a **minimum degree of care** has not been provided) on the part of a parent or caretaker which:
- Results in death, serious physical or emotional harm, or sexual abuse or exploitation.
- Presents an imminent risk of one of the above

Contention between different professionals arises because of discrepancy in interpretation of the above. CPS must be able to prove in family or juvenile court that a child is at **imminent risk of death, serious physical or emotional harm, or sexual exploitation** in order to supervise the family and compel family participation in needed services. Physicians should keep in mind that family laws have tried to balance the safeguarding of children **with** the privacy and self-determination of families.

The current circumstances, factoring in the age and capabilities of the child, will affect whether a caller's report is accepted and investigated. Some categories of conditions that will be investigated are:
1. **Visible injuries** and physical condition of child, especially if cause is unexplained
2. **Serious illness** of child **without necessary medical care** performed. This may be a one-time incident of grievous omission or commission, or it could be a pattern of repeated failures that cumulatively place the child at risk.
3. Child **inadequately supervised** or left alone. Whether this meets criteria depends on the length

of time, the age, and capacity of the child to be safe on his or her own, and the resources and persons available to the child.

4. Household **lacks adequate food, heating, and shelter**

5. Child **not adequately clothed** for protection from elements

6. Child **left in care of other child or person who lacks adequate competence** to protect and care for child. For example, a young child left with intoxicated boyfriend or irresponsible, acting-out teenage baby sitter.

7. **Violence or illegal activity** occurring in the home that placed the child in danger

8. **Caretaker capacity** to care for a dependent child greatly **diminished** by mental condition, substance abuse, and so on.

Problems negatively affecting children that can (but have not yet) lead to serious harm in the future can only be addressed on a voluntary basis by the family at these earlier stages. All social service programs, public and private, have a **voluntary intake office** (usually listed in the telephone book in the local government pages), which is, in fact, the method of access to services for most families.

Recent data have been reported by all 50 states to the **National Child Abuse and Neglect Data System (NCANDS).** Because these figures include only reported cases, it is thought that these numbers are probably conservative estimates. Nevertheless, they are seen as the most reliable figures available and reflect the magnitude of the problem. NCANDS statistics suggest that the **numbers of children and rates of maltreatment are high but have stabilized** over the past several years. Summaries of current results are found in Tables 8.1 through 8.5.

B. **The CPS investigation.** After receiving the report from the hotline, the CPS caseworker begins promptly to assess the degree of risk to the child. In emergency circumstances, law enforcement (i.e., the police) is immediately involved to protect the child. In the more

Table 8.1.   Overview of child maltreatment, 1999

Total case referrals	3 million
Accepted and investigated cases	1.8 million (60%)
Substantiated or indicated cases	560,000 = 826,000 children
	(29% of those investigated)
Boys:girls	48:52

Table 8.2.   Case distribution by type of maltreatment

Type	Total Cases (%)
Neglect	56.0
Medical neglect	2.4
Physical abuse	21.0
Sexual abuse	11.0
Multiple forms of maltreatment	25.0

Table 8.3.   Incidence and rates of child maltreatment by age, 1999

Age (years)	0–3	4–7	8–11	12–15	16–17
Number (thousands)	200.0	195.0	176.0	148.0	45.0
Rate/1,000	13.9	13.0	11.6	10.0	5.9

Table 8.4.   Child maltreatment fatalities, 1999

Total number of child fatalities	1,100
Boys:girls	53% to 47%
<1 yr	43%
<3 yr	70%
<6 yr	86%

Table 8.5.   Maltreatment perpetrator characteristics, 1999

Relationship to Child	Child Abuse and Neglect (%)	Child Fatality (%)
Either parent involved	87	81
Female parent alone	45	31
Male parent alone	16	11
Both parents	18	21
Female parent with other adult	8	16
Male parent with other adult	1	1
Other	12	—

typical nonemergent situation, the caseworker will contact the person making the report to the hotline and any other possible sources of important information about the current situation (e.g., teachers, doctors, relatives, neighbors, counselors). The caseworker will **contact** in person the parents and all the children residing in the household **within a prescribed time frame (e.g., 24 to 48 hours),** depending on the regulations in that state. Most laws require that **the investigation be completed swiftly (e.g., 60 days),** but regardless, the caseworker assesses from the first contact whether any safety intervention is needed, up to and including involuntary and urgent removal of the child from the home.

Three general outcomes to an investigation of a report are:

1. **Unsubstantiated,** meaning not sufficient evidence under state law or policy to conclude that maltreatment has occurred
2. **Substantiated,** meaning that the allegation was supported by state law or policy. In these cases, services can be offered on a **voluntary basis or can be court ordered.**
3. Some states allow for an **indicated or "reason to suspect"** status for cases that do not meet statutory requirements but significant evidence exists that the child has been maltreated or is at risk for such.

The CPS caseworker must make a legal determination regarding the report received, either that sufficient evidence was found to substantiate the caller's assertion, or that sufficient evidence was not found. "Unsubstantiated" does not mean the risk did not exist, only that sufficient evidence could not be established within the necessary time frame. Therefore, the PCP should be:

- **Specific in descriptions** and judgments about the dangerousness of the situation
- **Persistent,** as this report may be the only advocacy available to the child

If the PCP disagrees with the findings of the CPS worker, or if the PCP has not been included in the investigation as outlined above, the PCP can either write a letter to the CPS caseworker outlining the reasons for disagreement (with a copy to the Commissioner or other high-level person at the Department of Social Services) or call the local CPS office and speak with a supervisor or other higher-level administrator.

Depending on the legal findings and the child and family needs, the CPS can take a number of actions.

If the abuse or neglect is not substantiated, the CPS can provide information and offer a referral for voluntary services. If the case is substantiated, then an assessment of risk is made. In many areas this is done with the use of a formal rating instrument (e.g., Safety Assessment Instrument) that takes into account the history with the family, what the safety issues are, what solutions exist, and the amenability of the family to accept services. When the risk is judged to be mild and the parents are amenable to treatment, voluntary services will be offered to the family with continued monitoring of the situation. However, if the risk of abuse or neglect is serious and the parents' likelihood of following through with services and necessary safety steps is questionable, the caseworker will petition the family or juvenile court to order mandated participation in services and continued supervision of the home by CPS. If the risks are too great to leave the child in the unsupervised care of the parent or current caretaker, the child will be removed and placed in out-of-home care. The investigation and follow-up phase of CPS is typically 2 to 6 months, depending on the seriousness of the situation and the ability of other service providers to take over the monitoring of family improvement. If, however, a safety assessment determines that the child's risk of harm is not sufficiently reduced, CPS can stay involved (i.e., "keep the case open") on an ongoing basis until the risk is sufficiently reduced.

C. **Foster care prevention services.** If a child is at risk for removal from parents' custody, Foster Care Prevention Services (or "Preventive Services"), also known as Family Preservation and Reunification Services, may be offered. The purpose of these is to prevent the need to remove the child from the home or, if a child has already been removed, to hasten the safe return of the child back home. The services that can be provided to a family voluntarily or based on an order of the court include virtually any physical and behavioral health, social, and educational service available in the community. Child welfare services have various programs available to families that social services administer directly or through contracts with nonprofit community organizations.

D. **Out-of-home care: foster care, kinship care, group homes, and institutional placements.** When the situation warrants, CPS can remove children from their parents' custody. In 2000, approximately 581,000 children were in foster care and other placements, and these numbers have been increasing significantly over the past decade. Children can be removed from their home and placed with relatives, known as kinship care, or with foster parents who have been certified by the child welfare services organization or a not-for-profit service agency licensed to provide such care. Foster parents are given compensation for basic needs of the child (e.g., board, room, clothes) but are not paid wages. The amount of this varies from state to state, from lows of $200 to $300 per month per child to as much as $600 to $700 per month per child. Therapeutic or treatment foster homes are also available for children with serious emotional or behavioral disturbances. These specially trained and selected foster parents generally care for only one special needs foster child at a time and are paid a higher rate beyond the basic room and board rate of regular foster parents. They generally receive additional ongoing support and consultation from their sponsoring agency.

Alternatively, children can be placed in **community residences (or "group homes")** with 5 to 10 adolescents with emotional and behavioral problems living with 24-hour per day supervision by paid staff in a homelike setting, or **residential treatment centers** with an array of paid, multidisciplinary staff. These centers care for larger numbers of children (typically from 20 to 100 youth) in an institutional setting. Some programs focus on special populations (e.g., youth with sexual offending behaviors). The costs for these higher levels of services can range from $40,000 to $100,000 per year per child. Placement can be on a voluntary basis at the request of the parent, an involuntary removal by CPS, or a placement ordered by the family or juvenile court, based on the problem behavior of the youth. All types of placement must be brought before the juvenile or family court for approval. The court continues to have supervisory oversight throughout the life of the case until the child is retuned home or adopted. For older teens who will be going on to live independently after they leave foster care, the foster care system is required to prepare these youth for living on their own by providing **independent living services** until they are 21 years of age. For example, these youth may be offered case management, vocational readiness services, counseling, home and money management, and supervised housing.

E.   **Safety and permanency.** When a child is placed in out-of-home care, actual legal "custody" (or "guardianship," depending on the state's legal language) of the child is temporarily transferred to the social services department. Federal and state laws have been recently strengthened through the enactment of the **Adoption and Safe Families Act of 1997.** This Act calls for child safety and the establishment of caretaking continuity to be the paramount concern for all foster children. The law is clear that the social service system is to strive, from the first day the child is removed from their home, to ensure the best **permanent** home for this child. A formal review must take place after 6 months of placement, and a permanency plan established by 12 months. Unless reasons compel otherwise, the expectation is to either achieve reunification of the child with the family **within 15 months** or to begin the court process to terminate the rights of the parents on a permanent basis.

F. **Healthcare for foster children.** Children in foster care are at high risk for "falling through the cracks" and receiving inadequate pediatric care. Furthermore, these children have higher rates of serious emotional and behavioral problems, chronic physical disabilities, birth defects, developmental delays, and poor school achievement than children in the general population.

The American Academy of Pediatrics has published a **Policy Statement on Health Care of Children in Foster Care** that outlines standards for healthcare services, including:

1. Initial health screening before or soon after entering foster care
2. Comprehensive health assessment within 1 month of placement
3. Developmental mental health evaluation within 1 month of placement
4. Coordination with child welfare workers to assure treatment needs are met
5. Monitoring of children's health and mental health status at least twice per year in first year of placement, yearly thereafter

Understanding the child's comprehensive needs at the earliest possible time is also integral to determining whether the parent can learn to meet the child's needs and carry through with treatment within the new, pressing 15-month time frame dictated by the Adoption and Safe Families Act.

G. **Adoption and kinship guardianship.** When a foster child cannot be safely returned home, sufficient legal grounds may exist to permanently terminate the legal rights of the parents, thus freeing the child to be adopted. Two major routes exist to termination of parental rights: **voluntary surrender** of their rights by the parents or an **involuntary termination** when the child welfare agency successfully proves in the juvenile or family court that the rights of the parents should be permanently ended (see Chapter 9). The grounds for the involuntary termination of rights differ from state to state, but basically the social service agency must prove:

1.   Serious (and usually repeated) maltreatment, failure to meet the minimal basic needs of the child, or abandonment
2.   "Diligent" effort was made to provide each parent ample opportunity to participate in services that would remediate the original shortcomings in the parenting behavior
3.   The parent(s) did not or cannot make the needed changes to provide a safe home.

For example, a parent having a major mental illness or mild mental retardation does not create sufficient grounds for the parent to lose their rights. The parent would have had to fail repeatedly and consistently to demonstrate an ability to meet the needs of the child adequately, despite being offered opportunities to remediate the problems.

Once parental rights have been terminated (and only at that point), the child is eligible to be adopted. Parents who have been certified as an adoptive home can adopt them. Most children who have been in the foster care system, once freed for adoption, are adopted by their foster parents (national estimate of 75% to 85%). If an adoptive child is determined to be "hard to place" (i.e., children with emotional, behavioral, medical problems, are older, in sibling groups, minorities), the adoptive parents are eligible for the **federal adoption subsidy program.** The amount of this subsidy is often similar to what the foster family was receiving in foster care payments. Medicaid will also cover the child until 18 years of age (21 if handicapped) unless the child is not eligible for this federal program based on the birth parents' income level. Many states have state medical coverage programs to supplement those children not covered by the federal subsidy.

III.   **Income support programs.** Federal and state financed and regulated income support programs provide benefits based on income and other resources available to the child, family, or both. The amounts of the benefits vary greatly from state to state, and usually are adjusted for family size and current household income and resources. Programs include:

A.   **Temporary assistance for needy families (TANF).** This program, known as Aid to Families with Dependent Children before welfare reform or as "cash welfare," came into being with the 1996 **Personal**

Responsibility and Work Opportunity Reconciliation Act (PRWORA, also known as "welfare reform"). Only adults who live with dependent children are eligible for this aid, which provides money for (at a minimum) shelter and utility costs, clothing, and personal needs. If a family is eligible to receive TANF, it is usually also eligible to receive food stamps and Medicaid.

The new law created an expectation that welfare would be temporary, and that all clients receiving welfare prepare and accept paid employment at the earliest point possible. A 5-year lifetime limit exists for federal benefits (**Temporary** Assistance for Needy Families) for any adult and the covered family members. Many are wondering what will become of the children in these families should their parents lose TANF money. Each state is responding differently to this dilemma and the situation is evolving rapidly.

B. **Food stamps.** The funds can only be used for food (i.e., not for toiletries, clothing, liquor, and so on). In addition to those receiving TANF, families and individuals eligible to receive food stamps can be working, retired, or on disability.

C. **Home energy assistance**

D. **Childcare subsidy**

E. **Child support enforcement assistance** is available to any custodial parent without regard to income level.

F. **General assistance,** also known as Home Relief, Safety Net Assistance Program, and so on, grants cash support for people who are not part of a family and, therefore, not eligible for TANF. Many states abolished this non-federally funded program over the last several years, but some states have established partial support programs since federal welfare reform.

G. **Supplemental security income (SSI)** is the federally funded income support program for the **elderly and for disabled adults and children,** who meet specified financial need criteria. Children are deemed disabled and eligible for this category of income support if they meet all three of the following:

1. Medically determined physical or mental disorder
2. The condition has lasted or is expected to last at least 12 months or will result in death
3. The condition results in marked and severe limitation of functioning.

It is important to recognize that children who are disabled are **also eligible to receive Medicaid.** To apply for or gain further information about eligibility for this program contact the local office of the Social

Security Administration or call its toll free telephone number: 800-772-1213. Parents may wish to consult an attorney specializing in disability and SSI to obtain guidance about their child's eligibility.

IV. **Healthcare programs**

A. **Medicaid (may have a state name such as Medi-Cal in California).** This is the medical insurance program for low-income; disabled persons (adults or children); foster children; or persons with high enough recurring medical expenses that their income and other medical insurance does not cover all their costs. Covered services and reimbursement rates for these specified services are set by each state and vary widely.

B. **Medicaid waiver programs.** The federal government has approved Medicaid funding for a number of special medical and behavioral health programs for children by agreeing to waive usual Medicaid rules and allow payment for such services. A state petitions the Centers for Medicare and Medicaid Services (previously known as the Health Care Financing Administration) to pay for "waivered" services that are aimed at filling a gap in the service delivery system in a community. States are actively pursuing this avenue to support innovative programs. One example is the Care at Home Program for Physically Disabled Children in New York state where children who otherwise would need to be institutionalized can be cared for at home with home-based healthcare and home modifications.

C. **State Children's Health Insurance Program (SCHIP).** This federal program provided by all states (known by various names), covers more than 3 million children nationally who would otherwise not be covered. Typically, these children are in families that earn too much to be eligible for Medicaid but do not have private insurance.

D. **Medicare** provides health insurance for a very small number of children. It is the federal health insurance program intended to provide coverage for:
   1. Most **adults over 65 years of age**
   2. **Adults** who receive **Social Security disability** income for more than 24 months
   3. Any individual (including children) with **chronic renal disease** who requires dialysis or transplantation

   Medicare is not administered by a local or state social services agency but instead by the Social Security Administration. For more information, contact the local office of the Social Security Administration or call 1-800-772-1213.

E. **Early intervention program for infants and toddlers with disabilities.** Every state must provide early intervention services to both family and child from birth to 3 years of age when the child has a developmental delay or a diagnosed physical or mental condition that has a high probability of resulting in a delay. At its discretion, the state can serve children deemed to be **at risk** of developmental delay. The services covered can include comprehensive evaluation, parent training, counseling and home visits, special instruction in the care of the child, speech-language therapy, audiology, vision services, social work, occupational and physical therapy, psychological services, nursing, nutrition, transportation and related costs, and assistive technology devices and services.

V. **Summary.** The social services system oversees a large, broad, and multifaceted set of programs that are intimately involved in the daily lives of children and families. Because of the complexity of the organization of these services, it is difficult for the PCP to develop an overarching understanding of them. Knowledge of the array of services, how they operate and are funded, and how to access them is critical to the optimal health and mental health care of pediatric patents. It is also central to PCP's ability to advocate for improvements for children at the broader public (i.e., governmental) level.

SUGGESTED READINGS

American Academy of Pediatrics Policy Statement. Health care of children in foster care. *Pediatrics* 1994;93(2):335–338.

American Academy of Pediatrics Policy Statement. Identification and care of HIV-exposed and HIV-infected infants, children, and adolescents in foster care. *Pediatrics* 2000;106(01):149–153.

Simms M, Dubowitz H, Szilagyi MA. Health care needs of children in the foster care system. *Pediatrics* 2000;106(suppl. 4):909–918.

Szilagyi M. The pediatrician and the foster child. *Pediatr Rev* 1999; 19:39–50.

Web Sites

Adoption and Foster Care Analysis and Reporting System. A national data system under the auspices of the Children's Bureau. Available at www.acf.dhhs.gov/programs/cb/dis/afcars/index.html. Accessed on 6/25/02.

Children's Bureau, under the auspices of the US Department of Health and Human Services, is the overarching federal division involved in child welfare services. Available at www.acf.dhhs.gov/programs/cb/index.htm. Accessed on 6/25/02.

Centers for Medicare and Medicaid Services (previously known as the Health Care Financing Agency or HCFA) oversee Medicare, Medicaid, and the state children's health insurance programs (SCHIP). Available at www.hcfa.gov. Accessed on 6/25/02.

National Child Abuse and Neglect Data System Report 1999. Federal government agency that tracks most recent statistics. Available at www.acf.dhhs.gov/programs/cb/publications/cm99/index.htm. Accessed on 6/25/02.

National Clearinghouse on Child Abuse and Neglect Information, a general informational section of the Children's Bureau. Available at www.calib.com/nccanch/. Accessed on 6/25/02.

Office of Family Assistance, the branch of the federal Department of Health and Human Services that oversees TANF and PRWORA. Available at www.acf.dhhs.gov/programs/ofa. Accessed on 6/25/02.

Social Security Administration, which oversees the Supplemental Security Income (SSI) program. Available at www.ssa.gov. Accessed on 6/25/02.

9 ♣ The Legal System

Susan Vinocour and Paul D. Pearson

I. **Introduction.** This chapter provides a basic orientation to legal issues that can affect children, their families, and their relationship with their physician. Many aspects of family life are legally regulated, including marriage and divorce, child custody, adoption, protection from abuse or neglect, domestic violence, access to medical care and to education, and even some aspects of child behavior. Legal involvement can be stressful for families, children, and physicians. It often involves disruption or challenges to the organization of the family, and it can require additional role flexibility and support for the family on the part of physicians. The stresses and transitions that occur when a family is embroiled in court action require a primary physician to be honest, communicate clearly, and be emotionally supportive, even when engaging in behaviors the family may view as unwelcome (e.g., reporting suspected abuse or advocating for medical care against parental wishes).

This chapter addresses questions such as who has the legal right to make medical decisions for a child or to see a child's confidential medical records, what are your responsibilities as a physician if you suspect a child is being abused, what if parents will not give consent for a life-saving medical procedure for a child, who speaks for the child in court, and how can the court respond to a child who is out of control or refusing to attend school.

II. **Who is a "child"?** For legal purposes, a child is a person under the age of majority (18 or 21 years of age, depending on the state). The exceptions are adolescents who have:

A. Formally been **emancipated** by the court (declared to legally be an "adult," usually by virtue of the fact of their living independently from their parents or legal guardians, and being self-supporting)

B. Legally **married,** which confers adult legal status.

C. A person under the age of majority who has a child is regarded as a legal adult in so far as the relationship with the child is concerned. This means that a person under the age of 18 can consent to medical care for his or her own child.

III. **The court system.** It first would be useful to provide a basic orientation to the structure of the legal system, which can be confusing for physician and family alike. No one single court exists, but rather a variety of different courts and levels of courts. Each separate kind of court has its own specific jurisdiction and hears only certain kinds of cases.

For example, a designated **civil court,** which has different names in different states (e.g., Circuit Court, Supreme Court, Superior Court, Probate Court, or County Court), generally hears cases involved in divorce and custody, malpractice, personal injury, disputes about contracts and property, educational cases, psychiatric commitment proceedings, and the like. Criminal trials are held in **criminal court.** In many states a specialized **family court** was developed to handle issues relating to children and families and hear cases involving family support, abuse, and neglect; delinquency and incorrigibility; abandonment; foster care; termination of parental rights; adoption; and some types of family violence or requests for Orders of Protection. Some kinds of custody matters are also heard in family court. These include decisions about custody of children whose parents are unmarried, as well as cases seeking a change of the original custody decision, based on a significant change of circumstances. A variety of **specialty courts** hear only very narrow issues (e.g., Bankruptcy Court, Small Claims Court, and Surrogate's Court). In some jurisdictions, courts are now emerging that are specific to drug cases and domestic violence. Some people voluntarily agree to settle disputes through **arbitration and mediation,** rather than through the court system. Mediation can include all issues concerning children in the context of divorce.

Some court decisions can be reviewed by an **appellate court.** Appellate courts do not have witnesses appear and do not have juries. They merely review the legal record of a case to determine the existence of any procedural and legal defects in the original trial.

IV. **Representation of children in court.**

A. **Two types of representation.** The law recognizes that parents cannot always speak for their children in court, because the parents' wishes may be at odds with the child's needs or wishes. Therefore, children have their own spokesperson in court. The court appoints these people; parents do not hire them, so they can remain independent of parental pressure. Two types of legal representatives are seen for children in matters brought before the courts: **law guardians** and **guardians *ad litem*** **(GAL).** Law guardians are persons designated to represent a child in a family court matter or in a custody or visitation matter. In many states, but not all, law guardians are attorneys who specialize in representing children. GAL are appointed by the judge to investigate and recommend on behalf of a child who is not legally competent to act for him or her self because of infancy, intellectual impairment, or psychiatric disability, and whose parent cannot serve as an appropriate advocate for some reason. In most states, any person more than 18 years of age, or any parent (even if younger than 18) can serve as a guardian *ad litem.* No particular qualifications are required. Sophistication about child development, family interaction, psychopathology, and medical issues varies widely among these representatives.

B. **Tasks of the representative.** The fundamental task of a **law guardian** is to give a child his or her own voice in court, not to form an independent opinion about the best interests of the child and then advocate that position. The law guardian does not represent the opinions or positions of the parents or other adults. However, with very young children, law guardians can advocate their own opinions about what appears to be in the best interest of the child, instead of simply voicing the child's views, because the child is unable to come to a reasoned decision. In contrast, a **GAL** speaks on behalf of the child, representing the child's best interests, much as a parent might do.

Client advocacy by a law guardian often involves bringing important evidence to the court's attention, maintaining procedural safeguards (due process), raising relevant questions of law, and obtaining the assistance of experts in helping the court determine what is in the best interests of the child. Part of the job is to create a legal record that will clarify the child's needs and rights and the reasons for the court's decisions. Law guardians often petition the court to appoint a mental health expert to examine the child, parents, or both if psychological data are relevant to the child's position or best interests. They might also interview healthcare and education professionals who have contact with a child and they can review associated records. To view otherwise confidential records (e.g., medical records), they need either a signed consent (by the custodial parent or legal guardian) or a court order. The child's communications with his or her law guardian or GAL are confidential, protected by attorney-client privilege.

V. **Family court** is specifically designed to **address issues related to children and families.** Matters heard in family court include family support, allegations of child abuse and neglect, delinquency and incorrigibility, chronic school truancy, foster care, termination of parental rights, and adoption. Predivorce issues related to child custody and visitation are generally heard in civil courts, as are some issues related to domestic violence. Postdivorce custody and visitation issues are frequently heard in family court. Family court focuses is on keeping the family together, fixing problems, ensuring child safety, and rehabilitating delinquent or defiant youth, rather than on punishment. It is not a criminal court.

Jurisdiction may overlap with other courts, so that one aspect of an issue is decided in family court, whereas another aspect is separately addressed in a different court on a different time line. This can be confusing and stressful for families, as the courts are not well integrated. Some child issues (e.g., the right to a public and least restrictive education for disabled children) are not within the purview of family court, but are decided in the same court that hears general civil cases. Children involved in family court proceedings have law guardians appointed to represent them and speak for them in court. If the parents are charged (e.g., as in neglect or abuse proceedings), they will also be represented by attorneys. There are no juries in family court, but the court does call witnesses and take sworn testimony.

Family court has broad powers to place children out of the home (in foster care or detention facilities), terminate parental rights, finalize adoption, order counseling, modify terms of custody and visitation, designate who can occupy the family residence, and create or modify family support. However, it has **no direct authority over parents** when children are found to be delinquent, truant, or incorrigible; it only has authority over the youth in question. Its authority generally ends when the child reaches 18 years of age. The court has a limited ability to monitor compliance with its orders after a hearing. Another frustration for families can be the long waiting periods that often occur before a case is brought to completion. Although cases involving abuse and neglect, delinquency, and incorrigible behavior are generally addressed within a few months, cases requesting modification of custody orders can last 6 months to a year, or more, in some jurisdictions.

VI. **Divorce and separation**

    A. **Divorce.** Parental separation and divorce are major events in the life of a child, causing significant changes in the family, often affecting how much access a child has to each parent and the ability to maintain a strong, positive emotional connection to each parent. Divorce (or "dissolution of marriage") terminates marriage, and can alter the parents' relationships with their children, as well as with each other. The major issues in divorce relate to division of marital property, spousal and child support, and legal custody, residence, and time-sharing of any minor children. Usually also included are issues of insurance or payment for healthcare expenses, life insurance, and future education payments for children who are not yet legally adults and are still dependent on their parents.

        In some states, the traditional language of "custody" and "visitation" is giving way to the language of **parenting plans.** After divorce, each parent's rights and responsibilities toward any children must be formally spelled out, either in the form of an **agreement,** accepted by the parties and ratified by the court, or an **order** made by the court after the parties have litigated the issues. Divorce proceedings can be completed within a matter of months if the parents are able to reach an agreement without litigation. However, if the issues are contested and they cannot agree, the court will hear testimony to what is in the **best interests of the child** and make the final decision. This process typically drags on for 1 to 3 years, and is costly and stressful.

Previously, a legal presumption existed that mothers were better parents than fathers and should generally have preference in custody of the children, unless shown to be "unfit." That presumption is no longer part of the law, and mothers and fathers are now to be given equal consideration on their own merits, without regard to gender. Similarly, the laws of most states recognize that a parent's sexual orientation should not be a barrier to custody. In many states, judges are directed to at least take into consideration the expressed wishes of the child with regard to custody, where the child is 12 years of age or older. However, judges have much freedom in making custody determinations, and are not required to decide based on any one factor, including the child's wishes.

An important distinction is made between legal versus physical custody. **Legal custody** refers to the person(s) who has the right to make major decisions regarding the child (typically related to medical, educational, and religious issues). Legal custody may be "sole" or "joint" (sometimes referred to as "shared"). In sole custody, one parent has the unilateral right to make major life decisions affecting the child; in joint custody, both parents have the legal right to participate in decision-making. For joint custody to succeed and be a benefit to the child, the parents must be able to work cooperatively with each other regarding parenting decisions and tasks. They must be able to communicate effectively, to focus on the child's needs rather than their own disappointments or anger about their breakup, and to support the child in having a positive relationship with each other. Joint, or shared, custody is rarely granted in cases of a high degree of conflict between the parents. Where conflict is high and cooperation and communication are low, the court generally awards **sole** custody to one parent, putting that parent solely in charge of the child legally.

Physical custody merely describes where the child is physically situated, and has no bearing on the legal authority to make decisions about the child. A parenting plan should spell out the schedule of responsibilities, so that the parents and the children have clear expectations and understandings. Days regularly in each parent's responsibility; times of pickups and drop-offs, how these should occur; holiday schedules; and how information (e.g., school, medical) will be exchanged are usually written into the divorce agreement or order. Physical custody can take a variety of forms. For example, a father could have sole legal custody of the child, and also provide the child's primary residence. However, the mother might have visitation with the child in her home at times. During those visits, she has physical custody of the child, but this does not confer the legal right, for example, to authorize nonemergency medical care.

Unless otherwise stated in the divorce decree, a parent who is awarded sole, joint, or shared legal custody has authority to **consent to healthcare** treatment for his or her child following a divorce. That parent also has the right to see the child's medical records and to consent to release of the records to others. A parent who does not have **legal** custody cannot authorize medical or mental health care for the child or have access to the child's confidential records, without consent of the custodial parent. Having **physical** custody of the child does not give the parent the right to control decisions for the child; only a parent with **legal** custody has that right. In **sole** custody, the decisions are controlled **solely** by that one parent, who does not need the consent or knowledge of the other parent.

A child's physician must have the consent of the parent with legal custody before providing medical care. The terms of custody are set forth clearly in the divorce decree or order, using the words "sole," "joint," or "shared" legal custody. The decree often specifies which parent has the deciding vote on matters such as medical care, when parents with joint custody cannot reach agreement. The safest course of action, when in doubt, is to ask the parent to provide a copy of the custody portion of the order for your records. An exception in the case is a potentially life-threatening medical emergency, where preliminary care to preserve life can be provided without the consent of any parent and regardless of custody. Where parents have "joint legal custody," either one, individually, generally has the right to authorize care for the child, without the specific knowledge or permission of the other parent. However, it is generally good practice for the physician to obtain the support and agreement of both parents for medical care, where possible. This is especially true in situations involving the prescription of psychotropic agents, which are typically given for extended periods of time. In cases of routine pediatric care (e.g., prescription of an antibiotic), it is generally not necessary to obtain the consent of both parents.

Because many parents are distrustful of each other after divorce, some pediatricians have found that it helps increase medical compliance and cooperation if they communicate directly with each parent about diagnoses and treatment recommendations, rather than having one parent be the messenger to the other. In some cases, this can be accomplished with a simple post card. Other practitioners have an informational letter explaining how they will communicate with divorced parents that they give when new patients join the practice. This can help to clarify what the parents are expected to do and what the primary care physician (PCP) will do.

Judges have much latitude in designing **parenting plans** and making orders regarding custody, residence, and visitation. For example, physical custody could be as little as an hour a week, supervised by a third party, or as much as 50–50, alternating weeks, with each parent. A common arrangement is for the nonresidential parent to have the child alternate weekends and 1 or 2 evenings during the week. An attempt is made to tailor the parenting plan to the needs and vulnerabilities of the specific child, on a case-by-case basis, taking into account parent and child characteristics. No one kind of plan or arrangement is "best" for all children and families. Judges often rely on mental health experts to evaluate all the parties and make recommendations.

Studies have shown that **children's emotional adjustment** can be harmed by divorce and break-up of the family. Divorce has negative effects on even very young children. School-aged, and often older, children frequently believe they are to blame for the failure of the marriage. Especially following the actual separation (i.e., moving out of one parent) it is common to see signs of regressive, immature behaviors (e.g., enuresis), an increase in vague somatic complaints, mood symptoms (anger, anxiety, irritability, depression), behavior symptoms, and deterioration in school performance and attendance. These **symptoms generally peak in the first few months, but acute turmoil continues usually for around 2 years.** After this time, the general level of tumult has settled, although the damaging effects on the children often last for many years. Factors associated with child outcome are summarized in Table 9.1.

Table 9.1. Factors associated with child adjustment or outcome following divorce

Poor Outcome	Good Outcome
High degree of overt conflict after divorce	Parents able to cooperate in parenting Low conflict after divorce
Children triangulated and pressured to "take sides"	Maintenance of familiar routines and rules (e.g., stability of school, friends, and predictability of schedules)
No emotionally supportive adult figure	Positive relationship with both parents

Individual or couples work with a mental health professional can often help parents set aside their rancor and focus on creating two healthy homes for their child. Situations exist in which parents are unable to talk productively with each other. In these situations efforts to provide "marital counseling" or mediation for the couple is often fruitless; instead individual therapy, which is usually helpful, should be encouraged for the motivated parent. A clearly written parenting plan that minimizes opportunities for arguments and conflict is also essential in these cases.

Whether a party is entitled to be divorced depends on whether there are legal **"grounds"** (e.g., infidelity, spousal abuse, abandonment) for divorce under the laws of the state where the person seeking the divorce is a resident. Most states no longer require "marital fault" to be alleged, but allow **"no fault"** divorce in cases of irreconcilable differences, an irretrievable breakdown of the marriage, or the parties have been living separate and apart for 1 to 2 years. New York state is a notable exception, still requiring "fault" grounds unless a written, comprehensive settlement agreement has been in effect in excess of 1 year.

B. **Temporary orders.** In any divorce, separation, or family abuse action, temporary orders generally are available through the court to stabilize and protect adults and children in the initial stages of separating from each other. Such temporary orders can include the following:
  - Child support
  - Spousal support (alimony or maintenance)
  - Child custody, visitation, or access
  - Occupancy of the marital residence

- Uses of or freezes on marital assets and liabilities (including possible payment of initial counsel fees)
- Payment of existing or specified future bills (especially for healthcare)
- Orders of protection (see next section) to prevent harassment, threats, stalking, physical abuse, or communication between the parties or with children
- Appointment of a law guardian or attorney for minor children

Temporary orders can be an extremely effective tool at the outset of a domestic relations action. They are often the first "reality" experience the parties have with what can be reasonably expected from the legal system in their particular situation. Increasingly, states are implementing automatic temporary orders at the initiation of a domestic relations action (divorce, separation, custody) to maintain the financial, residential, and custodial status quo, until changed by agreement or later court order.

C. **Legal separation.** Most states provide for a process of formal legal separation for married persons who wish to live apart but do not wish to be divorced. The court can approve a formal, written settlement agreement between the parties that provides for terms of custody, visitation or access, healthcare, and family support in a manner similar to a divorce decree. If the parents later divorce, the terms of this parenting plan might be incorporated by reference into a divorce judgment or decree. However, a legal separation generally does not, unless the parties mutually agree, provide for a division or distribution of marital property.

Legal separation generally is considered by the parties only in cases wherein is seen a reluctance to proceed with divorce because of overriding religious objections, therapy is being attempted, reconciliation is hoped for, or one spouse does not want to subject the marital assets to division by court order and the other party does not have "grounds" (or does not wish) to compel a divorce.

VII. **Protection from abuse, threats, or harassment**

A. **Orders of protection.** Most states now have a court process that can be quickly and easily accessed, without the need of a lawyer, to protect adults or children from physical or mental abuse or threats and harassment from a cohabitant, whether a legal relative or not. Typically, such court orders can be obtained temporarily on an emergency basis just by the application of one party. This gives **immediate protection** to those allegedly subject to the abuse, with an opportunity for both parties to be heard within 1 or 2 days thereafter. The alleged abuser often is ordered to stay away from, vacate the home of, and desist from touching, threatening, stalking, harassing, or communicating with specifically named relatives or members of the household.

Local law enforcement authorities are often charged with informing alleged victims of their rights to obtain such orders or protection from either a family or divorce court or from a local municipal civil court. This is often done without notice initially to the defendant or alleged perpetrator. Many prosecutors (district attorneys) now have a policy of refusing to dismiss any criminal charges arising from domestic abuse calls to police, even at the request of the complainant, so prosecutions increasingly are proceeding based on the initial police report and complaint. This tends to eliminate the earlier experience of a victim seeking law enforcement protection or court protective or restraining orders, and then later seeking to have them dismissed on resumption of a relationship with the alleged perpetrator, only to start the cycle again before long.

B.   Restraining orders are also available, directing the respondent to refrain from certain specified actions involving particular persons or property. They are similar to orders of protection, but can be broader in scope and apply to even those who are not cohabitants. Temporary orders are also an option in these situations. Temporary orders can stabilize an entire family crisis in its early states. Orders of protection, to prevent physical or emotional trauma, often can be initiated through local law enforcement agencies or local (municipal) courts. Adults with a family crisis that requires legal intervention should be referred to a qualified attorney with experience in family or matrimonial law; in an emergency situation, the patient **should be referred directly to local law enforcement or to the local family or municipal court** for immediate relief.

VIII.   Child abuse and neglect. Provisions in the law provide protection for children who are being abused or neglected by their parents or other persons legally responsible for their care. A special case of neglect involves parental refusal, generally on religious grounds, to permit a medical procedure necessary to save a child's life. Courts can supersede parental authority and order care over parental objection, in appropriate cases, after a hearing. Physicians, nurses, and many other categories of professionals who come in contact with children are **legally mandated to report situations in which they have reasonable**

**cause to suspect that a child is being physically, sex-
ually, or emotionally abused** by a person responsible
for his or her care, or is being severely neglected. The
physician does not have to be able to prove abuse or neglect
is occurring; reasonable suspicion is enough to trigger the
requirement to report. An investigating agency exists
whose job it is to determine whether a foundation for the
suspicion is present (see Chapter 8).

A. **Mandated reporting of suspected abuse and
    neglect.** Abuse is defined to include significant phys-
    ical abuse, sexual abuse, or emotional abuse. Neglect
    includes a parent's failure to provide adequate basic
    necessities (e.g., food, shelter, and safety) as well as
    necessary medical or mental health care or education.
    The protection of the law generally applies to chil-
    dren up to 18 years of age. The abusive or neglectful
    acts must be by a parent or person in the role of par-
    ent. Assault or abuse by some other person would
    come under criminal law, and not be a child protec-
    tive matter, in most states. However, a parent who
    knows the child is being abused and fails to act to
    protect the child may be found to have neglected the
    child, even if that person had not behaved abusively
    toward the child personally. Because definitions
    and procedures differ from state to state, physicians
    should become familiar with the laws in their own
    particular state.

B. **Role of the physician.** Most states have laws re-
    quiring physicians and nurses, among others, to
    quickly notify a designated agency in cases where
    they have reasonable cause to suspect that a child
    is being abused. Many states also have laws that
    allow a physician to hold a child in emergency cus-
    tody, without parental consent, until police or child
    protective workers arrive, if the physician believes
    that the child would be at significant immediate
    risk if released to the parents. In some cases, physi-
    cians are also required to document visible injuries
    with photographs.

      If a physician reports in good faith, he or she will not
    be held liable for a report that is later not substanti-
    ated. Failure to report when required to do so is a mis-
    demeanor in most states, punishable by a fine. In addi-
    tion, failure to report can expose the physician to civil
    liability for damages if the child receives further
    injuries at the hands of the person in the parental role
    after the doctor should have reported but failed to do
    so. Note that, although medical records are generally
    confidential and cannot be disclosed without parental
    consent, the required reporting of possible abuse is an
    exception to confidentiality. It is a special challenge for

the medical professional that makes such a required report to speak to the family honestly and supportively about the need for the report.

C. **Possible outcomes.** A designated state agency investigates reports, and has the ability to bring the parents to family court by filing a petition of abuse or neglect against them when necessary to protect the child adequately. In some cases, the court can order a child removed from parental custody. In other cases, the protective agency can elect to provide services (e.g., counseling) on a voluntary basis to the family. Courts can also authorize needed medical or mental health care, against parental wishes. This requires sensitivity and care on the part of the physician, who is trying to maintain a working relationship with parents that can survive the immediate crisis of unwelcome legal intervention.

IX. **Guardianship, foster care, and adoption**
A. **Guardianship.** Parents, with court approval, can formally, legally designate another person—such as a relative or family friend—to be the legal guardian for their child. The guardian **functions as a parent,** with the same rights and parental responsibilities as a parent, as long as the guardianship is in effect. The guardian can give permission for medical care and make other decisions for the child that a parent ordinarily would make. The guardianship lasts as long as the parent wishes; it ends when the parent revokes it or when the child attains the age of majority (18 or 21 years of age, depending on the state). Typically, such a legal guardianship requires filing the designation document with the court. A guardian should be able to show the PCP a copy of the document appointing him or her. Parents often designate a guardian for their child when they are temporarily unable to parent because of illness or absence.

However, many "guardianships" are only informal, where a parent leaves a child temporarily in someone else's care. Informal guardianship, not approved by a court, does not confer legal authority on the guardian. In such cases, the guardian or caretaker can only authorize medical care for the child with a note, signed and dated by the parent, specifically allowing him or her to do so. These informal arrangements really do not provide adequately for the child, because the legal parent is absent and the informal caretaker does not have adequate legal authority to secure needed care for the child. Summer camp is one example of informal guardianship. Leaving a child with a stepparent, sibling, or extended family member is another.

B. Foster care. Children can be placed in foster care in a state-licensed home if the court feels it is necessary because of ongoing neglect, abuse, or parental abandonment, or if the parent–child relationship has broken down significantly and the parent is unable or unwilling to keep the child safely at home. Sometimes this is done with the parent's consent, but sometimes it occurs against parental wishes, as in cases wherein the court determines parental abuse or neglect. The **state has legal custody of a child in foster care,** and the Department of Social Services (DSS) (or commensurate agency) has the legal authority for making decisions authorizing any medical care when a child is in foster care; the Department's authority supersedes the parents' authority. The court periodically reviews foster care placements. However, children can be transferred from one foster home to another by the placement agency without court review or parental consent. Length of stay in foster care varies widely, but is changing because of the recent Adoption and Safe Families Act (Chapter 8).

Children in foster care usually have visitation with parents, and sometimes siblings. Foster care can lead to disruptions in medical care, as the agency or foster family may take the child to a different doctor while the child is in foster care. Although most foster homes provide well for children, they also vary widely in terms of quality of care and safety. Abuse occurring in foster care is not unheard of and is something to which the physician should be alert. Although parents can have positive feelings about a foster care placement, this is not always the case and tension may exist between parents and foster parents, which require extra flexibility and sensitivity on the physician's part. Children generally return to their parents after a period of placement, so the physician should attempt to maintain a positive relationship with the parents.

C. Adoption is a judicial process that creates a new, legal parent–child relationship where none existed before, while terminating any prior relationship between that child and any other parent. Adoption can be arranged privately by parents on a voluntary basis (**"surrendering"**), or can be by intervention of a government official or agency (**"termination of parental rights"**). It can occur shortly after a child's birth or any time thereafter.

When biological or birth parents decide voluntarily to surrender a child for adoption, arrangements for the placement with the adoptive parents may be made personally, in many states through a lawyer, or through a licensed intermediary agency that assumes temporary custody of the child and then facilitates the adoption. In the first case, often one or both of the biological parents and the adoptive parents know and are in direct contact with each other (an **"open adoption"**); they can have a wide variety of agreements about how the child will be raised, what the child subsequently will be told about the biological or birth parents, and whether the biological parents will maintain any presence in the child's life after the adoption. However, in many private adoptions and in all agency adoptions, the parents typically are unknown to each other, and the biological parents do not maintain any contact with the child after the adoption. Many states have laws that prevent the child and biological parents from ever knowing each other's identity without mutual consent or court order, although states are increasingly allowing an adopted child access to important healthcare information about the birth parents. Some states also provide an "Adoption Registry" to allow a birth parent and an adult adopted child to be identified to each other if both consent and register.

The laws regarding voluntary surrendering of parental rights vary somewhat from state to state. In general, laws require that, even for a child born out of wedlock, **both** biological parents (if known) be notified and given an opportunity to object or agree to the surrender of the child for adoption. Generally, a waiting period of up to several months is then provided before the adoption is finalized to ensure that the adoptive parents are capable. Some states may allow the biological parents to change their minds during this period and reclaim the child, even after physical placement of the child with the adopting parents. However, in such cases, if proper legal procedures have been followed, it will be difficult for the biological parents to revoke their consent and the court may determine that the "best interests" of the child warrant leaving the child in the adoptive home. Once the waiting period has ended, the adoption is final and permanent and cannot be revoked, even if the birth parents later have a change of heart, unless technical or procedural flaws were found in the adoption.

All states and many foreign countries have laws strictly regulating the nature of the reimbursement or other "valuable consideration" that can be paid to biological parents by adoptive parents or their agents in connection with the adoption. Family physicians, who often hear of adults interested in adoption or children available for adoption, can initiate contacts

concerning adoption, either directly or through a professional or agency, but **without** receipt of anything
of value relating to the placement or the adoption
itself. This means that a physician should not accept
any payment in connection with a potential adoption.

Not all adoptions are with the consent of the biological parents. The court can also terminate parental
rights in cases where parents abandon (extended failure to maintain contact or support) a child or permanent neglect or abuse is found. The exact criteria differ from state to state, but the essential feature is
that a petition is brought to court, usually by the local
DSS, alleging neglect, abuse, or abandonment by parents. If, after a hearing, the court finds sufficient evidence to support the allegations, the child is generally placed in foster care, while efforts are made to
rehabilitate the parents or correct deficiencies in
their capacity to provide adequate and safe care. If
they do not cooperate or the situation does not substantially improve, a petition can be brought to terminate their parental rights permanently. If the
court determines no reasonable prospect exists that
the child can be safely returned to the parents within
a reasonable time, parental rights can then be terminated and the child is eligible for adoption. Since the
passage of the federal Adoption and Safe Families Act
of 1997, increasing effort is being made to decide expeditiously whether children are able to return to their
biological parents or to pursue termination of parental
rights. As a result, the numbers of termination of
parental rights cases are increasing dramatically.

It does sometimes occur that only one parent's rights
are terminated, whereas the other parent's rights
remain intact. Similarly, one parent can voluntarily
give up parental rights permanently, in favor of the
other parent. For example, a biological father who has
no relationship with the child could agree to give up
parental rights, allowing a stepparent to become the
adoptive, legal parent. This also ends any financial
obligations of the biological parent to the child.

D.   Special issues. Foster parents can apply to adopt a
child who has been with them. Although some states
give foster parents a preference for adoption, it is not
a foregone conclusion that the court will place a child
permanently with the former foster parents. Courts
consider a number of factors in approving adoptive
parents for a child, including race, ethnicity, sometimes religion, whether the child has an emotional
attachment to the people applying for adoption, and
the general ability of those individuals to provide an
adequate home for the child. Judges have much lati-

tude in deciding how heavily to weigh each of these factors if they do not all lead to the same conclusion. Special federal statutes favor placement of Native American children with Native American adoptive families. Adoptions by unmarried or single adults, regardless of their sexual orientation, are increasing throughout the United States.

Stepparents' status with respect to children can be complex legally. The stepparent has married one of the child's legal parents. However, the stepparent has not legally adopted the child and, therefore, is not the legal parent to the child. Accordingly, a stepparent does not inherently have authority to be involved in healthcare decisions or consents for the child. The exception to this would be the situation in which the stepparent has adopted the child. The prerequisite for this would be that the rights of one of the legal parents had been terminated or surrendered. As a practical matter, PCPs may have frequent contact with a stepparent, who is acting on behalf of the child by authorization (expressed or implied) from the legal parent. It is generally advisable for the physician to obtain the consent of the legal custodial parent to delegate this authority to the stepparent. The presence of the legal parent is generally required for decisions regarding the initiation of psychosocial or psychiatric treatments.

X.   **Juvenile delinquency, incorrigible behavior and school truancy.** Sometimes children behave in ways that violate the rights of others, fail to attend school as legally required, or are "out of control," not responding to parental authority, and engaging in risky self-destructive behaviors. All states have laws allowing a family court to exercise control over youth who violate the law, are out of parental control, or refuse to attend school.

The court's procedures, rules, and authority are the same, whether a child is before the court for oppositional behavior or school truancy, or for delinquent or criminal acts (e.g., rape, murder, or arson). In either case, youth are assigned a law guardian to represent them in answering the charges in court. The child can be either detained or released to parents, to someone the parent designates, or to foster care, pending the hearing on the charges. A hearing is held with witnesses, but no jury. Medical and mental health records are often subpoenaed for such court hearings.

Those who commit what would be criminal acts if done by an adult are classified as **juvenile delinquents.** Family court generally handles delinquency charges against youth. This is based on the belief that young people, in their formative years, should be rehabilitated, rather than merely punished, and that they should not be held to the same standard as adults because they are not yet cognitively or psychologically mature. However, in some states, those as young as 13 years can be charged as **youthful offenders** if they are believed to have committed certain very serious crimes (e.g., murder). In such cases, they are tried in criminal court, rather than in family court, and sentenced as adults, if convicted.

Those who commit **"status offenses"** (acts that are only illegal for those with the status of being a juvenile) are often designated as **persons or children in need of supervision (PINS or CHINS)**. Status offenses include school truancy and "incorrigible" or "ungovernable" behaviors such as leaving home without permission, or refusing to submit to reasonable parental authority. In some states, a gap of several years (i.e., 16 to 18 years of age) exists during which parents are still legally and financially responsible for their child wherein the child can no longer be legally forced to attend school or comply with parental rules or remain at home. In this gap, parents do not have the leverage of charging the child with a status offense and getting the court's assistance in securing youth compliance with parental demands. This can be a frustrating, stressful time for parents.

If, after a hearing, the court determines that the child has violated the criminal laws, missed school illegally, or defied reasonable parental authority, it has the authority to order supervision (typically by a probation officer), psychotherapy, curfews, school attendance, foster care, or placement outside the home (including secure or nonsecure detention facility, foster care, and residential treatment programs). The court has the same power over a child who fails to attend school or follow parental rules as it has over children who commit criminal acts (e.g., armed robbery or murder). However, the **court has no direct authority to order the parents to do anything.** Its authority is only over the child in these cases, even if parental behavior is part of the problem. For example, parental substance abuse might be causing the child to act out, but the court cannot force the parents to become involved in substance abuse treatment.

XI. **Summary.** Many aspects of family life—relationships between parents and their children, and the welfare, education, and behavior of children—are legally regulated. Although family courts have been created specifically to address child and family issues, a number of other courts can also play a role at times.

In some cases, the court works to support parental authority over children who are engaging in inappropriate behaviors (PINS, CHINS, delinquency cases). In some cases, the courts intervene protectively on behalf of children whose parents are behaving inappropriately (abuse and neglect hearings, orders of protection, foster care placement, emancipation). The courts also redefine family relationships (divorce and custody, guardianship), sever old ones (termination of parental rights), and create new ones (adoption).

Many of these issues can have an impact on the child's mental health, as legal intervention in the life of a family is often a time of stress or crisis. Knowing what is going on with a family legally, as well as knowing how to access the legal system on behalf of a child, can assist the physician in identifying and meeting the needs of youthful patients and their families.

SUGGESTED READINGS

Ayoub C, Deutsch, R Maraganore A. Emotional distress in children of high-conflict divorce: the impact of marital conflict and violence. *Family and Conciliation Courts Review* 1999;37(3):297–314.

Galatzer-Levy R, Kraus L, et al., eds. *The scientific basis of child custody decisions.* New York: John Wiley & Sons, 1999:468.

Hetherington EM, Bridges M, Insabella GM. What matters? What does not? Five perspectives on the association between marital transitions and children's adjustment. *Am Psychol* 1998;53(2):167–184.

Journal of Mental Health and Aging 2000:6(4). Entire volume is devoted to issues of custodial grandparents.

Kelly J, Lamb M. Using child developmental research to make appropriate custody and access decisions for young children. *Family and Conciliation Courts Review* 2000;38(3):297–311.

Lamb M, Sternberg K, Thompson R. The effects of divorce and custody arrangements on children's behavior, development and adjustment. In: Lamb M, ed. *Parenting and child development in "nontraditional" families.* Mahwah, NJ: Lawrence Erlbaum Associates, 1999;vii:125–135, 365.

Wallerstein J, Lewis J. The long-term impact of divorce on children: a first report from a 25-year study. *Family and Conciliation Courts Review* 1998;36(3):368–383.

Woolraich M, Aceves J, et al. American Academy of Pediatrics, Committee on Psychosocial Aspects of Child and Family Health. The child in court: a subject review. *Pediatrics* 1999;104(5):1145–1148.

Web Sites

American Bar Association Center on Children and the Law. A wide-ranging Web site with extensive information about the law and court-related topics affecting children. Sponsors a paid monthly newsletter, the ABA Child Law Practice Newsletter. Available at www.abanet.org/child. Accessed on 6/20/02.

Bazelon Center for Mental Health Law. Legal advocacy site for individuals and families with mental disabilities. Special section on children's issues. Available at www.bazelon.org. Accessed on 6/20/02.

Office of Juvenile Justice and Delinquency Prevention. A division of the US Department of Justice, this Web site contains wide scope of information regarding juvenile delinquency and victimization. Available at www.ojjdp.ncjrs.org. Accessed on 6/20/02.

II

Common Clinical Problems in Child and Adolescent Mental Health

10 ♣ Aggressive Behavior

Christopher R. Thomas, Walter J. Meyer, III, and David L. Kaye

I. **Background.** Aggression is one of the more serious and upsetting behavior problems of childhood and adolescence. The term is used to describe a wide variety of behaviors, including tantrums, arguing, bullying, property destruction, and cruelty to animals as well as fighting. In the *Diagnostic and Statistical Manual of Mental Disorders,* Fourth Edition, Text Revision, these problems are generally subsumed under either conduct disorder or oppositional defiant disorder (ODD). Conduct disorder is reserved for those with serious and persistent aggression and other antisocial behaviors; milder, although typically just as persistent, defiance, arguing, and tantrums define ODD. Physical aggression toward others in childhood is predictive of other antisocial behaviors and problems. The dramatic increase in juvenile homicide during the late 1980s in the United States raised concerns about the problem of youth violence. Whereas juvenile arrests for violent crime decreased in recent years, reports by youth of their involvement in violent behaviors have not substantially changed. Health professionals can assist their patients and communities in dealing with youth violence through prevention and intervention.

To understand aggression in youth, it is important to remember the following:

A. **Aggression** typically does not appear overnight, but develops over time. Minor aggressive behaviors are commonly seen in toddlers, with tantrums, hurting others, or breaking things. It is usually the result of frustration and anger, and typically is directed toward caregivers or playmates. At this age, tantrums and aggression are of concern if:
   - Tantrums last more than 10 to 15 minutes or involve repeated destruction of property
   - Hitting, biting, kicking, and so on injures self or others

   This is an important stage when children are expected to learn more socially appropriate ways in managing their feelings. Most children are no longer aggressive by age 6. Those that show continued or increasing physical **aggression** toward others **after age 6** are at **grave risk for aggression during adolescence.**

B. **Boys** are more likely to be aggressive than girls. In addition, children with difficult temperaments, high activity levels, or intrusive behaviors tend to be at greater risk for aggressive behavior.

C. As with any other behavior, aggression is influenced by the consequences of caregivers (i.e., it can be reinforced or discouraged). Parental responses to early aggressive behavior, therefore, are very important.

D. **Exposure to violence** is a critical risk factor, including physical abuse and punishment, and witnessing violence at home or in the media. Children directly imitate behaviors they experience. In addition, exposure to violence can stimulate other aggressive behaviors.

E. Aggression can be a **symptom of other psychiatric and neurologic disorders,** especially those that affect the ability to control impulses, such as:
   - Attention-deficit/hyperactivity disorder (AD/HD)
   - Depression
   - Bipolar disorder. Aggression in these children is often a presenting problem and is described as "explosive," with limited or no provocation, and extreme in intensity (i.e., can include threats of homicide or severe destructiveness). These descriptors should alert the primary care physician (PCP) to this diagnostic possibility.
   - Psychosis
   - Traumatic brain injury, and other neurologic conditions that have an impact on executive functioning

F. **Substance misuse and abuse** disinhibits individuals and dramatically increases the risk of aggression and violence in adolescents.

G. Similarly, factors that **increase frustration** increase the risk of aggression.
   - Limited or delayed speech and language development, which reduces the primary avenue for appropriate expression of anger
   - Learning disabilities, which can lower self-esteem and increase negative feedback in school situational stressors
   - For a variety of reasons, growing up in lower socioeconomic conditions can also increase frustration and is associated with aggression and antisocial behaviors.

H. A particularly worrisome indicator is the child who shows no remorse or concern for others who have been hurt by them. These children have been described as **"callous-unemotional"** and are at high risk for serious antisocial behaviors persisting into adulthood.

II. **Practical office evaluation.** The first step in the evaluation of aggression is a **routine screening** for aggression and risk factors. General questionnaires such as the Child Behavior Checklist and Pediatric Symptom Checklist may be helpful for this screening. Although aggressive behaviors may never develop, monitoring at-risk youth can facilitate early intervention if problems are quickly identified. Typical questions to ask include:

1. Are there any problems getting along with others?
2. How does the patient handle frustration?
3. What punishments or rewards are used for discipline? (Is there a history of child physical or sexual abuse?)
4. Does anyone at home have a problem with temper or violence? (Have any problems with the law occurred? Does the family have a history of drug or alcohol abuse?)

If the screening questions indicate problems or aggressive behavior is the presenting complaint, then a more detailed interview is needed. A clinical questionnaire for parents may be an efficient way to obtain some of this detail (Fig. 10.1).

1. **What is the aggressive behavior?** Tantrums, arguments, threats, destruction of property, physical fights? Definitions of what is aggression and whether it is a problem can vary greatly, so it is best to obtain a detailed description of the behavior from both the parent and the child. It is important to phrase questions in a nonpejorative fashion, as children may be reluctant to talk about their bad behavior. "Your mother tells me there have been a lot of fights," is much better than "So why do you start all these fights." It also helps to begin with minor aggressive behaviors before asking about the more serious physical aggression. Sometimes, it is necessary to collect information from other sources such as a teacher. Typically, the greater the variety of aggressive behaviors, the more serious the problem.

2. **How severe are the behaviors?** With tantrums, you want to know how long they last or if anything is broken. With physical fights, it is important to learn if anyone is hurt or if any weapons were involved.

3. **When did the behavior(s) start?** Was there any change or stress at home or school? Typically, early onset and longer standing patterns of aggression are more serious problems. Aggressive behaviors can result from physical abuse or witnessing domestic violence, and from other extreme stresses as well (e.g., divorce, illness or death of a parent, family move).

4. **Does anything seem to provoke the aggression?** Although it is still alarming that a child will punch another after being called a name, it is different from incidents where the attack was unprovoked. Identifying possible precipitants helps in understanding potential causes and developing interventions.

5. **How is the aggression handled?** What has been tried? What do you do when you have been pushed

(*text continues on page 154*)

Name _____

Date _____

Filled Out By _____

Aggressive Episode Scale
Parent Response Form

1. Does your child have aggressive episodes (that is episodes of verbal threats, hitting, kicking, biting, throwing or destroying property, injury to self or others)?

    ___Yes   ___No

2. If your child has aggressive episodes, check off the behaviors that are typical:

    ___Hitting   ___Destroying property
    ___Kicking   ___Injury to others
    ___Biting   ___Injury to self
    ___Head butt   ___Injury to animals
    ___Throwing objects

3. How often does child show aggression in an average week?

    ___Many times per day   ___Once per week or less
    ___Every day (or nearly so)   ___At least 2-3 times per week
    ___One or two times per month   ___Less than once per month

4. Over the past 6 months, are these aggressive episodes

    ___Increasing in frequency
    ___Decreasing in frequency
    ___Stayed the same number

5. Has the child injured self___ or others___?

    ___Never   ___Many times
    ___Once or twice   ___Almost daily

6. How afraid are you that this child will hurt someone else?

    ___Not at all   ___Some
    ___Minimally   ___Very much concerned

7. How long does the child take to get back in control of themselves?

    ___Less than 5 minutes   ___30-60 minutes
    ___Less than 15 minutes   ___More than 1 hour
    ___Less than 30 minutes

A

Figure 10.1.   Aggressive episode scale parent response form.

8.   What helps the child calm down?

___Physical distance (for example time out)
___Physical closeness (for example restraint)
___Talking to child
___Other (please explain)

9.   Check all of the following that bring on aggressive episodes

___Transitions (changes from one activity to another)
___Changes in routine
___Limits (being told "no" or being asked to perform adult requests)
___Overstimulation (i.e., noise, crowds, etc.)
___Frustration with tasks
___Retaliation
___Self-esteem injured (name calling, embarrassment, shame, etc.)
___Upset over interaction with others
___Other (please specify)

10. In your opinion, why is this child prone to aggressive episodes? (Check all that apply)

___Genes	___Epilepsy	___Emotional Problems
___Diet	___Other medical illness	___Depression
___Poor sleep	___Evil or bad	___Other
___Stress	___Poor language skills	
___Brain damage	___Lack of discipline	
___Allergies	___Child abuse	

11. In your opinion, overall how well do the adults at home set limits?

___Very well   ___Lot of inconsistency
___Okay   ___No limits set

12. Do the adults make the rules clear to the child?

___Very clear   ___Not very clear
___Pretty clear   ___No rules at home

13. Do the adults agree on the rules and the consequences for misbehavior?

___Almost all the time   ___Not very often
___Most of the time   ___Never
___Some of the time

14. Do the adults follow through with the consequences when a rule is broken?

___Almost all the time   ___Not very often
___Most of the time   ___Never
___Some of the time

B

Figure 10.1. *Continued*

past your limits? Do you ever lose it with the child?
Inconsistent or overly harsh punishments can sometimes make matters worse.

6. **Are other antisocial behaviors seen** (e.g., lying,
truancy, running away from home, fire-setting, van-
dalism, or stealing)? Has there been any trouble with
the law? Are they involved with deviant peers or a
gang? Physical aggression can be a symptom of conduct
disorder. Peers are a strong influence on behavior during adolescence and gang members are especially susceptible to violence.

7. Is there any **evidence of other mental disorder**
(e.g., inattention, hyperactivity, depression, hallucinations, or substance use)?

8. Is there **access to lethal weapons?** Whenever threats
to use guns or knives have occurred, it is important to
assess if they are readily available and if any steps
have been taken to secure or remove them from the
home. Many parents believe their children do not
know where guns are in the home when, in fact, they
are aware. In addition, many families with guns in the
home have not taken reasonable steps to secure them
(e.g., locking them up, using trigger locks, or storing
them unloaded).

It is important to conduct a **general screening physical examination** to determine if any other medical (especially neurologic) disorders exist that may contribute to
physical aggression. **Laboratory tests (including com-
puted tomography, magnetic resonance imaging, and
electroencephalogram) are not usually indicated** unless warranted by physical signs or symptoms of another
medical condition.

III. **Triage assessment and treatment planning**

A. **General treatment planning.** Preventing serious
aggressive behaviors in children begins with **effective discipline.** It is important for clinicians to start
discussions around expectations and techniques with
parents early in their child's development. The American Academy of Pediatrics policy statement of Guidance for Effective Discipline (1998) outlines strategies
for effective discipline to help clinicians in advising
parents on discipline. The recommendation is for discipline measures that support a positive parent–child
relationship, use positive reinforcement to encourage
desired behaviors, and remove reinforcement or use
appropriate consequences to discourage unwanted
behaviors (Chapter 3).

A common question parents have about punishment
is the use of **spanking.** Recent research indicates that
corporal punishment has potentially deleterious effects
on child development and offers **no clear benefit in**

comparison with other more appropriate punishments. The American Academies of Pediatrics and Child and Adolescent Psychiatry strongly discourage the use of corporal punishment with youth.

It is also important to educate families about potential risk factors for aggression in their children. Numerous studies have shown the **negative influence of violent media** on aggressive behavior in children. Children become more violent in their play and interactions after viewing violent media and will also directly imitate acts they witness. Parents should be aware of the effects of exposure to violent media and video games for youth and encouraged to supervise the viewing habits of their children.

Guns within the home are another **potential deadly risk** for youth. Most parents believe that their children do not know where the gun is hidden or that it is safely out of reach. A gun in the home increases the risk of homicide threefold (Kellermann et al., 1993) and the risk of suicide fivefold (Kellermann et al., 1992). A study by Weil and Hemenway found that 30% of families with children kept loaded guns at home. In a subsequent article Hemenway et al. (1995) reported that 14% of gun owners with children at home kept the gun loaded and unlocked. Sixteen states now have laws that hold gun owners accountable for access to a gun that a child obtains and uses to harm themselves or others. Parents should be aware of the risks of gun ownership and, if they keep a gun, instructed to keep it unloaded and locked.

B. **Watching**
  1. **When to watch**
     a. Children with minimally aggressive behaviors that appear to be age appropriate should be monitored (e.g., a 3-year-old with occasional temper tantrums).
     b. Isolated, minor outbursts in the absence of a history of aggression or other behavioral and emotional problems should also be followed.
     c. Children who have been exposed to known risk factors (e.g., physical abuse or domestic violence)
     d. Children who have other disorders that place them at risk for aggressive behaviors (e.g., AD/HD, mood disorders, or neurologic disorders)
  2. **What to do while watching**
     a. **Psychoeducation**
        (1) Review history for psychiatric and neurologic risk factors (e.g., AD/HD, mood disorders, traumatic brain injury).

(2) Review history for social risk factors (e.g., poverty, maltreatment, parental substance abuse).

(3) Review history for cognitive and school-related risk factors (e.g., learning problems, held back, poor grades, truancy).

(4) Review parental expectations for confirmation of appropriateness within general community standards.

(5) Review parent's responses to child's misbehavior and discipline practices. Parents may need instruction regarding more effective strategies in dealing with aggression as well as how to encourage more desirable behaviors. For younger children, this would include instruction on use of time out, consistent response, and clear expectations for behavior. Positive behaviors should be rewarded and increased adult supervision and involvement provided.

(6) With adolescents, consequences for behavior should be discussed and decided on as a family in advance and then followed through when a behavior occurs. Although adolescents want increased independence, it does not mean they do not require parental involvement. Parents should continue to be aware of their teen's activities and friends. Excellent guides are available that describe effective parenting, including children with difficult temperaments (see resource list below).

(7) Encourage the monitoring and, if necessary, the curtailment of exposure to media violence (e.g., TV, movies, music). Whereas this exposure may have limited negative effect on normal children, for those at risk it can be a factor that precipitates aggressive or other antisocial behaviors.

b. **Advocacy** is generally not necessary at this stage. If aggressive behaviors are interfering at school, then more active treatment or referral needs to occur.

c. **Psychotherapy** is generally not necessary at this stage. Principles of good behavior management and discipline practices need to be reinforced as above.

d. **Medications** are not indicated at this stage.

e. **Laboratory and other evaluations** are not necessary, unless indicated by signs and symptoms of an underlying medical or neurologic condition.

f. **Follow-up** in 1 to 3 months to determine the evolution of the aggression. Parents can be encouraged to call in to the office to give a periodic update of the child's progress and to determine the need for earlier appointments.

C. **Intervening further**
   1. **When to intervene further**
      a. Children with frequent or severe tantrums
      b. Children with aggressive behavior that could result in physical injury to others
      c. Children with repeated incidents of physical aggression in or out of the home
      d. Persistent bullying or cruelty to siblings or peers
   2. **When intervening further**
      a. **Psychoeducation**
         (1) Explore the parents' views of the problems. Many parents appreciate that a problem exists and will make efforts to address them. Others, however, are in denial about the child's problems or their responsibility for such. In these cases, the PCP may need to persist in bringing up the topic and encouraging the parents to face the problems.
         (2) Explain the rationale for behavioral interventions to the parents and the child. The goal of positive discipline practices is to encourage the child to develop self-control and positive relationship skills. It is not primarily to "punish" the child so that "they learn." In fact, harsh practices generally do not produce positive results and control behavior only as long as the external threat is present; they serve mostly to promote efforts by the child not to be caught (i.e., by lying, hiding, avoiding). They do little to foster the development of the child's internalizing healthy ways of behaving and

relating to others. Parents and other adults cannot be ever-present to monitor and control the child. The child must learn to exert self-restraint. Positive behavioral interventions are best for accomplishing this.

(3) Instruction in behavioral interventions is indicated. Behavioral programs are more effective when they reward desired behaviors and provide consequences for negative behaviors. Parents will need to develop:

(a) A short list of **targeted discrete behaviors.** Desirable (e.g., cooperating, using calm tone of voice, waiting their turn) as well as undesirable (e.g., hitting, defiance) behaviors need to be identified. It is best not to target attitudes (uncooperative), intentions (mean), or generalizations (irresponsibility), which cannot be monitored (see below). Specific instructions should be given so that the child and parent will have no question what will happen when a certain behavior occurs. It is best to start with just one or two behaviors to train families on how to carry out the program and focus their efforts. Additional behaviors can be added later and parents usually generalize the techniques once they learn them. Children should be encouraged to take part in the planning of any behavior program as this promotes understanding and participation.

(b) A **consistent approach to monitoring** means that the parents must be able to monitor the targeted behaviors. If they cannot, then either a new plan needs to be developed or another behavior should be targeted. Parents who are unable to effectively monitor their children's behaviors with the support of the PCP should be referred for specialist mental health treatment.

(c) A **coordinated and realistic approach to providing rewards and consequences.** Parents or other responsible adults need to "be on the same page" about how to respond to children's behavior. When they cannot seem to make this happen, this is a reason to seek specialist mental health referral. In addition, the plan must be realistic (i.e., something the parents can actually carry out). Generally, this is best accomplished when the consequences are discussed, planned, and communicated to the child in advance. When parents respond in the "heat of the battle," they often make threats that they cannot or will not realistically follow through with (e.g., "Now you are grounded for the next month!"). Rewards need to be given as soon as possible following the desired behavior or reaching a certain goal. Often parents have a problem understanding why an expected behavior should be rewarded. They usually accept the explanation that their child is not showing that behavior now, this is a way to achieve it, and the rewards will not have to continue indefinitely. Sometimes, a sibling will undermine a behavioral intervention by provoking the patient into behavior that will be punished. The best way to handle this is to include the sibling in the program, making rewards and punishments based on mutual behaviors. Several excellent programs available to train parents in more effective discipline may be available through local community groups, schools, or agencies. Manuals also available for clinicians who want to carry out behavioral interventions are listed in the resources at the end of the chapter and also in Chapter 3.

(4) Monitor for signs of child maltreatment and make reports if necessary.

(5) Reinforce the negative effects of media violence as above.

(6) In adolescents, explore for substance misuse or abuse

(7) Look for positive avenues for the child to pursue (e.g., after school programs, Scouts, Boy's Clubs, interest groups, sports)

b. **Advocacy** is often needed at this stage, as school problems often have emerged. Assuring that the child or adolescent has had an appropriate evaluation by the school is paramount. The PCP can be helpful to the parents in advocating for the child's legitimate academic, emotional, and behavioral needs.

c. **Psychotherapy** with specialty mental health professionals should be considered at this stage. Parent training in behavior management should be a focal point of treatment. Cognitive-behavioral approaches in an individual format with the child, or in a group setting, are often helpful to address issues of anger management and social skills building. Psychodynamic approaches are helpful in selected cases but are not routinely recommended in the beginning stages of treatment.

d. **Medications** are indicated for comorbid, treatable conditions (e.g., AD/HD, mood disorders).

e. **Laboratory and other evaluations** are indicated only when signs and symptoms of an underlying condition warrant such.

f. **Follow-up** should take place in 1 to 2 months to monitor progress and assure parental pursuit of mental health treatment.

C. **Referring**
   1. **When to refer and transfer primary responsibility**
      a. Aggression that injures self or others

    b. Tantrums that include destruction of items of more than trivial value

    c. Aggression that is associated with other behavioral or emotional problems (e.g., aggression associated with other antisocial behaviors—fire-setting, cruelty to animals, or stealing)

    d. Aggression that continues despite appropriate parental intervention

    e. Aggressive children or adolescents who show "callous and unemotional" traits

    f. Aggression in which is seen imminent risk of harm to self or others should receive emergency evaluation and may require hospitalization.

2. When referring

    a. Psychoeducation

      (1) Challenge parental denial if present. This is often a problem that the PCP's persistent and firm raising of the issues can make all the difference in the world. The PCP should be prepared for angry denials in some cases, which can be unpleasant and are balanced only by recognition of the seriousness of the problem for the child and society, making the PCP's intervention necessary.

      (2) Reinforce behavior management principles as outlined above.

      (3) Continue to monitor for signs of child maltreatment.

      (4) Continue to discourage exposure to media violence.

      (5) Revisit the dangers of gun ownership. Especially in children in this high-risk category, access to guns needs to be diligently prevented. The best solution in situations at this stage is to remove firearms from the home entirely. Any other weapons (e.g., knives, brass knuckles) should also be removed.

      (6) Alert the family to legal options available to provide probationary supervision to the child ("Persons in Need of Supervision" or similar status; see Chapter 9).

      (7) Alert the family to emergency services available in the area. Families can be provided with the telephone numbers for crisis services, emergency psychiatric programs, or hospitals, and the police for situations in which is seen an immediate threat. The PCP should assure that parents are aware of their options in these urgent situations.

b. **Advocacy** remains important to assure that the child has had an adequate evaluation and is receiving sufficient support in the school setting to optimize chances for satisfactory progress and to prevent school from becoming a source of frustration fueling antisocial behaviors.

c. **Psychotherapy** should already be in place by this point. Usually, at this stage, the child and family are in need of more intensive treatment than is afforded by general outpatient approaches. Usually intensive, in-home programs are necessary to provide enough contact and leverage to have an impact on the situation. These programs can often intervene multiple times per week, are available in emergencies, and can access other support services on behalf of the child or family (e.g., respite, after school programs, job coaches). In these programs, a manager, usually assigned to oversee the case, can be a valuable contact for the PCP. A variety of these more intensive services are available in different parts of the country. Specialist mental health professionals should be familiar with the specific services available in a given locale.

d. **Medications** are indicated for underlying psychiatric and neurologic conditions. In addition, at this juncture child and adolescent psychiatrists would consider the use of nonspecific treatments with neuroleptics or mood stabilizers to improve impulse control or mood instability that may be contributing to the problem (see below).

e. **Laboratory and other evaluations** are warranted when signs and symptoms indicate a medical or neurologic problem.

f. **Monitoring** of the patient is primarily the responsibility of the treating mental health professionals. The PCP should remain available to the parents and child and bring them back in 1 to 3 months to monitor the situation and assure follow through with treatment. Phone calls from PCP office staff can be helpful in promoting optimal treatment.

IV. **Practical use of medications.** Medications are generally **not a primary treatment for aggression, unless it is related to a specific disorder** (e.g., depression, AD/HD, or seizures). In those cases, the indicated medication for the other disorder may reduce or control the aggression. Separate from this, are several medications that have shown some benefit in treating aggression unrelated to any other condition. Most studies on the pharmacologic treatment of aggression are with adults but some are with children and adolescents. Neuroleptics (antipsychotics, see Appendix C, D) and benzodiazepines (mostly lorazepam, see Appendix E) have been useful in controlling acute aggression and agitation, and are commonly used in emergency room settings. Numerous studies have shown **neuroleptics and mood stabilizers** (anticonvulsants and lithium) to be effective in treating aggression in certain cases, even without evidence of a comorbid psychotic, mood, or seizure disorder. Low doses of atypical antipsychotics (e.g., risperidone 0.25–0.5 mg initially, titrating to 2 mg/d) are commonly used clinically. Anticonvulsants and lithium are used at similar doses to those used in bipolar disorder. Promising reports have been issued on the use of **clonidine,** an α-adrenergic agonist, in treating aggression as well as symptoms of AD/HD. Dosing is similar to that used in AD/HD treatment. **Beta-blockers** have also been useful, especially as adjunctive treatment of aggression in the developmentally disabled. Because of the complexity and rapidly changing approach to the treatment of aggression, it is often preferable to refer these cases to a child and adolescent psychiatrist.

V. **Summary.** Violence is a major health problem for American youth, with homicide and suicide the second and third leading causes of death among adolescents. Identifying specific risk factors presents the opportunity for prevention through a public health approach. Pediatricians play a crucial role through patient education, screening for risk factors and early signs, primary intervention, and referral for additional services. Parents looking to pediatricians for guidance on child development and health need information on good discipline practices and factors influencing aggression. Routine screening and assessment of aggressive behaviors and risks provide the chance for early identification and intervention. Whenever a question arises regarding aggressive behavior, it is always useful to obtain a consultation. Behavioral programs, parent management training, and treatment for certain risk factors comprise the basic interventions that can be delivered in primary care for aggressive children.

Practitioners also play an important role in community efforts to reduce youth violence by providing valuable understanding and appropriate responses to schools or other agencies. Being aware of effective interventions informs this advocacy for child health. Many models of successful community programs incorporate public health in reducing youth violence and aggression (e.g., the Blueprints for Violence Prevention initiative). Working with families and communities, physicians have the opportunity to contribute to a safer and less violent future for youth.

SUGGESTED READINGS
Parent Guides on Effective Discipline

Faber A, Mazlish E. *How to talk so kids will listen & listen so kids will talk.* New York: Avon Books, 1982.

Kurcinka M. *Raising your spirited child.* New York: Harper Perennial, 1992.

Clinician Manuals on Behavior Management

Barkley R. *Defiant children,* 2nd ed. New York: Guilford Press, 1997.

Dinkmeyer D, McKay G. *Leader's resource guide: systematic training for effective parenting,* Circle Pines, MN: American Guidance Service, 1997.

Key References on Youth Aggression

AAP Task Force on Violence. The role of the pediatrician in youth violence prevention in clinical practice and at the community level. *Pediatrics* 1999;103(1):173–181.

AAP Committee on Psychosocial Aspects of Child and Family Health. Guidance for effective discipline. *Pediatrics* 1998;101(4):723–728.

Christoffel K, Spivak H, Witwer M. Youth violence prevention: the physician's role. *JAMA* 2000;283(9):1202–1203.

Christoffel K. Commentary. When counseling parents on guns doesn't work: why don't they get it? *J Am Acad Child Adolesc Psychiatry* 2000;39(10):1226–1228.

Frick P, Ellis M. Callous-unemotional traits and subtypes of conduct disorder. *Clinical Child and Family Psychology Review* 1999; 2(3):149–168.

Hemenway D, Solnick SJ, Azrael DR. Firearm training and storage. *JAMA* 1995;273(1):46–50.

Kazdin A. *Conduct disorders in childhood and adolescence,* 2nd ed. Thousand Oaks, CA: Sage Publications, 1995.

Kellermann AL, Rivara FP, Rushforth NB, et al. Gun ownership as a risk factor for homicide in the home. *N Engl J Med* 1993;329 (15):1084–1091.

Kellermann AL, Rivara FP, Somes G, et al. Suicide in the home in relation to gun ownership. *N Engl J Med* 1992;327:467–472.

Laraque D, Spivak H, Bull M. Serious firearm injury prevention does make sense. *Pediatrics* 2001;107(2):408–411.

Loeber R, Burke JD, Lahey BB, et al. Oppositional defiant and conduct disorder: a review of the past 10 years, part I. *J Am Acad Child Adolesc Psychiatry* 2000;39(12):1468–1484.

Searight H, Rottnek F, Abby S. Conduct disorder: diagnosis and treatment in primary care. *Am Fam Physician* 2001;63(8):1579–1588.

Waddell C, Lipman E, Offord D. Conduct disorder: practice parameters for assessment, treatment, and prevention. *Can J Psychiatry* 1999;44(suppl. 2):35S–40S.

Weil DS, Hemenway D. Loaded guns in the home: analysis of a national random survey of gun owners. *JAMA* 1992;267:3033–3037.

Web Sites

Blueprints for Violence Prevention. Available at www.colorado.edu/cspv/blueprints. Accessed on 6/20/02.

Centers for Disease Control and Prevention, Safe USA, Youth Violence. Available at http://www.cdc.gov/safeusa/youthviolence.htm. Accessed on 6/20/02.

National Youth Violence Prevention Resource Center. Available at http://www.safeyouth.org. Accessed on 6/20/02.

11 ♣ Anxiety Disorders in Children and Adolescents

Cynthia W. Santos and Michelle S. Barratt

I. **Background.** Anxiety disorders are among the most prevalent forms of psychopathology in children and adolescents, occurring about as frequently as asthma in the pediatric population. Although everyone experiences anxiety at some point, children with anxiety disorders **experience tremendous and persistent distress, and the anxiety impairs their day-to-day functioning in a significant way.** Children with anxiety disorders are often described as **"worriers,"** although they often present to their primary care physician (PCP) with **somatic complaints** of headaches, stomachaches, or fatigue. Because these children have fewer disruptive behaviors and, in fact, may seem eager to please others, parents, teachers, and physicians easily overlook their problem. On the other hand, some anxious children when pressed to face **avoided activities** have tantrums or "freeze," leading to the conclusion that the children are oppositional or disruptive. Their need for avoidance and control can also be frustrating to those around them. Children with anxiety disorders often experience an array of other symptoms including shyness, social withdrawal, lack of self-confidence, dysphoria, and hypersensitivity to criticism or rejection. At least one third of children with anxiety disorders meet criteria for two or more anxiety disorders. **Comorbidity with major depression and attention-deficit/hyperactivity disorders (AD/HD)** is also common.

Anxiety disorders commonly run in families, so clinicians often find that anxious children have anxious parents. Although older models of psychopathology have focused on the role of parenting and life experience, current models of anxiety disorders have focused on the functioning of the γ-**aminobutyric acid (GABA), norepinephrine, and serotonin systems.** Although we are far from a detailed understanding of the pathophysiology, the consensus in the field is that in cases of a clinical disorder, an alteration exists in one or more of these systems. Whereas **life events and parenting are important factors** in the development of anxiety disorders, **genetic factors** influencing these neurotransmitter systems appear to be **critical** (i.e., necessary but perhaps not sufficient) in the development of these disorders. In the case of **obsessive-compulsive (OCD)** particular interest has arisen in the role **of insufficient serotonin and the caudate nucleus of the basal ganglia.** Much of this has stemmed from observing the association between group A beta-hemolytic streptococcal infection and the onset of some cases of OCD. This has led to the concept of **PANDAS** (pediatric autoimmune neuropsychiatric disorders associated with streptococcus), which has now become an area of intense research interest and may lead to a deeper understanding of all anxiety disorders.

Because anxiety is associated with an array of physical symptoms (Table 11.1), these children commonly present to PCPs. Similarly, many medical problems or medications can be associated with anxiety (Table 11.2). A careful medical history and examination are important in the evaluation.

Many anxiety disorders can present in childhood. These include separation anxiety disorder (SAD), panic disorder (PD), generalized anxiety disorder (GAD), phobias, OCD, posttraumatic stress disorder (PTSD), and acute stress disorder. Because trauma-related problems are addressed in another chapter, these are not discussed here.

A. **Normal fears and anxiety.** Virtually **all children experience fears, anxiety, or both** at different points in their lives. Fear is seen as the subjective distress response associated with external threats. Anxiety is the neurobiologic response to anticipated threat; to a significant degree, it is internally driven. The focus of fears of normal children are included in Table 11.3. As children grow older the content of their fears changes, the number of fears increase, and the fears become more complex. It is the unusual child who denies any fears or worries. The following are helpful in distinguishing disordered from normal fears and worries:

1. **Content** of fears that are not developmentally appropriate (i.e., separation fears in a 7-year-old)
2. **Subjective distress** that bothers the child or leads to somatic complaints that interfere with the child's quality of life
3. **Impaired functioning** at school (usually seen in falling grades, school refusal, or poor concentration), home (i.e., family conflict caused by "defiant" or "controlling" behaviors), or with peers (avoidance, restrictions of activities)

Table 11.1. Somatic and cognitive manifestations of anxiety

Restlessness	Palpitations
Headaches	Hyperventilation
Stomachaches (or "butterflies")	Dizziness
Fatigue	Tremors
Sleep problems	Poor concentration and memory
Muscle tension	Irritability

Table 11.2.   Medical problems or medications that can be associated with anxiety

Medical Problems	Medications or Drugs
Hypoglycemia	Caffeine
Hyperthyroidism	Nicotine
Cardiac arrhythmia	Antihistamines
Pheochromocytoma	Antiasthmatics (theophylline)
Seizure disorders	Marijuana
Migraine	Sympathomimetics
Brain tumors	Stimulants (including cocaine)
Hypoxia	Steroids
	Antipsychotics (akathisia)
	Selective serotonin reuptake inhibitors (SSRIs)

   B.   SAD is characterized by excessive anxiety about separation from parents or other attachment figures. Separation anxiety is a normal developmental phenomenon in infants and young children. By the time children are 2 or 3 years of age, they should be able to separate from their primary caretaker for brief periods (i.e., hours) and manage their anxiety. Under stress, it is common for normal children to become temporarily more clingy. In contrast, children with SAD have **difficulty with most separations from caretakers;** they become clingy and fearful that harm or death will befall themselves or their parents.

Table 11.3.   Content of normal fears and anxiety

Age	Fears
Infancy (4–8 mo)	Strangers, loud noise, startled
Toddlerhood—preschool (6 mo–4 yr)	Separation, loud noise
Later preschool (3–5 yr)	Separation, monsters, the dark, animals, imagined and supernatural threats, physical well-being
Elementary school	Physical well-being or injury, social exclusion or teasing, natural events
Adolescence	School performance, psychological well-being, social acceptance

Their distress appears **excessive in intensity and duration.** This leads these children to refuse or strenuously **resist attending school, sleeping in their own bed, or attending social functions such as camp** or spending the night with a friend. **Nightmares** with the theme of separation occur frequently. **Somatic symptoms** are very common, particularly at times of separation. It is not unusual for SAD to begin following a stressor (e.g., parental separation, death or illness in a family member). Typically, the onset of the disorder is in **middle childhood (ages 7 to 9 years),** but can also manifest in adolescence, although this later presentation is often secondary to another disorder such as depression. The disorder occurs more frequently in girls. Sometimes the clinician finds that the **parent** is the one most anxious about separation, and this anxiety gets communicated to the child, who then avoids separation. Children with SAD are at **higher risk for developing panic disorder in adolescence or adulthood.**

C. **PD** appears to be related to SAD, with similar genetic loading. It is highly **unusual in very young children, but is not uncommon in adolescence** and has a peak age of onset between 15 and 19 years. As with most other anxiety disorders, it is more common in **girls (2 to 3:1).** PD is defined as the occurrence of unexpected, recurrent panic attacks, with or without agoraphobia. Panic attacks involve **discrete episodes of intense fear** or discomfort that **rapidly escalates,** and may last from minutes to hours (although typically <30 minutes). The episodes usually include a number of the following symptoms:
1. Palpitations
2. Sweating
3. Trembling
4. Shortness of breath
5. Feeling of choking
6. Chest pain
7. Nausea or abdominal distress
8. Dizziness, feeling faint
9. Derealization (feelings of unreality) or depersonalization (being detached from oneself)
10. Fear of losing control or going crazy
11. Fear of dying
12. Numbness or tingling
13. Chills

Panic attacks can occur spontaneously and without obvious precipitant, or can have clear triggers. Panic attacks can occur as part of virtually all other anxiety disorders, as well as some medical conditions (e.g., mitral valve prolapse). Adolescents with PD often

develop anxiety about having panic attacks (anticipatory anxiety), which leads them to **avoid places or
situations where a panic attack might occur,** or
where escape might be difficult or embarrassing. This
leads to increasing restriction of their life, which
when severe and generalized is called agoraphobia.

D. Children with **GAD** worry excessively about all kinds
of things. They find it difficult to control the worry,
even when reassured, and experience physiologic
symptoms of anxiety (e.g., restlessness, fatigue, irritability, muscle tension, and trouble with sleep and
concentration). They may **worry about performance
in school or sports, the future, punctuality,** or a
variety of catastrophic events. Although they **may
worry about separations,** their worries are not con-
fined to these situations but instead are generalized.
They tend to be **perfectionistic and overly con-
forming** as well as unsure of themselves. They constantly seek approval and reassurance, which can be
exasperating for parents. Boys and girls appear to be
equally affected. **Peak incidence is between 12
and 19 years of age.** Parental expectations of high
achievement or situations where parents consistently
yield to the child's demands can contribute to the
development of GAD in children. Children with GAD
often have other anxiety disorders or depression. Children with pervasive developmental disorders are at
risk for the development of this disorder.

E. **Specific phobias** are commonly seen in children,
especially those of preschool age. A specific phobia is
an excessive and persistent fear of an object or situation, which leads to avoidance of the phobic stimulus.
Usually they are **transient** and do not cause demonstrable impairment, so treatment is not necessary.
When the phobia does not subside over time and evidence is seen of substantial interference with a child's
functioning at home, school, or in the community, the
phobia should be considered a disorder and treated.
Typical specific phobias in preschool children include
fears of separation, needles and bodily harm, loud
noises (including thunderstorms), monsters or ghosts,
animals, and insects. School-aged children are often
fearful of being alone, burglars, bodily injury, illness,
failure, and punishment. Adolescent fears take on
more of a social dimension as they become focused
on appearance, peer scrutiny, school performance, and
social embarrassment. Children with **social phobia**
are afraid of social or performance situations where
they may be embarrassed. They may avoid speaking
in class, using a public restroom, or eating in public (e.g., the school cafeteria). Typically, adolescents

express the anxiety in the form of somatic complaints, freezing, crying, avoidance, or panic attacks. A related phenomenon is **selective mutism,** where younger children refuse to speak in certain settings, usually outside the home or family (e.g., school).

F. **In OCD,** children experience obsessions, which are persistently recurring thoughts, impulses, or images that are experienced as intrusive, inappropriate, and distressing. These are different from normal or even excessive worries about real problems. Common obsessions in children include **fears of contamination, harm toward parents or themselves, aggressive or sexual themes, or a need for symmetry.** These obsessions often lead to **corresponding compulsive behaviors or rituals such as washing, checking, counting, ordering, repeating, touching, and hoarding.** The **mean age of onset is 10 years,** with boys tending to be affected earlier. A small group of patients with OCD develop their symptoms in association with group A beta-hemolytic streptococcal infections as well as Sydenham's chorea. These are considered to be part of a syndrome called PANDAS, which are characterized by an abrupt onset, neurologic abnormalities (e.g., choreiform movements or tics) and exacerbation of symptoms following a streptococcal infection.

II. **Office evaluation.** Because anxiety and fears are a normal part of development, the first step in evaluation is determining whether anxiety symptoms are "normal," or represent pathologic dysfunction. Normal fear in children often serves a purpose of mastery—that is, children become anxious or fearful of a particular stimulus, work to overcome it, and feel proud of their accomplishment. It is also an important biological function that warns of impending danger. Transient rituals are seen in normal children to help bind mild anxiety (e.g., bedtime routines). It is normal when children respond temporarily to stressful life events (e.g., death, divorce, separation, trauma) with increased signs of anxiety. **When the anxiety is overwhelming to the child, disrupts his or her life, is persistent, and interferes with functioning, then a clinical disorder exists.**

Key areas for assessment of anxiety in children include:

A. Is the anxiety normal and appropriate to the child's age and situation?

B. Onset of anxiety symptoms: was there a psychosocial precipitant? Especially important, is there any sign of **child abuse or domestic violence?**

C. Did the child recently develop a **medical illness?** Does the child show signs or symptoms of an active medical condition? Is the child taking a new medication or an increased dose of a standing medication?

D. Is the child **avoiding situations** that might produce anxiety? Does it interfere with normal social or peer relationships?

E. What is the impact on functioning at home? What is the impact on the **family?** Have they had to **rearrange their lives to accommodate** the child's anxiety? How have they tried to help the child cope?

F. What is the impact on functioning at **school?** Are there **attendance** problems? Is academic functioning impaired?

G. Development of anxiety symptoms. Does the anxiety occur in response to a specific stimulus; does it occur spontaneously; or does it occur in anticipation of a specific situation?

H. Is evidence seen of common comorbid conditions (e.g., other anxiety disorders, depression, AD/HD; and with OCD, tic disorders?)

I. **Family psychiatric history.** Who else suffers from anxiety disorders? Any other psychiatric disorders?

J. Mental status examination. Does the examination reveal any objective signs of anxiety? For example, is there a worried look, rapid speech, agitation, appearing frazzled, or tense?

III. **Triage assessment and treatment planning**

A. **General treatment planning.** Assessment focuses on understanding the intensity of symptoms, the distress of the child and family, and the functional limitations imposed by the symptoms. General principles of treatment follow here. **Medication** (see next section) can play an important **adjunctive role** in the overall management, but **should never be seen as a stand-alone treatment.** It must be integrated into a broader treatment plan that attends to the child's and family's management of the distress, as well as school, family, and peer functioning. The **first step** in any management of anxiety disorders is **educating the child and parents.** The important concepts to understand are as follows:

1. **Anxiety responses** are **involuntary** response patterns. Children have no more control over their anxiety than they do over their blood pressure or heart rate! Two caveats:

a. As with your blood pressure or heart rate, an individual can do or not do many things that influence the anxiety response.

b. Anxiety responses can, and do, become embedded in behavioral or interpersonal patterns so that they can take on a flavor of willfulness or "manipulativeness." It is important, however, to be reminded that the primary response of the child is not conscious or under voluntary control.

2. **Anxiety,** as with all feelings, **has a "life."** It has a beginning, a middle, and, importantly, an end. Think of it as a bell-shaped curve. Generally speaking the middle (peak) period lasts only a limited period of time because of the finite amount of stored epinephrine necessary to generate this feeling state. It will pass!

3. When anxious, **avoidance** of (or retreat from) a feared situation or stimulus provides immediate relief. In the long run, however, it **"short circuits"** the natural resolution of anxiety. This effectively raises the curve and actually raises the intensity of future anxious responses.

4. **Successful treatment requires** facing the feared situation or stimulus (*"in vivo* exposure"*) and "keeping your feet moving" until the anxiety completes its natural course and subsides. The best way to understand *in vivo* exposure is to consider the behavioral treatment of an elevator phobia. One can talk for a long time about the advantage of using elevators, but the only effective treatment is to get the individual actually into an elevator and have that person use the elevator long enough for anxiety levels to be reduced by at least 75%. If the individual flees the elevator before anxiety has adequately reduced, the response of avoiding the elevator will be reinforced and the symptoms worsened. Therefore, it is helpful for parents or caretakers to accompany their children for *in vivo* exposure treatments. Parents or caretakers can be taught to help the child rate anxiety levels and ensure that the child remains in the feared situation long enough for anxiety to be reduced adequately. Having the parents or caretakers fully understand the psychological mechanisms for symptom formation is essential if they are to be "co-therapists" who can facilitate the treatment of the child and prevent a worsening of symptoms. *In vivo* exposure treatment is usually not initiated until the child has experienced considerable success in the desensitization through imagery process.

5. A helpful way to quantify anxiety in a given individual is to have him or her rate the level of distress in any given situation ("subjective units of distress" or **SUD**) from 0 to 100. As noted, before leaving a feared situation an

individual should have **decreased** SUD **by
at least 75%.** For example, a child afraid of
dogs should stay in proximity to the dog until
anxiety has dropped by at least 75%. Then the
child can leave the scene without the anxiety
response being reinforced.

6. The **parents' job** is to **reassure and support**
    the child to gain the courage to face the feared
    situation or stimuli until the anxiety has sub-
    sided. It is best for them to calmly and lovingly
    (i.e., without being judgmental or critical—which
    of course can be quite difficult!) cheer the child on
    to overcome the fears. Punishments or restric-
    tions of privileges have little place in the treat-
    ment of most anxiety disorders, and should only
    be considered in unusual circumstances.

    These treatment principles are the basis of
    the **cognitive-behavioral treatment (CBT)**
    of anxiety disorders. Every psychotherapeutic
    approach to anxiety should, and generally does,
    include such a pragmatic and focused component
    of its treatment. Substantial improvement can
    be expected within 3 to 6 months in most cases
    of moderate severity or less. **Psychoanalyti-
    cally,** informed treatment has been and contin-
    ues to be commonly used. Proponents of this
    approach note that anxiety disorders are typi-
    cally chronic conditions and that frequently self-
    esteem and relationship issues require atten-
    tion. For lasting and optimal results, they would
    argue one needs a psychoanalytic approach.
    Clinical research has supported the efficacy of
    the more easily evaluated therapies such as
    CBT. Many children with anxiety disorders have
    school-related problems. An important compo-
    nent of treatment is to provide liaison to the
    schools to assist with attendance problems and
    classroom functioning. As noted, an important
    principle with school attendance problems is to
    aid the child in returning to the school setting
    as soon as possible (i.e., getting back on the
    horse sooner rather than later). At times it is
    best to do this in a graduated way. For details
    on getting back to school see Chapter 18.

    The above principles apply to most situations
    in which PCPs may find themselves. More spe-
    cific recommendations are as follows:

B. **Watching**
    1. **When to watch**
        a. Symptoms are only mildly distressing to
            the patient

  b. Symptoms are recent and a reaction to a known stressor (other than child abuse or domestic violence)

  c. Child continues to function adequately, even if mild decrease from baseline

  d. Family conflict is mild to moderate

  e. Family able to respond productively consistently to child's distress or needs

2. When watching

  a. Psychoeducation

   (1) Education of child and parents about the nature of anxiety and the role of exposure in overcoming, as described above

   (2) Remind parents that **behavior is fundamentally not willful** or "manipulative." Fears are real to the child, although not realistic.

   (3) Reassure the child that parents will work with the child to overcome fears. Do not expect the child to overcome fears immediately. Aim for gradual improvement.

   (4) Expect normal behavior from the child so as to convey a hopeful and positive attitude (versus pessimistic communication that the child "can't" do it). Use praise and, with limits, reinforcers for successfully facing fears.

   (5) Reassurance that the course of mild anxiety disorders, especially when in response to a clear stressor, is likely to be time limited.

   (6) Guidance about separations, sleeping routines, and so on. Transitional objects (e.g., teddy bears, blankets) can be reassuring for younger children at bedtime and in the face of separation stress. Normal separation experiences (e.g., sleepovers) should be encouraged.

  b. Advocacy. In mild situations, little involvement with the school is generally necessary.

  c. Psychotherapy is not necessary at this stage. Guidance of the parents and patient in the general principles of anxiety management (as above) is generally sufficient.

  d. Medications are generally not indicated in mild cases. If sleep is disrupted so that functioning is impaired oral Benadryl (25 to 50 mg at bedtime) may be helpful for a **few days.** Parental demand for stronger medication is generally an indication for a referral to a child and adolescent psychiatrist.

e. **Laboratory and other evaluations.** A complete physical examination is indicated to rule out possible medical conditions contributing to anxiety. Laboratory workup is generally unnecessary unless indicated by physical symptoms or examination.

f. **Monitoring.** Follow-up phone call in 4 to 6 weeks to monitor progress. Follow-up visits as necessary if symptoms progress.

C. **Intervening further**
  1. **When to intervene further**
     a. Symptoms are moderately distressing to patient
     b. Functioning is impaired mildly to moderately
        (1) Family conflict or turmoil is mild to moderate
        (2) Minimal school missed (i.e., <2 weeks)
        (3) Mild-moderate restriction or avoidance of peer activities
     c. Symptoms may be more longstanding (i.e., few months)
     d. Minimal or no comorbid conditions
     e. Family able to respond productively to child's distress or needs most of the time
  2. **When intervening further**
     a. **Psychoeducation.** Education and reassurance as above
     b. **Advocacy**
        (1) Child should be **urged to continue to go to school** unless overwhelmed and unable to function. If this is the case, then refer the child to a child mental health professional.
        (2) Suggest parents arrange for **additional psychological support** from school personnel (e.g., guidance counselor, social worker, friendly teacher).
        (3) Scheduling a time when the child can contact the parent(s) during the school day can also help to bind anxiety.
        (4) Establish **in-school plan** to support the child and handle somatic complaints:

        (a) If the child develops symptoms during school he or she can go to the nurse's or other appropriate administrator's office.

        (b) Encouragement should be given to return to class as soon as possible but maximally within 15 to 30 minutes.

        (c) If the child has fever or the nurse's judgment is that the child is ill then, and only then, should the parents be notified and asked to pick up the child.

  c. **Psychotherapy.** Referral to a child mental health therapist is often warranted at this stage.

  d. **Medications** may be indicated (see next section) at this point. Psychotherapeutic approaches should generally be tried first, with medications reserved for situations in which these approaches offer insufficient help after a reasonable period of time (i.e., 3 to 6 months).

  e. **Laboratory and other evaluations.** Once an anxiety disorder has been established, no additional examinations or laboratory workup is necessary unless symptoms change and suggest a specific medical condition.

  f. **Monitoring.** Return to clinic in 2 to 4 weeks. If no improvement in 3 months or child deteriorates, then refer to child and adolescent psychiatrist for evaluation and perhaps treatment.

D. **Referring**

  1. **When to refer and transfer primary responsibility**

    a. Symptoms are severe

    b. Functional impairment is at least moderate

      (1) Family conflict or turmoil is moderate to severe or family overwhelmed

      (2) Substantial school missed (>2 weeks)

      (3) Moderate to severe restriction or avoidance of peer activities

    c. Symptoms are longstanding (i.e., >3 months)

    d. Current active child abuse or domestic violence

    e. Existence of significant comorbid condition (e.g., AD/HD, mood disorder)

      f. Minimal or no response to 3 months of primary care treatment

      g. Family unable to respond without fueling child's anxiety

  2. **When referring**

    a. **Psychoeducation. Reinforce** patient and family's understanding of anxiety and principles of treatment.

    b. **Advocacy**

      (1) Families may need the PCP to provide required documentation to the school for **medical clearance** to participate in physical education or other school activities.

      (2) Conversely, it is often appropriate to provide medical notes for children with moderate to severe anxiety disorders to be **excused** from standard physical education. In these cases, it is often preferable to arrange for an alternative curriculum, rather than have them excused altogether.

    c. **Psychotherapy**

      (1) Referral to a qualified child mental health professional should have occurred by this point.

      (2) A **cognitive-behavioral approach** is generally recommended.

      (3) **Psychoanalytically oriented** therapies may be useful, especially for more chro-nic conditions that have an impact on the child's self-esteem and ability to form peer relationships.

      (4) **Family involvement** in the therapy is almost always necessary for successful treatment.

    d. **Medications** are often indicated at this stage in conjunction with psychotherapy approaches (see next section).

    e. **Laboratory and other evaluations.** Further examinations and evaluations, beyond that initially done, are generally unnecessary in anxiety disorders.

    f. **Monitoring** to assure parental follow through with mental health treatment is critical; a telephone call in 2 weeks may be helpful reminder.

      (1) Follow-up appointment in 1 to 2 months.

      (2) Ask parents to have treating mental health professionals send written note regarding progress of treatment.

        (3) If no progress in 3 to 6 months, discuss the case with the treating mental health professionals before suggesting alternative treatments or second opinions.

IV. Practical use of medications. Many medications have been used to treat anxiety disorders in children and adolescents. Pharmacologically, the treatment for all of the anxiety disorders is fairly similar. Although the evidence for efficacy is not substantial (except in OCD) and US Food and Drug Administration (FDA) approval is present only for fluvoxamine (OCD ≥8 years) and sertraline (OCD ≥ 6 years), the consensus **first-line treatment** for anxiety disorders in children are the **selective serotonin reuptake inhibitors (SSRI).**

  A. SSRI. For a summary of SSRI see Appendix N. Adverse effects are generally mild and often subside within the first week, although children with anxiety seem more likely to experience these side effects. Practical recommendations for psychopharmacologic treatment are as follows:

    1. Regarding dosing, **start low** (2.5 to 5 mg daily of fluoxetine or equivalent for younger children, and 5 to 10 mg daily for adolescents) **and go slowly.** This minimizes side effects, especially anxiety or agitation, which can be a problem initially with these medications. Note that fluoxetine and citalopram are currently available as a liquid concentrate, which allows for greater dosing flexibility and tolerability.

    2. Some patients with severe anxiety may benefit from the short-term use of benzodiazepines (lorazepam or clonazepam suggested) while awaiting antianxiety effects of SSRI to take hold.

    3. **Treatment effects generally take 2 to 3 weeks, and at times 6 weeks,** to be noticeable. In OCD, effects may not be evident for 10 to 12 weeks.

    4. Be clear about target symptoms

    5. Although all SSRIs appear equally effective, some psychiatrists prefer paroxetine (more sedating) or sertraline (less activating) for treatment of anxiety disorders.

    6. Patients with concomitant chronic medical disorders, especially when requiring other medications, may be better treated with citalopram or sertraline because of minimal inhibition of the P450 system.

    7. Full therapeutic effects of a given dose are generally not seen until 6 weeks.

8. Therapeutic dose ranges for anxiety disorders other than OCD are 10 to 20 mg of fluoxetine or its equivalent; for OCD, dosages are typically higher (often 60 to 80 mg fluoxetine or equivalent).

9. Care should be given when prescribing SSRI to a child at risk for bipolar disorder because of a positive family history, as "switching" to a manic state can occur.

10. Although no data guide length of treatment, a reasonable approach is to **continue medications for 6 months after symptoms have remitted.** If a child has been on psychotropic medications for more than 2 years, it is reasonable to obtain a child psychiatric consultation.

11. When **discontinuing, SSRI should be tapered** over a number of weeks to minimize withdrawal symptoms (nausea, dizziness, headache), which tend to be most severe with paroxetine (the shortest half-life of SSRI). It is least problematic with fluoxetine and other longer acting SSRI.

B. **Tricyclics (TCA)** have been used for many years for anxiety disorders. For a summary of tricyclics, see Appendix P. They have **significant anticholinergic, antihistaminic, and anti–α_1-adrenergic activity.** This leads to important side effects (e.g., sedation, dry mouth, constipation, orthostatic hypotension, blurred vision, tachycardia, and cardiac conduction delays). These, along with a number of reports of sudden death in children taking desipramine, have seriously limited use of these agents in children. The best evidence for effectiveness is for clomipramine in the treatment of OCD. Because of strong anticholinergic effects and consequent side effects clomipramine is not used frequently in the United States at this time. Also, some evidence supports the use of imipramine in SAD. Again, because of adverse effects, this is not considered a first-line treatment for this condition. If prescribing these agents, obtain a **baseline electrocardiogram (ECG) and follow-up ECG after each dose increase above 2.5 mg/kg** (see Appendix P for details). For dosing see Table 11.4.

C. **Benzodiazepines** have been used for many years to treat anxiety disorders, despite lack of demonstrated efficacy in children. For a summary of these medications, see Appendix E. At this time, they **should not be considered first-line treatments** for the ongoing treatment of anxiety disorders. They can be helpful for short-term use (e.g., while awaiting the effects of SSRI to begin, or for anticipatory and **situational anxiety associated with medical procedures or**

Table 11.4. Dosing for treatment of anxiety disorders

Medication	Initial Dose	Maintenance**	Maximum
Selective serotonin reuptake inhibitors (SSRIs)*	Citalopram: 2.5–5 mg qd for younger children; 5–10 mg qd for adolescents	5–20 mg/d for younger children; 10–40 mg/d for adolescents For OCD: 20–80 mg/d	40–60 mg/d for children; 60 mg/d for adolescents
Tricyclic antidepressants (TCAs)	Imipramine: 10–25 mg hs for children; 25–50 mg hs for adolescents Clomipramine (for OCD): 10 mg for children; 25 mg for adolescents	Imipramine: 3–5 mg/kg/d as bid–tid Clomipramine: 75–150 mg/d as bid–tid for children; 100–200 mg/d as bid–tid for adolescents	5 mg/kg/d total dosage
Benzodiazepines	Clonazepam: 0.25 mg for children; 0.5 mg for adolescents	0.5–2 mg/d as bid–tid for children; 1–3 mg/d as bid–tid for adolescents	3 mg/d as bid
Buspirone	2.5 mg qd for children; 5–10 mg for adolescents	5–20 mg/d; tid for children; 30–60 mg/d as tid for adolescents	30 mg/d as tid for children; 60 mg/d as tid for adolescents

bid, twice daily; hs, at bedtime; OCD, obsessive-compulsive disorder; qd, every day; tid, three times daily.

*See Table A7 in the Appendices for dosing of other SSRIs.

**Total daily dose

travel). Clonazepam and lorazepam are currently the benzodiazepines most widely prescribed by psychiatrists. This is because of their intermediate half-life, which leads to less dependency or withdrawal than alprazolam and less accumulation than the older and longer acting, diazepam and chlordiazepoxide. For dosing see Table 11.4.

D. Buspirone is a **GABA inhibitor** that has been reported in small open-label trials and case studies to reduce anxiety in adolescents with generalized anxiety disorders. No controlled data are available for children. Psychiatrists often find this medication only modestly helpful and typically as an adjunct to other psychotropics. Hence, it is **not seen as a stand-alone or first-line treatment** for anxiety disorders. No specific laboratory work is required before beginning buspirone. For dosing, see Table 11.4. The anxiolytic effect takes 2 to 4 weeks to become apparent. Side effects are minimal and include gastrointestinal upset, nausea, dizziness, headache, and insomnia.

E. Other medications have been used to treat anxiety disorders in children and adolescents, including monoamine oxidase inhibitor (MAOI), antihistamines, beta-blockers, and antipsychotics. No efficacy has been demonstrated for any of these agents. **Antipsychotics** should be prescribed by the PCP only in the most unusual of circumstances (e.g., no child psychiatrists available in area and patient has severe disorder unresponsive to all aforementioned treatments). MAOI and beta-blockers also should not be used in children with these disorders. The **antihistamines** are a time-tested, although without controlled data, treatment for acute insomnia or situational agitation. It should also be appreciated that these agents disinhibit some children. They have **no place in the treatment of chronic disorders,** including anxiety disorders.

V. Summary. Anxiety disorders occur commonly in children and often present first to the PCP. Careful assessment, followed by a multimodal treatment plan involving parents, children, and schools is indicated. Although a role often is seen for pharmacology of these disorders, other treatment approaches should generally be used first.

SUGGESTED READINGS

For Physicians

AACAP Practice Parameters for the Assessment and Treatment of Children and Adolescents with Anxiety Disorders. *J Am Acad Child Adolesc Psychiatry* 1997;36(suppl. 10):69S–84S.

AACAP Practice Parameters for the Assessment and Treatment of Children and Adolescents With Obsessive-Compulsive Disorder. *J Am Acad Child Adolesc Psychiatry* 1998;37(suppl. 10):27S–45S.

Bernstein GA, Borchardt CM, Perwien AR. Anxiety disorders in children and adolescents: a review of the past 10 years. *J Am Acad Child Adolesc Psychiatry* 1996;35(9):1110–1119.

March JS, Leonard HL. Obsessive-compulsive disorder in children and adolescents: a review of the past 10 years. *J Am Acad Child Adolesc Psychiatry* 1996;35(10):1265–1273.

March JS, ed. *Anxiety disorders in children and adolescents*. New York: The Guilford Press, 1995.

Mental Health: A Report of the Surgeon General. Anxiety disorders. Available at http://www.surgeongeneral.gov/Library/mentalHealth/chapter3/sec6.html. Accessed on.

Swedo S, Leonard H, Garvey M, et al. Pediatric autoimmune neuropsychiatric disorders associated with streptococcal infections: clinical description of the first 50 cases. *Am J Psychiatry* 1998;155: 264–271.

Velosa JF, Riddle MA. Pharmacologic treatment of anxiety disorders in children and adolescents. *Child Adolesc Psychiatr Clin N Am* 2000;9:119–133.

For Parents and Adolescents

Chansky Tamar. *Freeing your child from obsessive-compulsive disorder: a breakthrough program for parents and children*. New York: Crown Publishing Group, 2000.

Rapoport JL. *The boy who couldn't stop washing*. New York: Plume, 1989.

Web Sites

American Academy of Child and Adolescent Psychiatry maintains an extensive set of parent handouts (Facts for Families) on a variety of child development and psychiatric topics. Available at http://www.aacap.org/publications/factsfam/anxious.htm. Accessed on 6/20/02.

Anxiety Disorders Association of America. Advocacy organization for adults, children, and families. Available at http://www.adaa.org/. Accessed on 6/20/02. Telephone (301) 231-9350.

Childhood Anxiety Network is an informal educational Web site for parents. Available at www.childhoodanxietynetwork.org. Accessed on 6/20/02.

Duke University Program in Child and Adolescent Anxiety Disorders maintains a Web site with information about pediatric anxiety disorders for parents and professionals. Available at www2.mc.duke.edu/pcaad/. Accessed on 6/20/02.

Freedom from Fear. An advocacy and support site mostly oriented to adults but with much good information. Available at www.freedomfromfear.com. Accessed on 6/20/02.

Kids Health. An extensive general pediatric education site for parents developed by the Nemours Foundation. Good sections on anxiety; other emotional problems written as handouts for parents. Available at http://kidshealth.org/parent/emotions/feelings/anxiety.html. Accessed on 6/20/02.

Obsessive-Compulsive (OC) Foundation, Inc., P.O. Box 70, Milford, CT 06460 (203) 878-5669. Advocacy and educational Web site about pediatric and adult OCD for parents. Available at www.ocfoundation.org. Accessed on 6/20/02.

Selective Mutism Group. An educational and support site for parents with children with selective mutism. Available at www.selectivemutism.org. Accessed on 6/20/02.

UCLA Department of Child and Adolescent Psychiatry maintains an educational Web site about anxiety disorders. Available at www.npi.ucla.edu/caap/default.htm. Accessed on 6/20/02.

12 ♣ Attention-Deficit/ Hyperactivity Disorder

Karen J. Miller and Stephen W. Munson

I. **Background.** Attention-deficit/hyperactivity disorder (AD/HD) is the most common significant pediatric behavioral disorder. The cluster of behaviors (behavioral syndrome) **appears early in a child's life** (typically in the preschool period) and usually persists throughout childhood and adolescence, with a **continuation into adulthood in up to 70%** of cases. The defining behaviors involve a persistent pattern of inattention, impulsivity, or both that is more frequent and severe than typically observed in individuals of the same age and gender. This is a syndrome marked by poor modulation of a number of adaptation systems and results in the child's **inability to stop, look, listen, and think.** Core symptoms and related problems occur along a continuum; they are manifest in various combinations and **across family, academic, and social contexts** (i.e., the symptoms are not just seen in problematic situations). The challenge for the clinician is to differentiate the primary attention dysfunction from normal variations and inattentiveness from other causes, including environmental factors and the contribution of related disorders. Because this disorder usually interferes with school function, it is important to differentiate AD/HD from other causes of poor school performance, including specific learning problems.

The prevalence of AD/HD among school-age children is between **3%** and **7%** with a **male** to female ratio of between 3:1 and 6:1. Multiple causative factors are implicated with strong evidence for a **genetic predisposition** that interacts with the environment to produce the clinical features. Evidence suggests that neurotransmitter dysfunction (involving **dopamine and norepinephrine**) impairs inhibitory systems. Neuroimaging and neuropsychological studies support the central role of the **prefrontal lobes and basal ganglia** in mediating AD/HD.

A. **Presenting problems**

1. **Inattention.** Children are described as having a short attention span, being impersistent, distractible, or both. They may not "stick with" activities requiring sustained concentration, especially difficult academic tasks. They may substitute daydreaming or social interaction for academic persistence.

2. **Hyperactivity.** The young child with AD/HD may be in constant motion, jumping about and unable to sit still for stories or meals. The school-aged child will often talk excessively, fidget, or

fiddle with anything within reach. Overt hyper-activity tends to decline with age, and adolescents may appear merely to be restless. Paradoxically, children of any age with this disorder can become glued to the spot for TV, video games, or computer activities, all of which provide a high level of intensity and rapidly shifting stimuli.

3. **Impulsivity.** Children with AD/HD have diffi-culty inhibiting responses. They become over-excited, grabbing, or touching even when told not to. They frequently interrupt others or act with-out thinking of consequences. Schoolwork is rushed or incomplete.

4. **Other related problems. Short-term audi-tory memory** is often impaired and, therefore, these children do not seem to listen or attend to verbal cues. They also have **difficulty control-ling their emotions** and can be easily angered or overly sensitive. Their tendencies to be impul-sively intrusive, noisy, impatient, aggressive, and insensitive to social cues result in difficulty in get-ting along with other children. With adults, they may be oppositional, defiant, and noncompliant. **Disorganization** often results in chaotic school desks and lockers, lost homework and assign-ments, forgotten appointments, missed dead-lines, and general messiness. Children with AD/HD often have **disrupted sleep, with diffi-culty falling asleep** being particularly common.

5. **Symptoms** typically **worsen:**
   a. When sustained, effortful attention is re-quired
   b. In unstructured situations with little adult supervision
   c. In group settings

6. **Symptoms often improve:**
   a. In one-on-one, structured interaction with adults (e.g., the doctor's office)
   b. In situations of high novelty (video games, sports events)
   c. In situations emphasizing active, rapid fire interaction (interactive seminars or games)

7. The current *Diagnostic and Statistical Manual of Mental Disorders,* Fourth Edition, Text Revision (DSM-IV-TR), practice is to categorize children into three diagnostic subgroups requiring six or more from a list of symptoms of either:
   a. Inattention (**AD/HD, predominantly in-attentive type**)
   b. Hyperactivity-impulsivity (**AD/HD, pre-dominantly hyperactive-impulsive type**)

   c. Both inattention and hyperactivity-impulsivity (**AD/HD, combined type**)
  B.   Differential diagnosis and comorbidity. AD/HD is frequently associated with other disorders and conditions. In some children, these disorders coexist with AD/HD, but can be the primary problem in others, producing symptoms that look like AD/HD but are not. The complexity of these interactions is summarized in Tables 12.1 and 12.2.

Table 12.1.   AD/HD "look-alikes"

Normal variation (e.g., toddlers and preschoolers)

Cognitive variation
  Mental retardation*
  Gifted*

Language disorder*

Learning disability*

Autistic spectrum disorder

Chromosome disorder (fragile X)

Emotional disorders
  Demoralization (chronic failure)
  Anxiety and obsessive-compulsive disorders*
  Depressive and bipolar mood disorders*

Behavior disorders
  Oppositional defiant disorder*

Medical disorders
  Sensory (hearing/vision)
  Iron deficiency anemia
  Undernutrition
  Medication side effect (e.g., antihistamines, sympathomimetics, benzodiazepines, carbamazepine, theophylline, phenobarbital)

Substance abuse

Sleep disorder

Environmental problems
  Child abuse/neglect*
  Stressful environment*
  Parenting problem*
  Parental psychopathology*
  Inadequate educational setting*

AD/HD, attention-deficit/hyperactivity disorder.
NOTE: Some conditions may present with AD/HD-like symptoms and therefore can be **confused** with AD/HD. Most of these are diagnosed **instead** of AD/HD, although some (denoted with an *) often coexist with AD/HD.

Table 12.2.   Medical conditions associated with AD/HD

Seizure disorder

Thyroid disorder

Traumatic brain injury

Neurocutaneous syndromes

Fetal alcohol syndrome and other *in utero* exposures (anticonvulsants; perhaps, cocaine)

Lead poisoning

AD/HD, attention-deficit/hyperactivity disorder.
NOTE: AD/HD frequently occurs in the context of these conditions, although
they account for only a **small portion** of the total cases of AD/HD. Each condition should be diagnosed separately.

> **Comorbidity** also has a substantial impact on
> functioning, treatment, and prognosis. Significant
> overlap exists between symptoms of learning dis-
> abilities, behavioral disorders, emotional problems,
> and AD/HD.
> 1. **Between 10% and 40%** of children with AD/HD
>   have **specific learning disabilities.** Particu-
>   larly common are fine motor coordination prob-
>   lems resulting in **dysgraphia.** Specific learning
>   disabilities can result in problems with academic
>   behavior that mimic AD/HD (Chapter 15).
> 2. **Oppositional defiant disorder** (ODD, Table
>   12.3) is a pattern of negativistic, hostile interac-
>   tions that occurs in **30% to 60%** of children with
>   AD/HD. Some children with AD/HD and ODD
>   are more likely to develop antisocial behaviors

Table 12.3.   Characteristics of oppositional defiant disorder

Oppositional defiant disorder consists of a chronic (>6 mo) and persistent pattern of hostile and defiant behavior that does not occur
exclusively in the context of a psychotic or major mood disorder.
Specific characteristics include at least four of the following:

Loses temper

Argues with adults

Defies or refuses to comply with adults

Annoys people deliberately

Blames others for mistakes or misbehaviors

Is touchy or easily annoyed by others

Is angry and resentful

Is spiteful and vindictive

(i.e., **conduct disorder**), leading to substance abuse and delinquency. Conduct disorder also frequently coexists with AD/HD, although not as frequently as ODD.

3. Although **depression** and **anxiety disorders** can present with impaired concentration and performance problems, they also commonly occur in children with AD/HD.

4. A small number of children experience **cycling** (i.e., **bipolar**) **mood disorders** with features of **mania.** Manic symptoms can mimic AD/HD behaviors, and children with comorbid AD/HD and mania are particularly difficult to treat.

5. Medical conditions such as **fetal alcohol syndrome** or central nervous system disorders can result in learning problems and AD/HD.

6. Children with **Tourette's syndrome** frequently have comorbid AD/HD; conversely, only a small number of AD/HD children have Tourette's syndrome.

7. **Psychosocial hardship,** including inappropriate parental expectations, inadequate school placement, stressful environments, trauma, and adverse social conditions (i.e., poverty, racism, violence), can produce behaviors that are mislabeled as AD/HD or can increase symptomatic expression of AD/HD.

II. **Practical office evaluation.** The office evaluation of AD/HD involves the collection of data from a number of sources, primarily the parents, other caretakers, the school, and the child. It is unusual for the child to display the same level of dysfunction in all settings or within the same setting at all times. In particular, the child may not demonstrate the symptoms in the primary care physician's (PCP) office. A **comprehensive, developmentally oriented history** is essential to define presenting problems, clarify diagnostic issues, identify related problems, and understand the child's academic and psychosocial context (Table 12.4).

A. **Parent interview**

1. About inattention:

Does your child have trouble finishing homework?

Does your child find it difficult to learn material requiring memorization?

Do teachers complain that they must constantly redirect your child to pay attention to the task at hand?

Does your child seem to drift off into a world of his or her own instead of attending to the academic work at hand?

Table 12.4. Sources of information

Parent interview

Chief concerns and history of core symptoms

Medical and developmental history

School history: remedial or special education; academic skills; classroom function

Social history: temperament; emotional status; relationships with adults and peers; stress

Current management strategies

Family history: AD/HD-like behavior; psychiatric and behavior disorders; academics; medical disorders, including tics

Child interview

Physical/neurologic (tics)/developmental examination

Child's perceptions of school function; behavior control; family and peer relationships

Mental status, including self-esteem, mood or affect, anxiety, thought and language

Level of activity and focus of attention (note, structured office visits may obscure manifestations of AD/HD)

School data

Teacher reports and observations

Report cards; psychoeducational evaluations; when indicated, speech and language assessment, occupational therapy

Reports of school mental health or special teams assessment

Behavior rating scales

Physical examination and laboratory testing (when clinically indicated)

Questionnaires

AD/HD, attention-deficit/hyperactivity disorder.

> *Does your child seem to be drawn to explore everything in a new environment, sticking with no single thing for very long?*
> **2.** About hyperactivity:
> *Is your child always a bundle of energy from the moment he or she wakes until crashing at night?*
> *Does your child seem to be impossible to keep up with because he or she never stops moving?*
> *Does your child never stop making noises and talking, humming, or singing?*
> *Does your adolescent seem constantly to be drumming or jiggling his or her hands or feet?*

Does the teacher complain that your child is unable to sit in his or her seat?

Does your child wear out baby sitters?

3.   About impulsivity:

Does your child seem to be lacking the fearfulness gene?

Does your child leap before looking?

Does your child speak before thinking, resulting in social awkwardness?

Has poor judgment resulted in more than the expected number of accidents or injuries?

Does your child have trouble on the school bus?

Has your child been in detention for misbehavior in school?

Can you take your child with you to the grocery store for weekly food shopping?

4.   About associated features:

a.   Poor listening skills:

Does it seem like your child never listens to what you tell him or her to do?

Does your child say he or she understands you but then act as if he or she didn't hear?

Do you "talk and talk" and it makes no difference to your child's behavior?

Do coaches complain that your child cannot follow directions?

Does your child seem to miss directions when given orally by the teacher?

b.   Poor management of feelings:

Does your child "fly off the handle" with little apparent provocation?

Does your child have a big temper?

Does your child seem to be upset by the smallest criticism?

c.   Social relationship problems:

Do your child's friendships seem brief and frustrating to him or her?

Do other kids try to keep away from your child?

Do teachers and peers see your child as the "class clown"?

Does your child needle and harass brothers and sisters?

Do you find your child stubborn or oppositional?

d.   Organization problems:

Does your child always lose important things?

Is your child's room a mess 5 minutes after you have cleaned it?

Does your child frequently miss deadlines even for things he or she cares about?

> *If you look in your child's backpack, do you find papers you should have received from school days or weeks ago?*

B. Child interview

1. About inattentiveness:

> *Do you have trouble paying attention when you have to study for more than a few minutes?*
>
> *Does your mind wander while you're reading and you find that you read the same thing over and over, and still don't remember what you read?*
>
> *Do you get bored when the teacher talks for a long time and then find yourself thinking about other things?*
>
> *Does the teacher often tell you to pay attention to your work?*
>
> *Do you feel that the teacher nags you about this?*
>
> *Do you find some subjects easy and some hard? Which ones?*
>
> *Do you start to do something and then find yourself doing something else before you finished the first thing?*

2. About hyperactivity:

> *Do you find it hard to sit still even when you try?*
>
> *Do people tell you that you talk too much or too loud?*
>
> *Do you have to play with things with your hands while you talk or listen?*

3. About impulsiveness:

> *Do you get in trouble before you know what happened?*
>
> *Are you a person who usually dares to do the unusual?*
>
> *Do you like to do things whenever you feel like it? Does this ever work out badly?*

C. School data. Information from the school regarding past and current functioning is essential. Review of **school records** (report cards and standardized testing) provides valuable information regarding the chronicity of problems as well as evidence of specific learning disorders beyond AD/HD. If a learning disability is suspected, either parents or physician can request the school perform individually administered assessments of cognitive ability (IQ) and academic achievement. Language and motor development assessments may also be indicated. In addition, **questionnaires** documenting behavior and approaches to academic work should be requested (see below).

D. Physical examination and laboratory evaluation. Sensory, **physical,** and **neurologic examinations** of children with AD/HD are **usually normal.**

However, such assessments provide opportunities to assess the characteristics of motor coordination, language skills, and social style. As noted, the behavior of children with AD/HD can appear normal in the PCP's office. However, over time, it is common to observe the defining symptoms, either in the examination room or the waiting room (sometimes as reported by support staff). Hyperactive and impulsive behaviors are often in evidence (e.g., touching things they should not, running all over, being loud, going into offices or drawers they should not). **Laboratory findings are usually normal** and, therefore, not necessary. However, lead levels and hematocrit should be considered in preschool children. Additional laboratory studies (e.g., thyroid screen or electroencephalogram) should be ordered in cases of clear clinical indications beyond symptoms of AD/HD. Although they are popular in research settings, computer-based continuous performance tests cannot be relied on to make a diagnosis. These studies are also too lengthy and cumbersome for office evaluation. Multiple factors affect performance on these tests and over-diagnosis is common (Table 12.5).

E.   **Questionnaires.** Although behavior rating scales cannot be used alone to make a diagnosis of AD/HD, they can be useful for data collection, monitoring treatment response, and screening for multiple disorders in addition to AD/HD. Numerous forms are available for parents, teachers, and youth. The PCP should become familiar with at least one of these standardized tools. The long forms of the **Conners** parent, teacher, and adolescent self-rating scales include DSM-IV criteria. Busy teachers may prefer the abbreviated form. The newly developed **Vanderbilt Rating Scales** incorporates DSM-IV criteria for AD/HD, ODD, conduct disorder; a screen for anxiety and depression;

Table 12.5.   Laboratory testing

Consider testing for:
  Hearing
  Vision
  Iron deficiency anemia
  Thyroid disorders
  Lead poisoning
  Chromosome disorders
  Substance abuse
  Sleep apnea

and a functional impairment scale. The **Clinical Attention Profile** (Fig. 12.1), a 10-item questionnaire for parents and teachers based on the Child Behavior Checklist (CBCL) is useful for monitoring treatment response. Because of its comprehensiveness the **Teacher Report Form** of the CBCL is often useful initially, although it is too lengthy for routine monitoring (see end of this chapter for references for other questionnaires).

F.   **Assessment of the family.** The reciprocal interaction between children and their environment is always important. The presence of a child who has AD/HD appears to increase family stress, feelings of parental incompetence, and marital conflict. However, an increased rate of psychopathology also exists in these families based, in part, on a genetic predisposition to the same problems that have affected the

---

Child's Name: _____   Today's Date: _____

Filled Out By: _____

Below is a list of items that describes pupils. Check whether each item is Not True, Somewhat True, or Very Often True for this child now or within the past week. Please check all items as well as you can even if some do not seem to apply to this child.

	Not True	Some-what or times True	Very or Often True
1. Fails to finish things he/she starts.			
2. Can't concentrate, can't pay attention for long.			
3. Can't sit still, restless, or hyperactive.			
4. Fidgets.			
5. Daydreams or gets lost in his/her thoughts.			
6. Impulsive or acts without thinking.			
7. Difficulty following directions			
8. Talks out of turn.			
9. Messy work.			
10. Inattentive, easily distracted.			
11. Talks too much.			
12. Fails to carry out assigned tasks.			

C. Edelbrock, Ph.D. 1986. In public domain.

Scoring:
Inattention (Sum #1, 2, 5, 7, 9, 10, and 12): 93rd percentile for Boys 9/Girls 7; 98%: B 12/G 10
Overactivity (Sum # 3, 4, 6, 8 and 11): 93rd percentile Boys 6/Girls 5; 98%: B 8/G 7
Total (Sum 1 –12): 93rd percentile Boys 15/ Girls 11; 98%: B 20/G 16

Figure 12.1.   Clinical attention profile (CAP) rating scale.

child. The causal direction is not always clear. The child's disruption may precipitate family turmoil but a dysfunctional family system can contribute to disorganized behavior in a child.

III. **Triage assessment and treatment planning.**
   A. **General issues.** Treatment planning and implementation involves a **team approach.** The team includes the child, the family, school personnel, and perhaps mental health professionals. It also involves a lot of information exchange and education. In particular, the Internet has allowed the dissemination of information about **fad treatments** (including effects of diet or sugar, use of herbal supplements, additives, allergies, and so on) that **lack scientific evidence.** A major role of the PCP is to establish a treatment plan with which the team can agree and for which good evidence exists for therapeutic success.
   B. **Watching**
      1. **When to watch.** Parents are often confused about appropriate levels of activity and intellectual ability in their children. **The key diagnostic question is whether activity levels and management of impulses are interfering with successful development.** For example, high activity levels that are not interfering with peer relationships or preschool adaptation can be noted and followed up when the child enters school. Similarly, because school-aged children vary in the degree of their activity, attentiveness, and aggression, those who are highly active and physical but are able to perform well academically and whose peer relationships are going well can be followed with supportive counseling for parents. Consultation with teachers can be helpful in deciding whether to press for more complete assessment and possible treatment when parents have raised concerns about high activity levels.
      2. **When watching**
         a. **Psychoeducation:**
            (1) Advise the parents about temperamental variation in children's activity levels and degree of emotional reactivity.
            (2) Enlist parents in monitoring the child's functioning at school, home, and in the community.
         b. **Advocacy.** Contact with school or after-school care providers to educate about normal variation in activity levels may be necessary.

  c. **Psychotherapy** is not indicated at this stage.
  d. **Medication** is not indicated at this stage.
  e. **Laboratory and other evaluations** are only necessary when indicated by clinical signs or symptoms.
  f. **Monitoring.** Establish a timetable for reassessment of the effects of the child's activity levels and approaches to school. If the child is currently doing well, make an appointment for the parents and child to return for assessment several weeks after the start of the next school year to assess adaptation to new levels of school work and new classroom environment.

C. **Intervening further**
 1. **When to intervene further.** It is time to consider treatment when the child's level of activity, inattentiveness, or impulsivity interferes with:
  a. Academic performance—failure to achieve at expected level, generally because of failure to persist and complete learning tasks, study, homework, and so forth
  b. Peer relationships—unable to maintain friendships usually because of impulsive, annoying behaviors
  c. Family function—behavior is a focal point of family conflict
  d. Emotional well-being—symptoms cause distress to child
 2. **When intervening further.** Establish a team approach that includes the family, primary physician, school personnel, and relevant other caretakers. The therapeutic alliance among all these parties has a substantial impact on adherence to recommendations. **The special case of the preschool child with AD/HD.** Although symptoms of AD/HD nearly always begin in the preschool period, they do not always require treatment. Whether to treat depends on the severity of symptoms, their interference with function and development, and the ability of the caretakers to adapt to and tolerate the child's behavior. First-line treatment should involve parent counseling and behavior programs. If these are not adequate, then low doses of psychostimulant medication can be given.
  a. **Psychoeducation:**
   (1) Counsel parents about the effect of AD/HD on behavior and response to discipline. This includes helping par-

ents to understand that much of the problematic behavior is **not motivated or willful behavior.**

(2)   Parents and children must understand that they **did not cause** this biologically based disorder. On the other hand, **they are responsible for its management.** Information sheets, book suggestions, and referral to parent support groups help to accomplish this goal.

(3)   Teach techniques of **behavior management,** including increased structure, giving clear directions, and using developmentally appropriate parenting techniques (Chapter 3).

(4)   If medication is introduced, education about expected effects and common side effects is essential. This should include discussion with the child as well as the parents.

b. **Advocacy:**

(1)   Parents and teachers alike need assistance in designing learning approaches that work best. Academic interventions include **appropriate academic planning, effective classroom management, and good communication with school personnel.** Most children with AD/HD can be served in mainstreamed classes but some will need tutoring, resource room support, inclusion or blended classrooms, or even self-contained special education. **Associated learning difficulties** must also be addressed and may require speech and language assessment and intervention. **Graphomotor, fine motor, or gross motor dysfunctions** are common and may require modified expectations or occupational therapy. **Technologic aids** (e.g., computers, calculators) may improve productivity. **In-school modifications** may be needed at the classroom level (e.g., writing assignments on the board, sitting near the front), at the task level (e.g., extended time), or at the individual level (e.g., private signal when teacher observes student off task).

(2) AD/HD is now considered a disability under the Individuals with Disabilities Education Act and **may qualify under the "Other Health Impaired" category for special education or related services.** Children with AD/HD who do not require special education services may qualify for appropriate accommodations under Section 504 of the Rehabilitation Act of 1973 (Chapter 7).

c. **Psychotherapy:**
   (1) **Supportive therapy,** which involves careful and empathic listening, can be usefully incorporated into primary office visits. Children and parents who are attempting to adapt to this set of problems need ongoing support in their efforts. **Support groups** (e.g., **Children and Adults with Attention Deficit Disorders [CHADD]) can also be useful.**

   (2) **Behavior therapy** can often be accomplished in the primary care office. Behavior modification is the systematic application of specific techniques that reward positive or adaptive behaviors and target maladaptive patterns. The most effective programs target a limited number of behaviors, provide prompt feedback, and are consistent across settings. Strategies include a combination of increased positive attention ("catch 'em being good"), punishment procedures (e.g., "time out") and "selective ignoring." Charts or point systems can be helpful in tracking specific behaviors. Behavioral interventions can result in short-term improvement in targeted behaviors but gains appear to be limited by the inability of a child to generalize skills to independent situations. Another problem is the adults' difficulty in sustaining behavior programs for long periods. Although the core symptoms of AD/HD respond much more to stimulant medication, behavior management combined with stimulant medication is more effective in addressing the

broader areas of difficulty (i.e., peer or social, family) seen in this group of children (see Chapter 3 for more detailed discussion of behavior management).

d. Medications:

(1) Stimulant medications, which have been extensively researched for the last 60 years, have been demonstrated to be a safe and highly effective treatment for AD/HD. PCPs are usually comfortable prescribing these medications. Their use will be summarized in section IV.

(2) Additional medications in the treatment of AD/HD include $\alpha\text{-}_2$ adrenergic agonists (clonidine and guanfacine), and some antidepressants (tricyclics and bupropion). Many PCPs are comfortable using these medications singly or in combination with stimulants. However, others prefer to refer to mental health specialists if stimulant medications are not sufficient to mange the problem (see section IV).

e. Laboratory and other evaluations:

(1) No specific laboratory measures are indicated, except when comorbid medical conditions or toxic exposure are suspected.

(2) Psychoeducational evaluation, including measures of ability (IQ) and performance, are helpful in monitoring treatment success over the long term. These are usually conducted by schools and can be requested by parents or PCPs (see Chapter 20 and Chapter 7 for further information about specific tests).

f. Monitoring. Follow-up must be frequent when initiating treatment for AD/HD. Parents are anxious and need support and medication effectiveness should be **assessed at least every 2 to 4 weeks when titrating doses.** Initial assessment and titration can occur with telephone contact, but the child should be **seen within 6 weeks** of initiating treatment. Side effects tend to occur early and children need support to "wait them out." On the other hand, when they persist, consider changes in medication. The alliance with the child will be improved if the physician is attentive to the child's experience with the medication. Once an effective medication dose and treatment plan is established, patients should be **seen a minimum of twice per year** for reassessment of medication and ongoing progress.

D. Referring

1. **When to refer and transfer primary responsibility.** Referral is indicated when:

   a. PCP treatment has not resulted in improvement in 3 to 6 months

   b. The comorbidity includes disorders that require mental health treatment beyond primary care office practice:
      - Mood disorders
      - Anxiety disorders
      - Severe oppositional behavior and conduct disorders
      - Aggressive behavior resistant to treatment

   c. Sometimes, parents or school personnel insist on treatment with medication despite little or no evidence of the AD/HD syndrome. When the PCP cannot convince the family that the diagnosis does not include AD/HD, then a referral to a specialist is indicated.

2. **When referring.** Continuing support for the child and family is an essential part of the PCP's role after referral for mental health treatment.

   a. **Psychoeducation:**
      (1) Education of the parents about the nature of mental healthcare, including the variety of medications and treatment approaches that can be offered, is important.
      (2) Helping the parents to accept and understand that this condition may well be a chronic condition that requires long-term management and support

   b. **Advocacy:**
      (1) Continuing involvement in school planning and advocacy for special educational modifications may be necessary to supplement what mental health specialists recommend. As children become older, this includes vocational training and support as well.

(2) Support for managed care payment for mental health services is especially important because many third party payers do not see the need for care beyond the primary physician's office.

c. **Psychotherapies:**
   (1) Beyond behavior modification and supportive therapy noted above, mental health providers can recommend family therapy to resolve family system complexity and group therapy oriented toward building social skills.
   (2) Specific therapies designed to treat comorbid conditions, including anxiety disorders and disturbance in mood and self-esteem, may be indicated. These may include cognitive behavior therapy and individual psychodynamic therapies. Refer to chapters on these disorders for detailed descriptions.

d. **Medications.** See section on medication treatment.

e. **Laboratory and other evaluations:**
   (1) Laboratory evaluations consistent with use of medication combinations (see section on practical use of medications)
   (2) Psychoeducational evaluations of ability and performance as noted above

f. **Monitoring:**
   (1) Communication with mental health providers and family members 4 to 6 weeks following referral to assure communication among team members and support for the referral
   (2) Follow-up with family and mental health provider in 6 months to assess treatment efficacy and compliance.

IV. **Practical use of medications**
   A. **Stimulant medications (Appendix O).** Stimulants should be considered the **first-line treatment for AD/HD.** These medications, which have been extensively studied for the last 60 years, have been demonstrated to be a safe and highly effective treatment for the condition. Stimulant use in the United States has almost tripled in recent years. This increase is largely caused by increased awareness of AD/HD, especially the inattentive subtype, as well as the increase in treatment of adolescents and adults.

Until the recent past, methylphenidate (Ritalin) accounted for more than 80% of stimulant prescriptions. Active marketing of a combination of amphetamine salts (Adderall) has somewhat changed this picture. Newer forms of methylphenidate have recently been introduced that administer the medication over longer periods in the day (Concerta and Metadate). Other stimulants include dextroamphetamine (Dexedrine) and pemoline (Cylert).

Stimulant medications act by **increasing the intrasynaptic availability of dopamine and norepinephrine** with resulting enhancement of attentional processes, sensitivity to reinforcement, and behavioral inhibitory controls. Stimulants do not have a paradoxical effect as individuals with and without AD/HD show qualitatively similar responses.

Stimulant medications **temporarily improve the core symptoms** of AD/HD:
- Increased attention span
- Normalized activity level
- Reduced impulsivity
- Improved academic productivity and performance
- Reduced emotional lability
- Reduced aggressive behavior
- Increased behavioral compliance

Some behaviors that **may not improve** with adequate stimulant treatment include
- Disorganization and messiness
- Forgetfulness

As noted, although increased focus and sustained attention often lead to improved academic productivity and achievement, stimulants **do not fundamentally improve reading or other learning disorders.** Special or remedial education services must be provided to address these issues.

Therapeutic response varies and approximately 70% will respond to the first stimulant tried. If alternative stimulants and a wide range of dosages are tried, the **response rate increases to 85% to 90%.** However, the response to medication cannot be used as a "test" for the diagnosis, because 10% to 30% of those appropriately diagnosed with AD/HD do not respond.

Common side effects include:
- Transient appetite suppression
- Weight loss
- Delay in sleep onset
- Rebound hyperactivity when the medication wears off

Stimulants can slow weight gain and growth velocity slightly but **no evidence of significant effect**

on adolescent growth or ultimate adult height
exists. If medication-related growth effects are suspected, modifying dosage or scheduling, increasing caloric intake, or medication-free periods may be appropriate. Routine "drug holidays" to prevent growth delay are not necessary.

Insomnia can be managed by structuring bedtime routines, eliminating an afternoon dose, or adding a dose if the child is unable to settle down because of the return or "rebounding" of AD/HD symptoms. A mild hypnotic (e.g., antihistamine) may be beneficial. Clonidine (0.05 to 0.1 mg every bedtime) is sometimes used in these situations.

Less common side effects:
- Stomachache
- Headache
- Moodiness or crying
- Fatigue
- Jitteriness
- Tics

It is advisable to take stimulants **with meals** to minimize stomachaches. Although tics and dyskinesias can develop on stimulants, no evidence indicates that stimulants produce permanent tic disorders. Approximately 50% to 60% of children with Tourette's syndrome also have AD/HD, which often presents 2 to 3 years before the onset of tics. Most children with tics and AD/HD obtain benefit on moderate doses of stimulants without unacceptable worsening of tics. At therapeutic doses, stimulants do not lower the seizure threshold but can alter blood levels of anticonvulsants. With careful monitoring, stimulants can be safely given to children with AD/HD and seizure disorders. Cardiovascular effects can include minor changes in pulse and blood pressure, although these are not sufficient to require monitoring beyond routine clinical practice.

Overmedication can result in fatigue, agitation, withdrawn behavior, or dazed appearance. Rarely, a toxic psychosis is seen at high doses.

No evidence exists that **substance abuse** results from properly prescribed stimulants in adolescents who have AD/HD. In fact, some evidence suggests that the adolescent with AD/HD who is appropriately treated with stimulants may be less likely to abuse substances. The risk of substance abuse in adolescence is increased when conduct disorder is comorbidly present. On the other hand, methylphenidate is increasing in popularity as a drug of abuse among teens. If misuse or diversion of methylphenidate by patient, peers, or family is suspected, an alternate form of the drug (Concerta, methylphenidate in a form that is difficult to abuse) or nonstimulant medication may be preferable.

Pemoline is associated with the risk of **toxic hepatitis,** which can occur in as many as 3%. Although this side effect is usually mild and reversible, fulminant and fatal liver failure has been observed. The onset of hepatitis cannot be predicted and may progress rapidly. As a result, the FDA has recommended monitoring of liver function every 2 weeks, and the Canadian government has prohibited its use entirely. We recommend that the PCP avoid the use of this agent at this time.

B. **Trial management of stimulant medication.** Appropriate management of medication begins with identification of the specific target symptoms that are expected to improve, discussion of limitations of medication with the child and parents, and arrangements for monitoring treatment responses. There are three stages of pharmacotherapy:

1. **Titration of medication**

   a. The most commonly used titration method is an **open trial** (nonblinded). **Placebo-controlled trials** can be useful in clinical practice especially when strong biases exist either for or against medication use. These are usually arranged through a medical center pharmacy.

   b. The **usual starting dose** (Table 12.6) for school-aged children is methylphenidate (5 mg/dose) or dextroamphetamine (2.5 mg) two times a day given at or just after meals. For preschool children, the usual starting dose of methylphenidate is 2.5 mg/dose. **Dosage adjustments** of 2.5 to 5 mg are made weekly until a therapeutic effect or adverse effects occur. Titration is best begun with short-acting medication. It is not unusual that a child may require a maintenance three times daily dosing regimen to address symptomatic behavior during the evenings (e.g., homework, and family and social activities). The third dose, when needed, can often be smaller than the other doses. This also minimizes the likelihood of the stimulant interfering with sleep initiation. When optimal dosage is achieved (usually 0.3 to 1 mg/kg/dose), a long-acting medication can be substituted at an equivalent total daily dose. Combined long- and short-acting stimulants can be useful.

Table 12.6. Summary of stimulant dosing

Medication	Duration of action	Initial dose	Maintenance	Maximum
Dextroamphetamine	4–7 hr	Preschool 2.5 mg; older 5 mg	10–30 mg/d as b.i.d.–t.i.d.	40 mg/d total
Adderall (1,d-amphetamine)	4–7 hr, XR longer	Preschool 2.5 mg; older 5 mg	5–30 mg/d as o.d. or b.i.d.	40 mg/d total
Methylphenidate (MPH)	3–5 hr	Preschool 2.5 mg; older 5 mg	10–40 mg/d as b.i.d.–t.i.d.	60 mg /d total
Concerta (MPH XR formulation)	>12 hr; peaks at 1–2, 6–8 hr	Not recommended for preschoolers; school age: 18 mg q.d.	18–54 mg q.d.	72 mg/d
Metadate (MPH XR preparation)	6–9 hr; peaks at 1.5, 4.5 hr	Not recommended for use in preschoolers; school age: 20 mg q.d.	20–40 mg q.d.	60 mg q.d.

q.d., every day; b.i.d., twice daily; t.i.d., three times daily.

Some children require medication only on school days, but most benefit from daily medication as their symptoms significantly impair functioning at home or with peers.

c. Monitoring of treatment response is critical. The initiation of medication can usually be managed over the **telephone.** Instructing the parent to call after 1 week of treatment allows the PCP to manage this initial titration efficiently. AD/HD-specific **rating scales** such as the **Conners Parent and Teacher Rating Scale, short form or The Clinical Attention Profile** can be completed by parents and teachers. It is important to obtain a **baseline rating** and assessments 5 to 7 days following dose changes during a trial. Narrative comments from teachers are often most informative. In secondary school, it is useful to obtain feedback from two teachers because multiple factors influence school behavior in adolescence.

d. Laboratory testing, including electrocardiogram (ECG), is not routinely necessary. Blood levels are not useful in monitoring stimulant medications.

2. **Maintenance phase**
   a. Children taking medications are often **seen every 3 to 4 months.**
   b. **Dosage should be continually reassessed and adjusted** in light of growth and weight gain as well as changes in academic requirements.
   c. **Review the child's and family's understanding** of medication as the child develops. Noncompliance in adolescence is significantly reduced when this step is followed.
   d. **Medical evaluation** at each visit includes:
      (1) **Height and weight**
      (2) **Blood pressure and pulse**
      (3) **Observation for tics**
   d. **Questionnaires.** Both parents and teachers should fill one of the above rating scales out **every 3 to 6 months.**

3. **Termination phase.** Treatment duration with medication is highly individualized and has lengthened as research has shown that AD/HD is commonly a chronic condition, and that stimulants continue to be effective in adolescence

and adulthood. Noncompliance and unsupervised termination is a significant problem in adolescence. Procedures for a trial off medication should be discussed routinely to prevent unsupervised termination. Trials off medication (2 to 4 weeks in duration) should not be conducted at the beginning of a school year or when other aspects of a child's life and treatment program are unstable. At times a placebo-controlled, crossover trial will be useful to determine the necessity of continuing stimulant medication. Clearly, demonstrable benefits should be present to warrant continued use of psychotropic medication.

C. **Nonstimulant medications** have been used in the treatment of AD/HD, but controlled studies are limited. They can be beneficial in children who respond poorly to an adequate trial of stimulants, experience unacceptable side effects, or have significant comorbid conditions. Consider referral to a developmental-behavioral pediatrician or a child psychiatrist for trials of these medications.

1. **Antidepressants.** Antidepressants that have been studied in AD/HD include tricyclic antidepressants (TCA; Appendix P) such as
   - Imipramine (Tofranil)
   - Nortriptyline (Pamelor)
   - Desipramine (Norpramin)

   As well as atypical antidepressants such as
   - Bupropion (Wellbutrin)
   - Venlafaxine (Effexor)
   - Serotonin reuptake inhibitor (SSRI) medications such as fluoxetine (Prozac)

   Tricyclic antidepressants have shown clinical efficacy in children who have AD/HD and can be useful when comorbid anxiety, depression, or tic disorders are present. Improvement in cognitive symptoms (inattention) has not been documented objectively, and effects can be short lived in some children. **Anticholinergic side effects** (dry mouth, constipation), cardiovascular, and neurologic side effects further limit the usefulness of TCA. Potentially **serious cardiovascular side effects,** especially the induction of **arrhythmias,** are possible and TCA use must be preceded by baseline ECG which should be repeated when dosage above 2.5 mg/kg is reached. The QT interval should not exceed 0.425 to 0.45 seconds. Because these concerns appear to be most evident with desipramine, we recommend using this agent only with great caution.

Monitoring of **blood levels** of nortriptyline can be helpful (therapeutic range reported as 50 to 150 mg/ml). TCA can **lower the seizure threshold.**

Bupropion (Wellbutrin; Appendix F) is a heterocyclic antidepressant with dopaminergic activity similar to stimulants. It shows modest efficacy in decreasing hyperactivity and aggressive behavior and can be considered a second-line treatment for AD/HD. Although the combination of stimulants with an SSRI should be considered first-line treatment for comorbid AD/HD with depressive disorders, bupropion has been used as a monotherapy with success in some of these cases. Bupropion can increase tics and **decreases the seizure threshold.** Rapid changes in blood levels of bupropion can result in seizures and the medication is not recommended for patients whose fluid volumes are not stable (e.g., eating disorders, substance abuse).

Venlafaxine (Effexor; Appendix R) appears as a promising second-line agent for AD/HD. This might be considered in children with comorbid anxiety or depressive disorders.

Fluoxetine (Prozac) and other SSRI medications (Appendix N) have generated interest, but little evidence of efficacy exists on the core symptoms of AD/HD. They may be used together with stimulants to manage comorbid depression and anxiety disorders.

2. α-2 Adrenergic agonists (Appendix A). Clonidine (Catapres) and guanfacine (Tenex) have been found to be effective in patients with AD/HD, although not as effective as stimulants. These medications can be useful in over-aroused, easily frustrated, extremely hyperactive, or aggressive individuals. They can be used as a first-line treatment in children with comorbid tics or Tourette's syndrome. They have been used clinically for AD/HD-related sleep problems and in combination with stimulants. Recently, the practice of combining stimulants and clonidine became controversial because of the report of three unexplained deaths in children treated with this regimen. Careful review of these cases resulted in the conclusion that their deaths were more likely caused by other factors and the use of stimulants and clonidine is once again considered safe. **Side effects** include sedation, depression, headache, bradycardia, and hypotension. Abrupt discontinuation can precipitate

tachycardia and hypertension. Parents must be fully advised and counseled regarding these potential problems and the need to take regularly (also **do not discontinue suddenly**). Patients in families who cannot follow this regimen faithfully should not be prescribed this medication. **Guanfacine** is a more selective α-2 adrenergic agonist and produces **less sedation.** Doses of these medications are determined by clinical response and side effects. Clonidine is usually started at 0.05 mg at bedtime (guanfacine 0.5 to 1.0 mg) and increased by 0.05 mg every 3 to 5 days, to a range of 0.2 to 0.4 mg clonidine in three or four divided doses (2 to 3 mg of guanfacine). The half-life of guanfacine is somewhat longer than of clonidine and may be effective in twice-daily doses. Clonidine is also available as a transdermal patch that is effective for 4 to 5 days. Skin irritation is a frequent problem with this.

3. **Miscellaneous medications**
   a. **Mood stabilizing medications** including sodium valproate (Depakote), lithium carbonate, and carbamazepine (Tegretol) can be useful in the treatment of comorbid bipolar disorder with AD/HD. Because of their potential for behavioral destabilization, unfavorable side effect profile, and need for frequent blood tests, these agents are not recommended in uncomplicated AD/HD.
   b. **Antipsychotic medications** (e.g., chlorpromazine, haloperidol, risperidone, ziprasidone) can be useful in unusual cases. They should be reserved for specialists treating this disorder as a last line of treatment of severely disruptive behavior. These medications have a risk for substantial and long-term side effects. See Appendices C and D for side effect profile of these medications.
   c. **Donepezil** (Aricept), an anticholinesterase first used in patients with Alzheimer's disease, has recently been tried in children with treatment-resistant AD/HD. At this point, it should be considered a speculative and adjunctive agent for this population.
   d. **Atomoxetine,** a nonstimulant inhibitor of the presynaptic norepinephrine transporter, is a new drug in investigational stages of development. It appears to be promising as an alternative to stimulants.

V. **Summary.** AD/HD is a common neurobehavioral syndrome with serious consequences for affected children and their families. The core symptoms of inattention, hyperactivity, or both often impair social and academic function. Well-established diagnostic criteria exist, but a thoughtful differential diagnosis and careful assessment for possible comorbid conditions is essential. Management includes education for the child and family, behavior management programs at home and at school, emotional support, academic intervention, and, most often, medication. AD/HD is a chronic disorder in most cases but successful adaptation to persisting symptoms and positive outcome can be achieved with appropriate support and management.

SUGGESTED READINGS

American Academy of Child and Adolescent Psychiatry. Summary of the practice parameter for the use of stimulant medications in the treatment of children, adolescents, and adults. *J Am Acad Child Adolesc Psychiatry* 2001; 40(11):1352–1355.

American Academy of Pediatrics. American Academy of Pediatrics clinical practice guideline: treatment of the child with attention-deficit/hyperactivity disorder. *Pediatrics* 2001;108(4):1033–1044.

American Academy of Pediatrics. Clinical guidelines: diagnosis and evaluation of the child with attention-deficit/hyperactivity disorder. *Pediatrics* 2000;105(5):1158–1170.

Barkley R, ed. AD/HD report. Comprehensive bimonthly newsletter edited by well-known expert in field. To order: (212) 431-7006 or www.guilford.com/periodicals/jnad.htm

Child and Adolescent Psychiatric Clinics of North America. July 2000. Entire issue devoted to AD/HD topics.

Dulcan M, Benson R. Practice parameters for the assessment and treatment of children, adolescents, and adults with AD/HD. *J Am Acad Child Adolesc Psychiatry* 1997;36 (suppl. 10): 85S–121S.

Jensen PS, Hinshaw SP, Swanson JM, et al. Findings for the NIMH Multimodal Treatment Study of ADHD (MTA): implications and applications for primary care providers. *J Dev Behav Pediatr* 2001;22:60–73.

Pediatric Clinics of North America. October 1999. Entire issue devoted to AD/HD topics.

Wender E. Managing stimulant medication for attention-deficit/hyperactivity disorder. *Pediatr Rev* 2001;22(6):183–190.

Web Sites

ADHD.com: the online community. A national education and resource site for families. Available at www.ADHD.com. Accessed on 6/20/02.

Children and Adults with Attention Deficit Disorder (CHADD). A national parent advocacy, education, and support site. Many communities have local chapters of this organization. Available at www.chadd.org. Accessed on 6/20/02.

National Institutes of Mental Health. 5600 Fishers Lane, room 7C-02, MSC 8030, Bethesda, MD 20892. Copies of the 1998 Consensus Conference on AD/HD, booklets on ADHD, LD and mental disorders available online or can be ordered (single copies free). Available at www.nimh.nih.gov. Accessed on 6/20/02.

Pediatric Development and Behavior web site includes the Clinical Attention Profile, multiple handouts, and hyperlinks to reliable sites. Available at www.dbpeds.org. Accessed on 6/20/02.

Books for Parents

Barkley RA. *Taking charge of ADHD: the complete, authoritative guide for parents, revised.* New York: Guilford Publications, 2000. Telephone: (800) 365-7006.

Hallowell E, Ratey J. *Driven to distraction: recognizing and coping with attention deficit disorder from childhood through adulthood.* New York: Pantheon Books, 1994.

Jones CB, Searight HR, Urban MA. *Parent articles about ADHD.* San Antonio: Communication Skill Builders (Psychological Corporation), 1999. Telephone: (800) 228-0752. Handouts to photocopy.

Nadeau K. *Survival guide for college students with ADD or LD.* New York: Magination Press, 1994.

Parker HC. *The ADD hyperactivity workbook for parents, teachers and kids,* 2nd ed. Available (in English and Spanish) through ADD Warehouse: Telephone: (800) 233-9273.

Questionnaires

Achbach T. *Teachers report form of the child behavior checklist.* Available from the author at www.aseba.org/index.html. Accessed on 6/20/02.

Conners CK. *Conner's rating scales.* Multi-Health Systems, 908 Niagara Falls Boulevard, North Tonawanda, NY 14120. Telephone: (800) 456-3003. Available at www.mhs.com. Accessed on 6/20/02.

Edelbrock C. *The clinical attention profile.* Available along with scoring instructions (in public domain) at Pediatric Development and Behavior website: www.dbpeds.org (click on "Handouts"). Accessed on 6/20/02.

Wolraich M. Vanderbilt rating scale. Available as free download http://peds.mc.Vanderbilt.edu/cdc/rating~1.html. Accessed on 6/20/02.

13 ♣ Eating Disorders

Carolyn J. Piver Dukarm and Stephen W. Munson

I. **Background.** Several types of eating disorders are seen: those resulting in increased weight, those leading to weight loss, and those associated with no change in weight. This chapter deals only with those disorders associated with weight loss or weight maintenance. Such **eating disorders** occur in an estimated **3% of women** in the United States, more than 90% of whom are **adolescents or young adults** and although the disorders occur in men, they are rare. Among those disorders, there are two types: **anorexia nervosa** and **bulimia nervosa.** The prevalence is significantly greater if important clinical variants (e.g., **binge eating disorder** and **eating disorder not otherwise specified**) are included. Eating disorders occur in **all ethnic groups and socioeconomic classes in the United States, but are more frequent among whites.** Internationally, they are more common in industrialized countries. The most frequent age of onset is in adolescence or young adulthood, but these disorders are found among preadolescents with increasing frequency.

   A. **Clinical characteristics**

      1. **Anorexia nervosa is characterized by:**

         a. The cardinal and defining feature of this disorder is the **restriction of intake and refusal to maintain body weight** above a minimum necessary for height. In early adolescence, anorexia nervosa can exist without a history of weight loss; instead, the individual fails to achieve expected weight gain during a period of growth.

         b. **Distorted body image** (i.e., feels "fat" even in face of strong objective evidence to the contrary)

         c. **Intense fear of weight gain,** which may be verbalized but is commonly inferred from the patient's food restriction and avoidant behavior

         d. **Dramatic change in eating habits,** including food intake restriction, often accompanied by significant alteration in treatment of food, obsessive cooking for others, cutting portions into tiny subportions rather than eating them, and limiting a variety of foods

         e. **Excessive and rigid exercise regimens** complementing food restriction are common.

         f. **Some** with this disorder **actively purge** (e.g., with self-induced vomiting or misuse of laxatives, diuretics, enemas).

         g. **Amenorrhea** (absence of three or more consecutive menstrual cycles) in postmenarchal females

    h. Reduced capacity for adaptation to physiologic stress; as weight loss persists, metabolic changes occur that reduce the body's capacity to respond to stress. This can result in intolerance to cold and exercise, or changes caused by mild illnesses.

  2. **Bulimia nervosa** is characterized by the following factors:

    a. The defining characteristic of this disorder is a pattern of **recurrent binge eating**—at least two times per week for 3 months (binge eating is defined as consuming an unusually large quantity of food in a discrete period of time and **feeling out of control** during the episode).

    b. **Recurrent purging, fasting, or excessive exercise** (at least two times per week for 3 months) are used as a **compensatory mechanisms** "not to gain weight" following an episode of binge eating.

    c. **Overall self-esteem is excessively dependent on body weight or shape.**

B. **Comorbidity.** Although anorexia nervosa and bulimia occur alone, in "pure" forms, it is **not unusual for a given individual to meet criteria for both diagnoses,** either at the time of presentation or over the course of time (i.e., diagnosed with anorexia at 15 years of age, and developing bulimia at 20 years of age). Eating disorders can occur in the context of virtually every psychiatric disorder. **Anxiety disorders and depression** are common comorbid experiences and can themselves influence the onset of disturbed eating behavior. **Obsessive-compulsive symptoms and personality traits** are especially common. Among those with bulimia, personality patterns consistent with developing borderline personality are frequent.

C. **Etiology.** The **cause** of these disorders is **multifactorial.** An increased rate of eating disorders in first- and second-degree relatives suggests a **genetic** influence, and serotonin imbalance can contribute in some cases. Also, clear **psychodevelopmental** factors are involved, including a search for autonomy and self-control. Many who develop these disorders have been unusually compliant with family and school expectations, meticulously performing academic tasks and striving for perfection in both performance and interpersonal relationships. Attempts to conform to external expectations can lead to inadequate attention to the development of self-perception and self-directed behavior. This insufficiently developed "self" has great difficulty negotiating the trials and tribulations of adolescence, which require a degree of freedom from others' expectations and emotional needs. The symptoms that emerge in the context of developmental pressure to differentiate from the matrix of family expectation can be seen as a **paradoxical attempt to both assert self-control and prevent psychological growth** toward adulthood. These conflicts between compliance and self-determination and the symptomatic attempts at their resolution are unconscious and only vaguely understood by the patient. The symptoms are often a **source of pride** ("I can do something others cannot," "I am stronger than they are") *in lieu* of the development of genuine self-esteem, which seems out of reach to them.

Because of the child's attentiveness to the expectations of others, his or her **responsiveness to family conflict** is high. Families with unresolved problems can seize on the young person's experiments with food and weight control as a distraction and increase the intensity of the child's internal struggle, thus perpetuating and exacerbating the behavior. Patients have nearly always experienced intense questioning and pressure from parents in response to their changes in eating and food-related behaviors, which has only served to intensify the problem and increase resistance to intervention.

In addition to the natural and ubiquitous experimentation with food among pubertal youth, **sociocultural influences** (e.g., an abundance of food and an emphasis on thinness) can play a role in the development of symptomatic eating behavior.

Outcome in **anorexia nervosa** is variable, with the usual course of recovery taking a number of years. The percentage that fully recovers is modest and good outcomes occur in less than 50%. Almost 25% have poor outcomes and approximately 5% die per decade of follow-up. Most continue into adulthood with morbid food and weight preoccupation. Individuals with **milder cases** (i.e., those not requiring hospitalization) may have a better prognosis, but often have long-standing disturbances with body image and eating patterns and psychiatric disorders later in adulthood. The lifetime prevalence of major depression and obsessive-compulsive disorder is high. For **bulimia,** much less is known about outcome. The prognosis appears better but high lifetime rates of depressive disorders, anxiety disorders, suicide attempts, and substance abuse are seen in these patients. For most of these patients, the bulimia resolves over time, although it is often after a protracted course involving relapses and remissions. As compared with anorexia, a much smaller percentage of patients have poor outcomes (10%) and the mortality rate is lower (1%).

II. **Practical office evaluation**

   A. **History.** The diagnosis is primarily based on history from the patient and family. Specific questions to include:

1. To assess any recent **changes in weight or weight loss,** ask:
   - **Have you lost or gained any weight in the past year? Did you intentionally lose weight? What were your highest and lowest weights?**
2. To assess **body image,** attitudes toward shape and weight, ask:
   - **What do you think when you look in the mirror? If gaining 5 pounds would eliminate all of your symptoms, could you tolerate the weight gain? What effect would weight gain have on your moods and self-esteem?**
3. To assess history of **restrictive intake,** obtain a detailed dietary history:
   - **Can you tell me what you eat on a typical day? What do you usually eat for breakfast, lunch, and dinner? How frequently do you skip meals? Do you ever eat snacks?**
4. To assess if **obsessive about exercise,** assess total amount of exercise for a typical day and week:
   - **How much exercise do you do each day? What types of exercise do you usually do? What would happen if you missed a day of exercise? Do you compete in any sports?**
5. To assess history of **amenorrhea** or **irregular menstrual periods,** it is important to keep in mind that healthy adolescents may have irregular periods during the first 1 to 2 years after menarche and amenorrhea or irregular periods may be seen in any instance of significant weight loss or high stress:
   - **When was your last menstrual period? Are your menstrual periods regular?**
6. To assess **physical symptoms** such as fatigue, cold intolerance, abdominal discomfort, constipation, headaches, syncope:
   - **How have you been feeling physically? Are you frequently tired?**
7. To assess for **mood changes,** including anxiety, depression, irritability, isolation from friends and family:
   - **Have you noticed any changes in your moods? Have you lost interest in your usual activities?**
8. To assess history of **purging** (self-induced vomiting, ipecac use to induce vomiting, laxatives, diuretics, appetite suppressants):
   - **Have you ever intentionally made yourself vomit after eating? What were you**

trying to do? Have you ever used laxatives as a way of trying to lose weight? Diuretics to lose weight?
9. To assess history of **binge eating:**
   * **Do you ever feel the urge to eat a whole container of food, for example ice cream or cookies? Do you ever give in to this urge and then afterward feel guilty? If this happens, how often?**
B. **Physical examination**
   1. Measure **weight and height;** calculate **percentage of recommended weight** for height; percentage of recommended body weight (%RBW) = weight/RBW. To estimate RBW for postmenarchal females: 100 pounds at 5 feet, plus 5 pounds/inch over 5 feet. %RBW < 90% generally requires attention.
   2. **Body mass index** (BMI): weight (kg)/height (m)^2; in anorexia nervosa, BMI ≤17.5
   3. **Vital signs:** hypotension, bradycardia, hypothermia, and orthostatic pulse changes
   4. **Skin:** dry skin, lanugo, alopecia, calluses or abrasions over the knuckles (secondary to self-induced vomiting)
   5. **Head and neck:** parotid gland enlargement (secondary to purging), dental enamel erosion (secondary to purging)
   6. **Extremities:** acrocyanosis, decreased capillary refill, edema, loss of muscle mass
C. **Laboratory data**
   1. Results of laboratory tests vary, depending on degree of malnutrition and presence or absence of purging.
   2. Laboratory tests in anorexia nervosa are often normal even with a significant amount of weight loss.
   3. No confirmatory laboratory test exists for anorexia nervosa or bulimia.
   4. Recommended laboratory tests and potential abnormalities
      1. Serum electrolytes
         * Hypokalemia
         * Hypochloremia
         * Metabolic alkalosis (associated with vomiting)
         * Hyponatremia
      2. Renal function tests
         * Blood urea nitrogen may be elevated (secondary to dehydration) or decreased (because of low protein intake)
      3. Complete blood count
         * Mild anemia
         * Thrombocytopenia

- Leukopenia (secondary to margination of white blood cells)
  4. Liver function tests
     - Elevated liver enzymes (most frequently ALT)
     - Elevated cholesterol
  5. Electrocardiogram
     - Bradycardia
     - Prolonged QTc interval (caused by electrolyte imbalance)
     - Nonspecific T-wave abnormalities
     - Low voltage
- D. **Additional medical complications**
  1. Cardiovascular: mitral valve prolapse, dysrhythmia, and ipecac-induced cardiomyopathy
  2. Gastrointestinal: constipation, delayed gastric emptying, esophagitis, hematemesis, including Mallory-Weiss tears (from excessive vomiting)
  3. Endocrine: growth retardation and short stature, delayed puberty
  4. Skeletal: osteopenia (from weight loss)
  5. Neurologic: peripheral neuropathy, cortical atrophy

III. **Triage assessment and treatment planning**
- A. **General treatment planning.** When assisting patients with these disorders, certain guiding principles apply to all situations: the **development of a trusting, confidential relationship with both the patient and the family is essential** and often complicated. As a part of this, the treatment approach must be a collaborative process, involving the patient, family, and any other provider.

  A key feature of many eating disorders, especially anorexia nervosa, is the **"ego syntonic"** nature of the symptoms; patients feel they "don't have a problem" and may see real or perceived **advantages** to some of their symptoms. Therefore, **denial and resistance** to change are often prominent features. Acknowledging this conflict and the difficulty of change can be beneficial. Bulimic patients, on the other hand, are frequently ashamed of their symptoms and very much want to be rid of them, if they only could. Consequently, once the symptoms are out in the open, they are motivated to engage in treatment.

  The complexity of these disorders often requires treatment by a formal or informal **treatment team.** Interdisciplinary collaboration and close communication is essential. Clinical improvement is gradual and often occurs with intermittent advances and regressions. This pattern leads to anxiety for the caregiver and the family. The primary care physician (PCP) should communicate with all members of the treatment team often and with candor.

When symptoms are severe and refractory to out-patient treatment, a higher-level intensity of services is necessary (i.e., day treatment programs or hospitalization). **Indications for hospitalization include:**
1. Severe malnutrition (<75% RBW)
2. Physiologic instability (including severe bradycardia, hypotension, hypothermia, or orthostatic pulse changes)
3. Acute medical complications (e.g., cardiac dysrhythmia, electrolyte disturbances, pancreatitis, dehydration)
4. Acute psychiatric emergency (suicidal ideation, acute changes in mental status; e.g., psychotic thought or delirium)
5. Acute, complete food refusal or rapid weight loss

B. **Watching**
1. **When to watch.** It is not unusual for adolescents, especially girls, to feel they are "fat" or to be concerned about their weight. Adolescents often experiment with diet, eating patterns, and changes in exercise with the goal of improving their attractiveness and acceptance among peers. Changes in these patterns without significant weight loss, obsessive preoccupation, anxiety or depression, or significant family conflict over eating warrant a "wait and watch" stance. If either the family or the PCP is concerned about these changes, a return appointment to monitor physiologic stability is warranted.
2. **When watching**
   a. **Psychoeducation**
      (1) **Educate the child and parents about healthy nutrition, eating habits, and caloric intake.** It can be surprising to see how little accurate information adolescents and their families have regarding these issues. Referral to a nutritionist is often helpful to prevent the emergence of a destructive pattern.
      (2) **Frame the issue as one of helping the adolescent to develop self-control.** Eating can be such a battleground for autonomy ("this is **my** body") that it is best to avoid words or statements that sound as if the PCP is attempting to correct or control the teen. Instead, the goal can be framed as one of developing self-control (i.e., learning to "eat when you are hungry and not to eat when you are not").
      (3) **Neutrally educate parents and adolescent about risks of eating disorders.** Generally, adolescents

do not respond well to stern admonitions or condemnations and, in fact, can be expert at casually frustrating adults who communicate this. Taking an educative stance can send a powerful message about the actual physical and emotional effects of weight loss and starvation. Describing the risks without overstating the case is more effective with the teen and does not escalate the parent's distress and anxiety, which in turn could exacerbate the situation.

(4) **Set up a plan of monitoring.** Parents should be discouraged from "micromanaging" a child's eating habits (e.g., minimize comments and arguments at the dinner table, avoid "knowing looks" as the child eats, weighing the child). It is better to have the PCP monitor the child's eating habits and weight (see below). This relieves the parents from this responsibility and allows some breathing room to prevent the type of standoff that usually leads to further difficulty.

b. **Advocacy** in the schools is generally not needed at this stage. Parents may have been in touch with the school, which is usually sufficient. It is important to remind parents that coaches and other adults involved in **weight-restricting activities** (e.g., gymnastics, dance, modeling, skating) can unwittingly promote eating disorders. These settings must be overseen to prevent this development.

c. **Psychotherapy** is generally not indicated at this stage.

d. **Medications** are not indicated at this stage.

e. **Physical examination and laboratory evaluation.** After the initial evaluation, as outlined earlier, teens who are "flirting" with eating disorders should have their vital signs, height, and weight routinely followed. Weight should be within the range of 90% to 110% RBW. If no laboratory abnormalities appear initially, then no additional laboratory study needs to be repeated. One exception would be ongoing purging behaviors, which may require continued monitoring of electrolytes and perhaps amylase. Another exception would be in the case of rapid weight loss. Decisions regarding laboratory monitoring need to be made on the basis of the clinical evaluation of the individual patient.

f. Monitoring. The patient should be brought back in 4 to 6 weeks to follow up on the status of the nutritional and physiologic status, weight loss, and eating habits. This conveys to the patient that this issue is taken seriously and is not one to be dismissed.

C. **Intervening further**

1. **When to intervene further.** Early treatment and prompt reversal of physiologic changes have been demonstrated to improve prognosis. The emergence of significant physiologic or psychological change beyond developmentally appropriate experimentation warrants active intervention as follows:

   a. Weight loss (or failure to gain in expected manner) of greater than 5 to 10 pounds and weight is <90% RBW

   b. Sustained insistence on adequate weight despite evidence to contrary

   c. Signs that the eating disorder is taking over the adolescent's life and impinging on the patient's life (school, peers, activities, family)

   d. Moderate family conflict over eating habits and weight

   Many PCPs are comfortable with early intervention techniques, including patient and family education, nutritional advice, weight monitoring, and patient advocacy. However, others prefer to refer to specialists as soon as they suspect the patient is developing an eating disorder. Two types of referral are typical (a) to collaborative mental health specialists who can provide family and individual counseling while the PCP monitors weight and eating patterns and (b) to an interdisciplinary team with expertise in managing adolescents with eating disorders. Interdisciplinary treatment is the modality most studied and most likely to be successful in more severe cases. An interdisciplinary team might include an adolescent medicine specialist, mental health provider, and nutritionist.

2. **When intervening further**

   a. **Psychoeducation**

      (1) **Continue to educate about nutrition, the risks of weight loss and starvation, and healthy eating habits (as above).** If not already done, **referral to a nutritionist** should take place to address these

issues more intensively and also to help in structuring meal planning.

(2) **Discuss directly** with the adolescent **the emotional effects** of the weight loss. Adolescents are typically ambivalent about their weight loss. It can be helpful for patients to identify and discuss **both** the advantages and disadvantages of their illness. It can also help to explore personal values and whether the symptoms of the eating disorder are consistent with or inconsistent with the patient's own values.

(3) **Firmly emphasize** that the patient's **weight loss is concerning** to the PCP. Although the patient should not be condemned or seen as "bad," the PCP can deliver the message as part of his or her responsibility to promote the child's health in the long run.

(4) If appropriate, **giving a specific diagnosis (e.g., anorexia nervosa)** can be helpful in challenging the patient's denial and also in broadening the family's understanding of the problem as more than "just needing to eat more."

b. **Advocacy.** Intervention in the school is an important element in the treatment of these disorders. Teachers, school nurses, and peers are all confused and upset by eating disorders and can inadvertently complicate the treatment. Some interventions include:

(1) Identify a **contact person** at the school with whom students can speak confidentially

(2) Focus on the issue of health not "labeling"

(3) Maintain **confidentiality.**

(4) Avoid treating the student differently and, therefore, stigmatizing the individual or creating a contagion effect if other students perceive preferential treatment being given to a student with an eating disorder

(5) Be supportive and express concerns objectively based on facts

(6) Educate teaching and athletic staff about warning signs

(7) Encourage activities, clubs, and so forth, which help build skills, relationships, and self-confidence without emphasis on physical appearance.

c. **Psychotherapy.** Regardless of whether mental health referral is made, a **behavior management plan** needs to be implemented at this point. These techniques can be crucial in helping the patient face the objective reality of behavior and, hence, **increase motivation to change** eating patterns and stabilize weight. Operant conditioning with rewards for positive change and restriction of activities and privileges for weight loss is a common approach. The plan need not be extensive or detailed but must provide a tangible response to the eating disordered behaviors. Requiring a child to return for a follow-up appointment within a short period of time is a behavioral intervention and sends the message to the adolescent that this issue is serious and should not be dismissed. Another example would be for the PCP to agree to sign off medical clearance for a school athletic team only if the child were at a specified weight. This kind of plan must be developed with the close involvement and input of the parents. Although it is unusual for a child to participate productively in the development of a behavior management plan, also include the child if she or he is willing.

   Referral for psychotherapy by a qualified mental health professional is often warranted at this point. It is not unusual for a patient to participate in two or more of the following types of therapy, either simultaneously or in sequence, especially when the symptoms become more severe or chronic.

   (1) **Cognitive-behavioral** therapy focuses on **identifying** dysfunctional thinking patterns that determine behavior and **restructuring** these thinking patterns. Research has focused on group therapy using these techniques. However, individual therapy with these techniques is helpful, either alone or in conjunction with group participation.

   (2) **Individual dynamically oriented therapy** focusing on themes of improving self-esteem, control, reducing perfectionism, improving interpersonal relationships, and resolving family conflicts is also useful. With this therapy, particular emphasis is placed on helping the patient effectively express feelings and ideas.

> > > (3) **Family therapy** emphasizes the identification and modification of family stressors, patterns of interaction, and belief systems that influence the development of and maintenance of the eating disorder.
> >
> > d. **Medication** is generally not indicated at this stage unless a treatable comorbid condition (e.g., anxiety or depressive disorder) has emerged.
> >
> > e. **PE and laboratory evaluation.** Close monitoring of physiologic status is necessary at this stage. Additional laboratory evaluation would follow from the clinical examination findings.
> >
> > f. **Monitoring.** Patients at this stage require monitoring of physiologic status and weight every 1 to 2 weeks.
>
> D. **Referring**
>
> > 1. **When to refer and transfer primary responsibility.** If the patient's weight loss persists or evidence exists for physiologic instability, referral to specialists is advisable. If such specialists are not available, hospitalization may be indicated.
> >
> > 2. **When referring**
> >
> > > a. **Psychoeducation**
> > >
> > > > (1) **Continue to educate and discuss the situation to enhance motivation to change.** This also promotes an orientation to external reality that helps to counter the teen's inner gratification at being able to do something others cannot (i.e., not eat).
> > > >
> > > > (2) **Remain available and maintain positive relationship with the adolescent while mental health treatment becomes central.** The PCP should take a stance of continued interest and "cheering on" in the hope that the adolescent will overcome the eating disorder sooner rather than later.
> > >
> > > b. **Advocacy** is generally managed by other members of the treatment team (i.e., mental health professional, nutritionist, psychiatrist). The PCP may be of critical importance in advocating for adequate insurance coverage for treatment, which is generally lengthy (i.e., years) and may require high-level intensity services.
> > >
> > > c. **Psychotherapy** is carried out by qualified mental health professionals. Usually the therapy will include individual and family therapy components. Groups may also be

available and can be helpful. When standard outpatient treatment is unsuccessful, the patient may require a **partial hospital or day treatment program.** Patients attend these programs usually every day for several hours each day. Cognitive-behavioral and behavior management approaches are used in individual and group formats. Family therapy, nutritional guidance, and medical monitoring are also often included in the treatment package.

d. **Medications** are often used at this stage (see next section for discussion).

e. **PE and laboratory evaluations.** Continued close (i.e., every week) monitoring of weight and vital signs is required at this stage. If the patient becomes physiologically unstable hospitalization is required (see above).

f. **Monitoring** as above. A particularly difficult issue is when the parents question the adequacy of the mental health treatment. Because of the often-slow pace of improvement, families may look to the PCP for other referrals or to grumble about the professionals involved, which can be difficult to evaluate in a balanced manner when hearing from only one perspective. It is recommended that the PCP hear the parents out while trying to maintain an objective stance about the mental health treatment. At times, a poor match is made between a given mental health professional and the patient or family. On the other hand, these patients are renown for being challenging! In general, it is best not to rush to judgment and make a recommendation the first time parents bring this issue up. Rather, agree to consider the issues, monitor the situation, and talk again about it.

Ideally, the PCP has a good working relationship and sense of trust in the mental health professional before the treatment begins. When this is not the case, it is imperative to discuss the problems raised with the mental health professional to come to an agreed on course of action.

IV. **Practical use of medications.** No medications target the core symptoms of anorexia nervosa. However, medications have a place under other circumstances. For patients with comorbid depression and anxiety, selective serotonin reuptake inhibitor (SSRI) antidepressants can be useful. Fluoxetine has also been found helpful for many patients with bulimia, and some studies have indicated its usefulness in

the **maintenance** of weight gain in patients with anorexia nervosa. The decision to use medications in these situations depends on:
- Severity of symptoms (the more severe, the more likely to use medications)
- Response to psychological treatments (i.e., a medication trial is reasonable in cases of failure to respond to reasonable efforts lasting 3 or so months)
- Patient and family preferences

Uncommonly, symptoms of eating disorders appear in patients with psychotic disorders. In such cases, treatment of the comorbid psychosis with appropriate mood stabilizing or neuroleptic medications is indicated. Most likely, a psychiatrist or developmental pediatrician with special interest and expertise will provide such treatment.

A. **Selective serotonin reuptake inhibitors**
   1. In patients with **bulimia,** fluoxetine has been shown to be effective in decreasing the frequency of binge eating by >50% The usual dose is 20 mg in the morning, but some patients require 40 to 60 mg. Some patients find this medication activating and it may interfere with sleep. Other SSRI are probably also effective.
   2. Antidepressant medication for **coexisting depression** or anxiety disorder is usually one of the SSRIs (e.g., fluoxetine, or paroxetine). Refer to the chapters on depression and anxiety for a detailed account of the use of these medications. In general, the principle is to start slowly with half the usual adult daily dose and increase over 5- to 7-day intervals to avoid side effects.
   3. Psychopharmacologic agents have not been shown to be effective in reducing the primary symptoms of anorexia nervosa during the acutely malnourished state; fluoxetine may help stabilize recovery in patients with anorexia nervosa who have regained to >85% RBW

B. **Hormonal therapy**
   1. Treatment of amenorrhea with estrogen or progestin must be individualized and should be considered investigational with respect to its effects on bone density in anorexia nervosa.
   2. Patients with anorexia nervosa who are on oral contraceptive pills may have a "false sense" of health as they have monthly menstrual bleeding even at low weights.

C. **Supplements.** Supplementation with calcium (1000 to 1500 mg/day) and a multivitamin including vitamin D (400 IU/day) is recommended in patients with eating disorders.

V. **Summary.** The disorders discussed in this chapter are common, and represent a substantial level of suffering and disability among young girls and women. It is not unusual for patients and their families to experience a prolonged course. However, if patients are treated early and with both vigor and sensitivity, the outcome can be good. The treatments are primarily psychosocial, and generally require a multidisciplinary team. When used, medications play an ancillary role. Success depends on patience, persistence, genuine optimism, and excellent communication among the multiple participants.

SUGGESTED READINGS

American Psychiatric Association Practice Guideline for the Treatment of Patients with Eating Disorders. *Am J Psychiatry* 2000; 157(suppl. 1):1–25.

Becker AE, Grinspoon SK, Klibanski A, et al. Eating disorders. *N Engl J Med* 1999;340(14):1092.

Fisher M, Golden NH, Katzman DK, et al. Eating disorders in adolescents: a background paper. *J Adolesc Health* 1995;16:420–437.

Kreipe RE, Dukarm CP. Eating disorders in adolescents and older children. *Pediatr Rev* 1999;20(12):410–421.

Mehler PS, Anderson AE. *Eating disorders: a guide to medical care and complications.* Baltimore: Johns Hopkins University Press, 1998.

Web Sites

AnorexiaSurvival.com provides an excellent "educational coaching" newsletter for parents looking for ways to help their child with an eating disorder. Written by a psychologist who specializes in eating disorders, the e-mail newsletter is available free of charge. Available at www.anorexiasurvivalguide.com. Accessed on 6/29/02.

Gurze Books is an online bookstore specializing in eating disorder publications and educational materials. Lots of links to related organizations, self-help, and national referral sources. Available at www.gurze.com. Accessed on 6/29/02.

Mirror. Mirror is a Canadian-based web site dedicated to education, support, and prevention of eating disorders. It has much that parents and teens will find helpful, along with an excellent list of links. Available at www.mirror-mirror.org/eatdis.htm. Accessed on 6/29/02.

National Association of Anorexia Nervosa and Associated Disorders (ANAD) is the oldest support and advocacy group for families and patients with eating disorders. Available at www.anad.org. Accessed on 6/29/02.

Something Fishy web site on eating disorders is a support and education site for those struggling with eating disorders and their families. This is an unusually good site with many moving personal testimonials about the nature of eating disorders and recovery. Provides tremendous insight into the psychology and experience of having an eating disorder. Much is available in Spanish and French. Available at www.something-fishy.org. Accessed on 6/29/02.

14 ❧ Feeding and Sleeping Problems of Infancy and Early Childhood

Bruce Bleichfeld and Maureen E. Montgomery

I. **Background.** As most primary care providers are aware, many of the common problems faced by parents of infants and young children center around feeding and sleeping. Most infants experience some degree of unpredictability, irregularity, and irritability in the first weeks to months of life. These problems can improve or resolve, reappear in another form later, or progress and become severe and chronic. The challenge is to understand the natural history of normal feeding and sleeping behavior in these age groups, and to distinguish between those that are benign and self-limited and those that will likely require therapeutic intervention. Always **consider each family's unique cultural values and expectations** as well as the context of normal early childhood development when assessing sleeping and feeding disorders. The social needs and values of the parents have a major impact on child rearing. For example, in western cultures where considerable value is placed on the development of independence, learning to sleep alone at an early age is important. In other cultures where a premium is placed on cooperation, sleeping in a family bed is more likely to be the norm. Neither of these should be considered abnormal, but rather variations in emphasis. Problems for the child certainly can arise, however, in cases of a mismatch and the values and expectations of the parents are too much at odds with those of the dominant culture.

Primary care physicians (PCP) are experts at early identification of developmental delays in motor, language, and social skills in children. Child mental health experts have focused on understanding regulatory disturbances and the need for relationship assessments in infants and toddlers. The development of self-regulation is a dynamic process involving the continuous back-and-forth transactions between the infant and caregivers (transactional model). Sleep and eating difficulties need to be understood within this unfolding context. During the **first few months of life, the developmental task** of infancy is to achieve **homeostasis,** or physiologic balance, which produces periods of **quiet alertness** throughout the day. Achieving homeostasis allows the infant to learn from, and interact with, the environment and to organize a pattern of behavioral responses to experience. Cycles of hunger-satiety and sleep-wakefulness are examples of behavioral patterns associated with successful integration of repeated experiences and self-regulation. A child who has difficulty establishing homeostasis subsequently will have difficulty performing critical developmental tasks.

By **3 months of age,** the full-term infant can be expected to have developed many of the skills required for **state regulation.** Feeding and sleeping patterns are generally becoming regular and predictable and caregivers can recognize and discriminate many of the baby's signals (e.g., hunger, fatigue, distress, discomfort). It is important to note that the behavior of the caregiver, as well as the infant's own neurobiologic characteristics, including temperament (see below) and neurologic integrity, can interact to either promote or impede this process.

Attachment refers to the affectionate and interactive ties that an infant forms with the primary caregiver between the ages of 3 and 6 months. It is this attachment that **mediates emotional regulation** in the infant. When the attachment process goes awry it is difficult for the baby to establish the ability to self-soothe. This, in turn, can interfere with the development of regulated sleeping and feeding patterns. In most situations, the most powerful impediments to secure attachment are **caretaker factors** (especially maternal depression, substance abuse, and maltreatment or neglect). Child factors (e.g., neurologic integrity, prematurity, chronic disease, developmental disabilities or delays), or dyad factors ("poor fit" between child and parent) also contribute in some circumstances.

Patterns of early attachment (i.e., at 12 months) have been shown to be clinically meaningful, and the PCP often intuitively assesses the quality of this relationship during office visits. In practice, the attachment process can be described as a series of reciprocal exchanges between the child and parent. Specifically, a child gives a signal (e.g., hunger, discomfort) that may or may not be (a) age appropriate (verbal or nonverbal) or (b) easy to decode, and to which the parent may or may not respond. Securely attached infants and their parents successfully negotiate these interactions in a mutually meaningful and satisfactory manner, smoothly integrating the day's activities (eating, sleeping, playing). The PCP can be a resource and "coach" to caregivers of young children by offering specific suggestions and observations that emphasize the importance of this interaction.

Temperament refers to the child's biologically endowed tendencies of action and mood, or behavioral style. Babies differ virtually from birth in these "styles," or how they tend to engage with the world, although experts disagree with respect to precisely what characteristics constitute temperament, their stability over time, and to what degree they respond to the environment. Major dimensions of temperament include activity, reactivity, emotionality, and sociability. For example, some babies have high activity levels; they are highly reactive, emotionally intense, and socially careful. This **"difficult temperament"** which can be manifest from the first weeks to months, can interfere with a child's ability to self-regulate. At the same time, this style is in continuous interaction with the environment. Although it is easier for parents if a "goodness of fit"

(Chess and Thomas, 1986) exists between their own temperamental characteristics and those of their child, it is the capacity of the parents to accept and respond to the child's temperament that is crucial to the outcome for the child.

Development of normal eating and sleeping patterns depends on the development of self-regulation. The most important factors in this process are (a) the development of homeostasis and state regulation; (b) secure attachment and emotional regulation; and (c) the optimal channeling of temperamental styles. These are not just qualities a baby is born with, but rather require "good enough" (Winnicott, 1965) interaction between the baby and caregivers. Disruptions in any of these can produce feeding and sleeping problems in young children.

II.   **Feeding.** Successful feeding depends on the child's ability to master both motor and social skills. Integrity of the gastrointestinal (GI) and neurologic systems is required, as is competence in social interaction with the caregiver. Using a transactional model, a feeding can be viewed as a series of complex interactions between the child and the caregiver that requires the child to signal personal needs and wants (e.g., hunger, satiety, distress) and the caregiver to read these cues and respond appropriately.

Childhood **feeding disorders** are common. In this chapter a **feeding problem** is defined as a deficit in any aspect of nutritional intake that results in undernutrition, poor growth, or stressful meal times for the child and family. Using this definition, it is estimated that **25% to 40%** of healthy infants and young children experience **mild symptoms.** More **serious problems** occur in less than **1% to 2%** of children. Young children with **developmental disabilities or GI disorders are at substantially higher risk** for both mild and severe problems. The pediatric literature has historically used the term **failure to thrive (FTT).** This has had various definitions, but usually refers to a child whose growth has decelerated and fallen below the 3% to 5%, or who has had a change in growth that has crossed two major growth percentiles (Behrman, et al., 2000). Traditionally, FTT has been divided into "organic" and "nonorganic" types, with "nonorganic" types accounting for at least 50% of all cases. However, this classification has been misleading in that many, if not most, cases have multiple factors involved in their cause. The *Diagnostic and Statistical Manual of Mental Disorders,* Fourth Edition, Text Revision (DSM-IV-TR) classifies these problems as **feeding disorders of infancy and early childhood.** This diagnosis requires a "persistent failure to eat adequately, with significant failure to gain weight or significant loss of weight over at least 1 month"—not caused by an associated medical condition. Chatoor has proposed a clinical typology of these serious feeding disorders:

A.   **Feeding disorder of homeostasis** (0 to 3 months) is manifested from the first weeks of life by difficulty establishing a regular, calm feeding pattern with adequate or appropriate intake. Intake quantity can vary, and timing and duration of feedings are unpredictable. The baby is often irritable, sleepy, or fatigues easily during feedings. Child and caregiver factors can contribute to the development of this disorder. Because medical or developmental factors are often present, this can lead to an escalating cycle of anxiety in both parent and child, which leads to greater feeding difficulties. Nevertheless, the ability of the caretaker to read and respond to the cues of the infant or young child is crucial. Treatment often involves referral to a feeding disorders clinic or involvement of a similar multidisciplinary team.

B. **Feeding disorder of attachment** (3 to 6 months) is characterized by a lack of engagement and pleasure between baby and caregiver. Frequently, the caregiver lives in adverse conditions (i.e., poverty, unemployment, community violence) and has serious mental health problems, including depression and substance abuse. Generally, involvement and affection toward the baby are lacking (e.g., bottles propped for the baby to feed). The caretaker's needs appear to take precedence over the baby's. This leads to depressed responsiveness by the baby and subsequent developmental delay and growth failure. This type of feeding problem usually appears between 2 and 6 months. Often, these cases present to an emergency department with an acute illness, during which the child is then discovered to be seriously underweight. Once admitted to the hospital, these babies quickly begin to gain weight and affectively perk up with the responsive care given by the hospital staff.

C. **Feeding disorder of separation/individuation** (6 to 36 months) is manifested by struggle or conflict during mealtimes as the child moves toward becoming more independent. Caregivers often interpret these normal developmental strivings for independence as "difficult" or "stubborn," resulting in major conflict and efforts to force feed the child. Food refusal (e.g., refusing to open mouth, spits out food or spoon) characterizes this disorder, which generally occurs in the context of otherwise normal development. Mothers are often anxious and insecure about their effectiveness, which can interfere with their accurate reading of the child's feeding cues. Their anxiety worsens as their child continues to refuse to eat. Temperament factors can also be relevant, with these children being described as interpersonally sensitive (i.e., tuned into external cues in environment versus internal cues) and persistent. This type of feeding problem becomes apparent between 6 and 36 months of age. Treatment generally involves outpatient parent–child psychotherapy to help the parent learn to read the child's cues and to structure mealtime routines.

Chatoor also describes a **posttraumatic feeding disorder** that has its onset following an incident of choking, gagging, or vomiting that may be associated with medical conditions or procedures. This can occur from infancy on and is manifested by an acute phobic avoidance of eating. This may complicate any of the above clinical typologies. Feeding problems can range from mild and transitory to severe and life threatening. As noted, treatment approaches vary, depending on the type of problem, but require a comprehensive understanding of the child's medical history, temperament, attachment status, and parent–child interaction surrounding feeding.

III. Sleeping

A. **Normal development.** Children typically require decreasing amounts of sleep as they get older (Table 14.1). Nighttime sleep gradually becomes consolidated into longer periods of time, so that **by 4 months of age, most infants sleep 6 to 8 hours without interruption,** and by 6 months, babies usually sleep up to 10 or 12 hours. Between 4 and 6 months of age, infants who had developed consolidated patterns of sleep often experience a new onset of **nighttime waking.** This waking is brief and transitory if caregivers allow the baby time to learn to self-soothe and settle before intervening. Nocturnal arousals for feedings are normal for full-term infants up to the age of 3 to 6 months, and brief arousals (usually, five to eight per night) are a part of normal sleep at all ages. A clinical problem exists when the child is unable to return to sleep following these arousals. Hence, the developmental task for the child is to learn how to go back to sleep after these arousals. Developing this ability requires an intact central nervous system, physical comfort, unfettered breathing, and also the *opportunity* to "build the muscles" of falling back asleep. Parents need to support the child's "exercising these muscles" (often by not intervening and allowing the child sufficient time to fall back asleep

Table 14.1.   Total hours of sleep (including naps)

Age	Hours/Day
Newborn	16
3 mo	15
12 mo	14
5 yr	10–11
10 yr	10
14 yr	9
18 yr	8

on his or her own) so that the child is able to learn to do this without being overwhelmed.

From the age of about 6 months to 2 years, the infant becomes less dependent on the caregiver for meeting basic needs such as feeding and sleeping. The developmental task of separation or individuation in which the child is engaged at this age can be confusing, stressful, and problematic for both the child and the parent. This can be seen in struggles related to many behaviors, including feeding, sleeping, and discipline. Allowing the child a degree of autonomy and control, within appropriate limits, is central to the management and prevention of these problems. As these issues of separation come to center stage, struggles over bedtime often intensify.

B. **Sleep problems** are broadly classified into:

1. **Dyssomnias** are a disturbance in the amount or timing of sleep. Dyssomnias can be classified as intrinsic (e.g., obstructive sleep apnea, narcolepsy) or extrinsic (related to environmental factors or parenting practices). These typically present with chief complaints of **nighttime waking** (nocturnal arousals), **difficulty falling asleep,** or **bedtime refusals** (struggles around going to bed). It is estimated that up to 40% of young children experience at least mild symptoms of dyssomnia. Dyssomnias are unlikely to improve without appropriate treatment.

2. **Parasomnias** are behaviors that intrude into sleep during partial arousals from the deepest, slow-wave, nonrapid eye movement (NREM) sleep (i.e., the first 1 to 3 hours after sleep onset). These include **sleep terrors, confusional arousals, sleepwalking, sleep talking,** and **rhythmic movements** (head banging and body rocking). Although their eyes are open, they are not awake. In contrast, **nightmares** occur during REM sleep, so that these occur more towards morning (REM periods begin after 90 minutes of sleep and lengthen as sleep continues). Children will be awake when they fearfully approach their parents. Parasomias rarely occur in young children (<5% of infants <1 year of age) and become more frequent in the preschool years (up to 40% of 4-year-olds). Over-tiredness and anxiety (including that caused by maltreatment or other stressors) contribute significantly to the development of parasomnias. Parasomnias are generally self-limited and resolve spontaneously in otherwise normal children.

C. The key to **prevention** of most sleep problems in children is the early establishment of **good sleep hygiene,** appropriate to the developmental stage and cultural norms of the family. Successful sleep patterns are best fostered by:

- **Regular bedtime rituals and schedules**
- **Avoiding excessive nighttime feedings**
- **Avoiding excessive parental interventions in the process of falling asleep**
- **Avoiding overstimulation immediately before bedtime**
- **Appropriate limit-setting**

  Instituting these practices may be the only intervention required when minor sleep disturbances arise.

IV. Practical office evaluation. The American Academy of Pediatrics recommends at least six office visits during the first year of life and not fewer than three visits during the following year. Over the course of these visits, the PCP is in the unique position of being able to observe multiple child–caregiver (usually the mother) interactions. As a trusted expert, the PCP can provide anticipatory guidance about issues in normal child development, thereby **preventing** many of the common problems of sleeping and feeding encountered in young children. If a problem does develop, a successful intervention acknowledges the complex issues involved in these disorders and incorporates techniques that can be implemented by both the child and the family.

The **basic principles** involved in the assessment of eating and sleeping disorders in young children are:

A. A **comprehensive,** developmentally oriented **history** of the problem (Tables 14.2 and 14.3)

B. A thorough **physical examination,** with special emphasis on the respiratory, GI, and central nervous systems. Although behavioral and interactional issues account for most feeding and sleeping problems encountered in young children, medical conditions must be considered. A careful and complete physical examination, looking especially for signs of acute or chronic illness, growth failure, or airway obstruction will identify those children who require more extensive and immediate laboratory evaluation. Measurements of the child's growth parameters is essential.

  1. Respiratory system. Look for signs of acute or chronic disease that cause symptoms of airway obstruction, pain or fever (urinary tract infection, otitis media, acute asthma or laryngotracheomalacia, enlarged tonsils or adenoids). Any of these conditions can cause sleep disturbance.

  2. GI system. Look for signs of gastroesophageal reflux or congenital anomalies of the GI tract (clefts, tracheoesophageal fistula, pyloric stenosis). A child with an organic illness commonly exhibits slow weight gain, or even weight loss. However, the converse is not true; the differential diagnosis of failure to maintain a normal growth rate is not limited to organic conditions.

Table 14.2. Comprehensive feeding history

Presenting symptoms. Is the problem primarily one of food refusal, lack of interest, food selectivity, or disruptive behavior, or is it a combination? Is the appetite sufficient to support growth (i.e., is caloric intake sufficient)? Is the child growing satisfactorily? Does the child gag, cry, refuse to chew or swallow, or show lack of awareness or feeling of hunger?

Onset of feeding problems, age of the child, contributing factors. When did the problem begin? What else was happening in the child's life at the time? Inquire about changes in family structure, routine, illness, out-of-home care. Any history of physical or sexual abuse? Did the child experience a frightening episode (e.g., choking, with a feed)? Has anyone else in the family had eating difficulties or disorders (e.g., anorexia nervosa)?

Changes in feeding problems over time. Are there some foods or liquids that the child previously accepted but now refuses? Has there been a change in appetite? What feeding milestones have been achieved (bottle, cup, solid food, feeds self)?

Feeding environment. Who primarily feeds or eats with the child? Where does the child eat (lap, infant seat, high chair, couch, floor, TV table)? Is the child overstimulated while eating (i.e., too much noise, activity, talking)? Describe the typical meal schedule (time of day).

Mealtime habits. How regularly does the child eat? What is the child's "style" of eating: Rapid? Slow? Picky? What foods does the child usually accept or reject? How much does the child feed him or her self?

Parent expectations, response, and feeding techniques. What do the parents think the child should be doing? How is that different from what is occurring? How did they develop this expectation? What strategies have been tried to solve the problem? Does the caregiver coax, praise, offer rewards or bargain with the child to eat? Does the caregiver distract the child with toys or allow the child to eat almost continuously throughout the day in order to get the child to "eat enough" (grazing)?

---

3. **Central nervous system.** Look for hyper- or hypotonicity, seizures, integrity of the suck-swallow mechanism, microcephaly, prematurity.

C. An assessment of the **parent–child interaction** ("dyadic fit"), especially **around feeding.** For most feeding problems encountered in young infants, observing a feeding in the office is extremely useful to the diagnosis and treatment. Integrity and proficiency of the infant's suck-swallow abilities, adequacy of milk production in breast-feeding mothers, and quality of the infant–mother interaction can be readily assessed. The characteristics of specific concerns ("spitting"

Table 14.3.   Comprehensive sleeping history

Presenting symptoms. What is the total number of hours of sleep the child receives in a 24-hour period, and how is the time divided into naps and nighttime? Does the child refuse to be put to bed or does the child wake up frequently during the night? Do the parents report snoring or symptoms of sleep apnea? Is the child tired and irritable during the day? Is the child ill?

Onset of sleeping problems, age of the child, and contributing factors. When did the problem begin? Any previous episode of similar problems? Has anything changed in the child's life: Family structure, new siblings, routine, illness, out-of-home care? Any history of physical or sexual abuse?

Changes in sleeping problems over time. Has the child ever slept through the night without difficulty? If so, when? For how long? Are the child's sleep cycles now, or were they ever, regular and predictable?

Sleep environment. Is the home and neighborhood sufficiently quiet for the child to fall asleep? Is it safe enough?

Establishment of good sleep hygiene. Is the child put to bed awake? Is the child fed during the night? Where does the child sleep? Does the child sleep in his or her own bed?

Parental expectations and response. Are bedtime and bedtime expectations appropriate to the age of the child? Are there other problems with the child's behavior which the parents report? Are parents able to set limits, teach discipline, develop consistent patterns of expectation? Does the infant's sleep schedule conform to the family's schedule in a socially appropriate way? What have the parents tried to do to solve the problem: Bringing the baby into their bed, rocking the baby to sleep, allowing the child to fall asleep on the couch, and then putting the child to bed?

---

vomiting, choking) may be observed and discussed with the mother. When a sleep problem exists, observing the interaction is also helpful to assess the comfort of the parent in holding the baby and soothing the baby; and whether separation problems exist. It is also helpful to inquire what other sources of information or assistance the caregiver has sought and found useful (or not useful) in dealing with the sleeping or feeding problem. Answers provide insight into the family support system and the child-rearing beliefs.

V.   **Triage assessment and treatment planning**
   A.   **General issues.** Mild feeding and sleeping problems are extraordinarily common in young children. The children appear healthy and happy, and are growing and developing well. The reported problem is not interfering substantially with either the child or the family's life. These mild problems (**perturbations**) are gener-

ally treated by the PCP with a combination of education, anticipatory guidance, support, and reassurance. Problems of more moderate difficulty (**disturbances**) can also be handled by the PCP, but require a specific treatment or intervention strategy and frequent follow-up and monitoring. Typically, these disturbances cause significant distress (physical, behavioral, or psychological) to the child or family, but are not interfering with the child's health or development. In severe cases (**disorders**), the problem is clearly interfering with the child's health and, usually, the family functioning. The child has signs of failure to maintain a normal growth rate or has lost weight, or the family exhibits signs of extreme distress or discord. Treatment of these problems requires a multidisciplinary approach with cooperation between experts in early childhood development, child and family mental health, and often medical experts from the fields of neurology, otolaryngology, or gastroenterology, and related healthcare professions. This is generally best accomplished by referral to a specialist (e.g., feeding or sleep disorders) clinic with expertise in this area. If these outpatient services are not readily available and the child's health is at risk, hospitalization for initial assessment, stabilization, and treatment may be recommended.

VI. **Feeding**
   A. **Watching**
      1. **When to watch (perturbation)**
         a. Symptoms are mild or of brief duration (lasting less than 30 days). Examples include:
            1. The baby "spits up a lot"
            2. The baby seems "gassy"
            3. The toddler "is a picky eater," or "won't eat vegetables (fruit)"
            4. The toddler who "doesn't eat enough"
         b. Growth rate is normal or exceeding expectations
         c. Physical examination is normal
         d. Parents not distressed or only mildly distressed
         e. Absence of additional risk factors (e.g., maternal depression, attachment disorder)
      2. **What to do when watching**
         a. **Psychoeducation of parents**
            (1) **Reassure the parents about the child's health.** It is important to review the growth chart with parents and demonstrate to them that, although their concern is taken seriously, the child's health and well-being is not in danger. Making a follow-up appointment further reassures parents by letting them know that their concern will not be

forgotten or ignored. This often decreases parental anxiety enough to interrupt the development of more serious difficulties.

(2) **Educate about developmental variation.** Babies all develop in different ways, and frequently **not** "according to the book." Maturation and integration of the various neurologic pathways involved in eating takes differing amounts of time in babies. This is normal!

(3) **Accentuate the positives.** Always point out emerging and developed skills or achieved milestones. This further decreases parental anxiety, a major factor in many eating problems.

(4) **Encourage the parents to work together to solve any problems.** Consistency in approach among caregivers and commitment to regular schedules are important for the development of healthy eating patterns.

(5) **Review baby's diet.** If the symptoms are mild, it is generally **not** recommended to change formula or discontinue breast-feeding. Some breast-feeding infants will exhibit sensitivity to specific foods (often caffeine or dairy products) in the mother's diet, which can be given an elimination trial, if appropriate.

(6) **Explore parental concerns.** Understanding the source of parental anxiety is often helpful. This must be done in a way that does not diminish the parent, but rather as genuine curiosity or interest. Asking the parent "what do you worry will happen if this continues?" can be clarifying.

b. **Advocacy.** PCPs may offer to speak to spouse, grandparent, or daycare center staff.

c. **Psychotherapy** not indicated.

d. **Medication** not indicated.

e. **Laboratory and other evaluations.** If possible, a feeding is observed in the office. No laboratory testing is indicated.

f. **Monitoring.** The child should be given an appointment to return to the office within 4 to 8 weeks, to monitor weight gain, and family functioning. This also lets the family know that their concern is taken seriously. It is optimal if both parents come to this appointment.

B. Intervening further
  1. When to intervene further (disturbance)
    a. Symptoms are moderately severe or of longer duration (1 month to 3 months). Examples include:
      1. "The baby is always fussy" or "cries all the time"
      2. "The baby spits up everything she eats"
      3. "The baby is always hungry" or is described as "greedy"
      4. The older infant shows a lack of pleasure with eating or lack of appetite
      5. The toddler is "is frequently throwing food" or "won't sit at the table"
      6. The toddler "**drinks** more than she **eats**"
    b. Growth rate is normal or has decelerated **slightly.**
    c. Parents exhibit moderate degree of frustration, distress or worry.
    d. Additional risk factors may be present (parenting style or expectations are inappropriate to developmental age of the child, marital disagreement, or discord around parenting issues).
    e. Physical examination is normal.
  2. What to do when intervening
    a. Psychoeducation
      (1) Encourage parental teaming. To prevent a negative feeding cycle to persist or develop into a disorder, both parents must actively participate and support each other.
      (2) Nurture an emotionally neutral tone at mealtime. Often these situations have escalated into a battleground, which creates tremendous tension and exacerbates feeding problems. Instructing the parents to take an emotionally neutral stand with the child and to de-emphasize over involvement in the feeding process removes the emotional overlay that often accompanies mealtime struggles.
      (3) Provide instructions for **food rules** at mealtime:
        (a) All meals should be **regularly scheduled,** including snacks.
        (b) Meals should **last only 10 to 25 minutes,** depending on the child's behavior. If the child throws food, the meal should be terminated. If the child shows no interest after the first

5 minutes, the meal should be terminated. These techniques aim at promoting appetite.

(c) Meals should **take place in the same location,** with optimal seating for feeding and with no environmental distractions (no TV, radio, or toys). Offer **developmentally appropriate menu,** with appropriate portion size, and repeatedly offer new or less preferred foods.

(d) Emphasize appropriate education about children's caloric dependence on **adequate dietary fat** for optimal brain development.

(e) **Limiting fluids to after meals** and not **before** or **between** meals often increases a toddler's appetite. The Academy of Pediatrics recommends that children be weaned from the bottle after the age of 12 months. This strategy often eliminates excessive fluid intake. Cultural and personal preferences need to be considered to assure that this guideline is implemented flexibly.

(f) Parents should **attend and respond to the child's hunger and satiety cues and not force feed.** A bottle or food should only be presented if the child gives eye contact or opens his or her mouth. Meals should be pleasant and emotionally neutral, with minimal discussion of the child's eating or not eating.

Note: Inability to carry out these suggestions is frequently an indicator of family dysfunction or psychopathology and a referral to a feeding specialist is indicated. If the family is consistently following the rules and symptoms do not improve, an undetected physical problem may exist (often, mild gastroesophageal reflux).

      b. Advocacy. It is important to identify the social supports for the primary caregiver and to stress that no one person should be solely responsible for *all* the feedings (except in the case of breast-feeding infants in the first few months of life). A referral to a home health agency for visiting nursing services with pediatric expertise can be helpful to monitor weight gain and to provide education and support.

      c. Psychotherapy. A referral to a psychologist, social worker, or other mental health expert who specializes in early childhood behavior can be helpful to provide assistance with problems in parent–child interaction. Referral sources need to be able to recognize the presence of maternal depression as a contributing factor, which requires appropriate referral.

      d. Medications. No appetite stimulants are recommended for treating feeding disorders in infants. Some medications are known to interfere with appetite (antibiotics, cimetidine, ranitidine). Parents often inquire about the need for vitamins or **high-calorie supplements** (Pedia-Sure, Ensure). These **are not indicated for mild to moderate feeding problems** unless a specific deficiency is documented (e.g., anemia).

      e. Laboratory evaluation. Targeted laboratory investigation is indicated for signs or symptoms suggestive of a specific disease. For example, if the dietary history suggests a risk for anemia (usually excessive milk intake), obtain a hematocrit.

      f. Monitoring. Schedule appointments with specialists early in the course of treatment if a referral seems highly likely. Often, specialists' offices or clinics have a long waiting list and the appointment can be canceled if primary care treatment is successful. It is important that the primary caregivers (i.e., both parents) attend office visits if at all possible. This implies that the problem is important and that it requires more than one caregiver to be actively involved in its treatment.

C. Referring

   1. When to refer and transfer primary responsibility (disorder)

      a. Symptoms are severe or longstanding (>3 months), or interventions have failed

and symptoms are worsening. Examples include:
1. Complete food refusal
2. Severe mealtime struggles or food restriction

b. Growth rate has significantly decelerated, with evidence of FTT.

c. Parents unable or unwilling to comply with treatment plan or exhibit extreme distress

d. Abnormality on physical examination with respect to swallowing and sucking

2. **What to do when referring.** Generally, young children with severe feeding disorders require referral to a specialized feeding disorder clinic. If this is not available, the components of a feeding disorder clinic team need to be assembled. Typically, this team includes the following:

- Pediatric gastroenterologist
- Psychologist or child and adolescent psychiatrist
- Social worker
- Nutritionist
- Occupational or physical therapist
- Pediatric ear nose throat (ENT) specialist, for consultation

a. **Psychoeducation**

(1) **Prepare family for referral.** It is important to inform caregivers that referral to a specialist clinic requires an intense level of involvement for both the family and the physician. Most children require frequent weight checks—initially, at least weekly. The solution to the problem often involves collaborative problem-solving by the specialist and the family, with a trial-and-error treatment approach before the child begins to gain weight and responds to treatment. This will generally take a number of months and often progress does not occur in a straight line of improvement. The family or the specialist may call on the PCP for interval weight monitoring, and reinforcement of treatment approaches.

(2) **Destigmatize treatment** by suggesting that family or parent–child therapy often assists the caregivers in their efforts to read and respond to their children's signals.

(3) **Support the treatment** and monitor the situation. Helping the parents remain persistent in their

treatment efforts is crucial. Frustration can mount and, if it escalates, can lead to requests or demands for another referral.

(4) Monitor for signs of maltreatment. Although most feeding problems do not involve child abuse, some do, which requires the involvement of Child Protective Services or a commensurate agency.

b. Advocacy. Child Protective Services may need to be involved in some situations.

c. Psychotherapy. The feeding clinic or specialist often refers a family to a child mental health expert, preferably one with experience and competence in working with infants and younger children. General child mental health specialists often do not have experience with this population.

d. Medication. Currently, no medications are recommended to stimulate appetite. The specialty team may recommend calorie-dense foods and supplements (e.g., Pedia-Sure, Ensure), and vitamin supplements. Gastroesophageal reflux is often discovered and should be treated routinely, typically guided by the feeding clinic specialist.

e. Laboratory evaluation. Basic screening tests are helpful to assess nutritional status before referral to a feeding clinic. Tests include a complete blood count, basic metabolic panel, urinalysis, and thyroid function tests. If no organic cause is suggested, no further testing is recommended before referral. If the physical examination is abnormal, initiate targeted laboratory and radiologic evaluation.

f. Monitoring. During the referral period, the PCP should be involved with office follow-up visits in collaboration with the specialty clinic. The PCP may only need to see the patient every 3 or 4 months during treatment. When the patient is discharged from the specialist, the PCP should schedule visits more frequently to monitor weight gain and support continued treatment strategies in the home.

VII. Sleeping
  A. Watching
    1. When to watch (perturbation)
      a. Symptoms are mild (e.g., one episode of nighttime waking or refusal to go to bed per week) or of brief duration (<30 days)
      b. Physical examination is normal

2. **What to do when watching**
   a. **Psychoeducation**
      (1) **Review normal sleep expecta-tions for age, including preva-lence of sleep problems.** Discuss normal sleep requirements and pat-terns in children with parents.
      (2) **Articulate the benefits of attend-ing early to perturbations.** The goal is to prevent minor problems with falling asleep and nighttime waking from becoming patterns of behavior that persist and worsen.
      (3) **Review principles of sleep hy-giene.** The key to solving minor sleep problems in infants and toddlers is to educate and support caregivers in the establishment of good sleep hygiene. Good sleep hygiene involves:
         (a) A **regular schedule** of bed-times, naps, and morning wak-ing. This can be difficult for families to do consistently. Pediatricians need to be per-sistent in supporting consis-tency. Parents need to be in synch with each other regard-ing approach to sleep. If they cannot accomplish this with PCP coaching and support, they should be referred to a child mental health specialist.
         (b) A consistent **sleeping envi-ronment**—preferably a cool, dark room, and a bed or crib in a room separate from par-ents. Cultural considerations need to be taken into account here. It is important for the PCP to explain clearly the ra-tionale for sleeping in a sepa-rate room to avoid parents feel-ing misunderstood or merely criticized. Reassuring parents that this will not damage or harm their child may help.
         (c) A **regular** bedtime routine:
            • No vigorous activities in the hour before bedtime
            • Consistent soothing, calm-ing rituals (stories, bath)
            • No frightening TV, videos, or stories

- Child put to bed **awake,** from early infancy

(4) Use of **sleep aids** the child can control (pacifiers, thumb sucking, or transitional object; e.g., blanket, bunny). Children should **not use bottle feedings to fall asleep.** If the child has been accustomed to falling asleep while being fed, the caregiver should begin a very gradual decrease in the volume of feeding. The amount in the bottle can be decreased by 2 ounces every 2 days, until the bottle is discontinued completely and the child is put to bed awake. A transitional object can be introduced at this time, if this has not already occurred.

(5) **Strategies for waking.** See "When Intervening Further" for more detailed discussion of this. When the child awakens during the night (e.g., **night waking**), encourage parents to **wait** before making contact with the child. The child can be allowed to "cry it out" if the parents are comfortable with this or, alternatively, the time interval can start with a brief period (a minute) of waiting and gradually lengthening until the child falls back asleep on his or her own. For **night thrashing and terrors,** the child should **not** be awakened. The child is not awake during these episodes and awakening will exacerbate the problem. If left to him- or herself, the episode will run its course and the child will fall back asleep. If parents are uncomfortable leaving the child during this, they can stay close enough to observe the child, but should not intrude and awaken the child. For **sleep walking,** the same general principles apply, although the child's safety must be assured. This may require door alarms under some circumstances.

(6) When nightmares occur, parents should provide comfort and reduce precipitating daytime stress that could be contributing to nightmare frequency.

b. **Advocacy.** The PCP can offer to speak to all the caregivers responsible for caring for the child throughout the day (e.g., grand-parents, spouse, daycare center, partner) to discuss the importance of good sleep hygiene and open communication to prevent excessive daytime napping.

c. **Psychotherapy** is not necessary at this stage unless parents are unable or unwilling to consistently follow recommendations.

d. **Medications** are not indicated.

e. **Laboratory evaluation.** No medical workup is indicated for mild sleep difficulties, unless suggested by other signs and symptoms.

f. **Follow-up.** Telephone contact within 2 to 4 weeks to assess status of the problem. If improvement is noted, another phone contact can be arranged at increasing intervals. If no improvement is seen, a follow-up appointment should be made. Both parents should be expected to attend this appointment.

B. **Intervening further**
   1. **When to intervene further (disturbance)**
      a. Symptoms are moderate (e.g., child experiencing nighttime waking, tantrums, or stalling tactics at bedtime, up to four times per week) or the symptoms are of longer duration (at least 1 month).
      b. Caregivers have been unable to establish good sleep hygiene practices with PCP guidance and support.
      c. Family functioning is not significantly impaired.
   2. **What to do when intervening**
      a. **Psychoeducation**
         (1) **Review normal sleep patterns and expectations.** Explain normal sleep patterns and behaviors at all stages of development to parents before initiating a treatment plan. In addition, the PCP will need to identify all the caregivers involved with the child throughout the 24 hours of a day.
         (2) **Reinforce good sleep hygiene (as above)**
         (3) **Explain relationship between many sleep problems and separation issues, if appropriate.** Address the concept of sleep-onset associations and identify separation concerns. It is helpful to explain to caregivers that toddlers frequently resist being put to bed by making

frequent requests for parental attention (e.g., a drink, another trip to the bathroom, a kiss). Parents may acknowledge that it is often difficult to tell whether the needs are situationally based, anxiety based, or simply oppositional in nature.

(4) **Explore parental responses to problem.** Ask the parents what they believe is the cause of the problem and what strategies they have already tried to alleviate it. It can be helpful to ask them if they have received any advice from others (e.g., grandparents) on what they should do. Then ask what approaches they have tried and what the child's responses were, which allows you to better tailor responses and guidance. It can also help pinpoint where difficulties are arising.

(5) **Strategies for bedtime struggles and nighttime waking.** Treatment strategies vary widely and not all interventions will be therapeutic for all children and their families. Often, the PCP needs to discuss some or all of the following options with the family to decide what intervention will be most appropriate.

    (a) Use of a **sleep log** to identify the child's sleep patterns and the parents' responses. A sleep log is kept for each day of the week, documenting times the child is put to bed (naptime and nighttime), struggles and solutions attempted around settling issues, and nighttime waking (times and lengths of waking and parents' responses).

    (b) In young children, most bedtime refusal appears to be predominantly the result of fears or separation anxiety, and parents can begin a program of **gradual separation** from the child at nighttime. A chair (or mattress on the floor) can be placed in the child's room where the parent can quietly wait for the child to fall asleep. Over a period of a few weeks, the chair can be moved gradually closer to the door until it is no longer in the room.

(c) An alternate approach to addressing separation fears in young children is the widely recognized **Ferber method** (see *Suggested Readings*), which consists of the caregiver leaving the child awake in the bed, then checking on the child at regular intervals throughout the night. This method (desensitization) involves gradually and progressively lengthening the times of reentry in response to the infant's crying.

(d) For the **older child** who refuses to stay in bed, the caregiver should inform the child that the door will be closed until he or she gets into bed. When the child remains in bed, the door will be opened and will remain open if the child stays in bed. A night light is helpful to some children.

(e) For persistent night waking, when caregivers appear exhausted and frustrated, some experts recommend simply allowing the child to "cry it out" for several consecutive nights (i.e., reducing the positive reinforcement of a parent's presence in response to a child's crying). This approach generally results in the disappearance of night waking within a week. This technique can work for families who can remain neutral (i.e., avoid carrying out angrily, as a "punishment") and agree to make such a commitment. In cases where the child is likely to hurt self or persistently vomit, this strategy could lead to endangerment of the child and therefore should not be implemented).

(6) **An approach to sleep terror and sleep walking.** Elements of the approach to parasomnias include:

       (a) Unless arousals are persistent, special intervention is not necessary.

       (b) Children normally outgrow these episodes.

       (c) Reassurance and explanation for the child and family is usually adequate.

       (d) Brief 30- to 60-minute naps in the late afternoon may help to reduce stage IV NREM sleep later.

       (e) Parents should remain with the child to prevent possible self-injury.

       (f) Parents should not attempt to wake the child.

  b. **Advocacy.** Intervention is needed only if child maltreatment is suspected as a contributing factor to the sleep disturbance.

  c. **Psychotherapy.** At this stage, a referral to a mental health specialist is often helpful. If family dysfunction is interfering with establishing and maintaining a consistent treatment plan, a referral for family or marital counseling may be helpful. When problems occur because the *child* is unable to respond, refer to a child therapist experienced in treating sleep problems.

  d. **Medication.** Although medications can be helpful in the short-term treatment of sleep problems, most sleep experts do not recommend their routine use.

  e. **Laboratory evaluation.** A complete physical examination should be performed to rule out organic illness as a cause of the sleep disturbance. As noted, any condition that impairs respiration (e.g., enlarged tonsils or adenoids, acute upper respiratory infection, asthma) or causes pain or fever can disturb a child's sleep. If no medical condition is suspected, no further laboratory work is indicated.

  f. **Monitoring.** Regular (i.e., at least every 2 weeks initially) follow-up for infants and children with significant sleep problems is recommended. Much of this can be done through brief phone contacts. Sleep problems do not resolve easily or quickly, and caregivers benefit greatly from support and "coaching" by the PCP. A face-to-face appointment with both parents should be scheduled in 1 to 2 months, or fewer, if the family has been referred for mental health treatment.

C. **Referring**
1. **When to refer and transfer primary responsibility (disorder)**
   a. Symptoms of nighttime waking or bedtime refusal have been present at least five times a week, for at least 4 weeks.
   b. Caregivers are unable to implement the treatment recommendations, despite persistent PCP support over at least 3 months.
   c. Family is severely disrupted or is distressed because of the child's sleeping difficulties.
2. **What to do when referring**
   a. **Psychoeducation**
      (1) **Explain the rationale for the referral.** In addition to addressing the issues discussed in sleep disorders, explain the need for the involvement of experts in the fields of child development and mental health for children with severe sleep disruption problems. The family should be referred to a specialty sleep disorders clinic, if such is available. If not, then refer to a child mental health professional with expertise in this area. Most families will welcome expert assistance because sleep problems in children usually have a major impact on the health and well-being of all other family members.
      (2) **Be alert to signs of maltreatment.** Although most young children with sleep problems will not have a history of maltreatment, some will. Remain attentive to signs of child abuse or neglect and contact Child Protective Services or commensurate authority, if necessary.
   b. **Advocacy.** Contact the leader of the sleep disorder clinic or the individual therapist to whom the referral is being made, to facilitate the transition of care for the child and family. Explaining to the family that all relevant information regarding the diagnosis and previous therapeutic interventions will be discussed with the therapist should reassure them that you will remain actively involved in the management and treatment of the problem.
   c. **Psychotherapy.** Depending on the nature of the problem, individual or marital counseling may be helpful to parents. The role of

the PCP is to inform caregivers of this possibility. Experts who treat severe sleep disorders in young children can make referrals to adult mental health providers when maternal depression, marital discord, or other mental health issues in the family are identified as contributing to the child's sleep disturbance.

   d. **Medication** can be helpful on a short-term basis. However, most experts do not recommend use for longer than 2 weeks. Specific medications are discussed in the following section.

   e. **Laboratory evaluation.** Unless a specific organic cause for sleep disturbance is suspected (e.g., obstructive apnea), no laboratory testing is recommended before referral to a sleep disorder clinic.

   f. **Follow-up.** Close monitoring and follow-up are essential in the treatment of severe sleep disorders. Once the multidisciplinary team is managing the child's treatment, the PCP can follow on a less frequent basis, usually every 3 months with phone contact, and every 6 to 12 months for appointments.

VIII. **Practical use of medications**

   A. **Feeding problems**

   1. **Psychotropic medications should not be used** in the treatment of feeding disorders in infants and young children.

   2. Certain medications (notably macrolide antibiotics) can decrease appetite.

   3. **Nutritional supplements** (e.g., **Ensure, PediaSure**) are not routinely indicated unless a specific deficiency is discovered.

   4. Contributing conditions, most notably gastroesophageal reflux, should be treated routinely.

   B. **Sleeping problems.** Medications rarely have a role in the management of sleep problems in young children. First-line treatment includes behavioral interventions and establishing good sleep hygiene. On a short-term basis (not longer than 2 weeks), some experts recommend the use of sedating **antihistamines** (e.g., diphenhydramine 1 to 2 mg/kg) at bedtime for children who are experiencing **severe** bedtime struggles or night waking. It is important to advise parents that some children will experience agitation or arousal when given these medications. **Benzodiazepines,** at low doses, are also used in cases of severe parasomnias. Although **tricyclics** have also been used for parasomnias and enuresis, these medications should be used with great caution in younger children because of the risk to toddlers and small children of accidental overdose. Even seemingly "tiny" or innocuous overdoses in very young children have been associated with fatality. It is important to stress that these medications should be securely stored so young children do not have access to them. For children whose sleep disturbance is severe enough to use medication beyond a few weeks, it is recommended that the PCP enlist the assistance of a child and adolescent psychiatrist or other expert in early childhood sleep problems.

IX.   **Summary.** Feeding and sleeping problems, which often commonly present within the first 3 years of life, can potentially have serious consequences for both the child and the family. The core symptoms for feeding and sleeping disorders often impair state, growth, and parent–child relationships. Well-established diagnostic criteria exist for both feeding and sleep problems and careful assessment must consider both biologic conditions that can contribute to the problems and the nature of the child–parent relationship. Both problems can potentially have a severe impact on future emotional and social development and should be viewed from a transactional perspective. In most cases, feeding and sleep problems are often transitory, during the first 3 to 4 years, but without proper support and management they can develop into chronic problems or disorders.

SUGGESTED READINGS

Feeding Disorders

Behrman R, Kliegman R, Jenson H. *Nelson's pediatrics.* Philadelphia: WB Saunders, 2000:120.

Benoit D. Feeding disorders, failure to thrive, and obesity. In: Zeanah CH, ed. *Handbook of infant mental health,* 2nd ed. New York: Guilford Press, 2002:339–352.

Bleichfeld B. Contributing author to: Psychological aspects and behavioral issues in pediatric feeding. In: Arvedson JC, Brodsky L. *Pediatric swallowing and feeding,* 2nd ed. Albany, NY: Singular, 2002:563–605.

Chatoor I. Feeding and other disorders of infancy or early childhood. In: Tasman A, Kay J, Lieberman J, eds. *Psychiatry.* Philadelphia: WB Saunders, 1997: Chapter 37.

Manikam R, Perman J. Pediatric feeding disorders. *J Clin Gastroenterol* 2000;30(1):34–46.

Satter EM. The feeding relationship. In: Kessler, Dawson P, eds. *Failure to thrive and pediatric undernutrition: a transdisciplinary approach.* Baltimore: Paul H. Brookes, 1999:121–144.

Schwarz SM, Corredor J, Fisher-Medina J, et al. Diagnosis and treatment of feeding disorders in children with developmental disabilities. *Pediatrics* 2001;108(3):671–676.

Sleep Disorders

Anders TF, Eiben MS. Pediatric sleep disorders: a review of the past 10 years. *J Am Acad Child Adolesc Psychiatry* 1997;36:9–20.

Anstead M. Pediatric sleep disorder: new developments and evolving understanding. *Curr Opin Pulm Med* 2000;6(6):501–506.

Chess S, Thomas A. *Temperament in clinical practice.* New York: Guilford Press, 1986.

Dahl R. The development and disorders of sleep. *Adv Pediatr* 1998; 45:73–90.

Ferber R, Kryger M, eds. *Principles and practice of sleep medicine in the child.* Philadelphia: WB Saunders, 1995.

Stores G. Children's sleep disorders: modern approaches, developmental effects, and children at special risk. *Dev Med Child Neurol* 1999;41(8):568–573.

Winnicott D. *The maturational process and the facilitating environment.* New York: International Universities Press, 1965.

Parent Support Resources

Feeding and Nutrition

Macht J. *Poor eaters: helping children who refuse to eat.* New York: Plenum Press, 1990.

Satter E. *How to get your child to eat—but not too much.* Palo Alto: Bull Publishing, 1987.

Wilkoff W. *Coping with a picky eater.* New York: Fireside, 1998.

Sleep

American Academy of Pediatrics. Guide to your child's sleep. New York: David McKay, 1999.

Ferber R. *Solve your child's sleep problems.* New York: Simon and Shuster, 1985.

Mindell J. Sleeping through the night. New York: Harper Collins, 1997.

Web Sites

America On Line. The Health section leads to several accessible resources regarding feeding and sleep. Available at www.aol.com. Accessed on 6/20/02.

American Academy of Child and Adolescent Psychiatry. This site makes available Fact for Families Sheets on a variety of pediatric subjects including feeding and sleep problems. Available at www.aacap.org/. Accessed on 6/20/02.

Sleep Home Pages has extensive links and information regarding sleep and sleep disorders. Available at www.bisleep.medsch.ucla.edu/. Accessed on 6/20/02.

15 ♣ Learning Disorders

Mary Ellen Gellerstedt and Stephen W. Munson

I. **Background.** School performance is one of the most important aspects of the life of children and adolescents. Among the many factors relevant to a child's achievement in school are abilities, motivation, family support, educational opportunity, and the school environment. When any of these factors is amiss, a child's learning is negatively affected. Over the years, a particular set of children has been the focus of much attention. These are the children who, despite sufficient overall intelligence, motivation, family support, and opportunity, have significant problems learning in one or more academic areas. Although variability in natural aptitude between academic areas is common in a given child, for some this variability results in significant learning problems.

A. **Descriptors and definitions.** Educators and psychologists have designated these difficulties **learning disabilities.** Within schools and under the laws establishing special educational services, this is the label that is used. It is also the language with which most parents are familiar. On the other hand, neurologists often use the terms **dyslexia, dyscalculia, or dysgraphia** to describe these children. Problems exist with each of these labels:

- Stigmatization (**disability** implies a fixed deficit that may become embedded in self-concept; **dyslexia** "medicalizes" a variation of normal)
- Arbitrariness (learning disability is a legal or education term for which the definition varies from state to state, and at times, from school to school)
- Inflation of the state of our knowledge (**dyslexia** implies a precise and specific neurologic disorder that does not capture complexity or limitations in our knowledge base)

The *Diagnostic and Statistical Manual of Mental Disorders,* Fourth Edition, Text Revision (DSM-IV-TR), as well as the international ICD system, attempts to solve these problems by using the simple label "learning disorders." In this chapter, the term **learning disorders** refers to these problems, recognizing that others may be more comfortable using alternative labels. However, the primary care physician (PCP) should be familiar with the broad spectrum of labels.

School districts often use performance norms (e.g., the child's academic skill as measured by educational testing is at least 1.5 standard deviations below **grade** level expectation) to identify students to be labeled "learning disabled" and to receive special attention. A more flexible approach is to assess the child's overall ability (full scale IQ) and compare that ability with academic achievement. Thus, a child with an IQ of 140 who reads at or just below average would still be seen as having a learning disorder because reading ability is so far below the child's general potential. Although this is clearly an instance of a learning disorder, school districts often will not recognize or provide services for a student whose performance is not below the mean for age and grade. Similarly, a child with an IQ of 70 whose ability in reading is significantly below what is expected is also seen to have a learning disorder. However, this system also presents problems because children with lower IQ are often not evaluated for specific learning disorders because their learning problems are assumed to generally stem from poor ability. They, therefore, miss the opportunity for special services they so badly need.

DSM-IV definitions call for a discrepancy of two standard deviations below that which is expected, based on the child's age, schooling, or intellectual ability, combining many of the criteria noted above.

B. **Epidemiology of learning disorders.** Regardless of how these learning problems are defined, substantial agreement exists that the school experience of a large number of children is affected by learning disorders. Although prevalence of learning and language disorders varies among studied populations, it is generally estimated that from **10% to 20%** of children and adolescents experience a defined learning problem (Beitchman et al., 1997). The US Department of Education (1995) reports that more than **10% of children receive special education,** of which half experience learning disorders and about a quarter have language disorders. In general, studies have reported a higher incidence of learning disorders among boys, but this gender discrepancy may be the result of sampling errors.

Learning disorders often occur together, for example, reading disorders and spelling problems. Nearly **80% of all learning disordered children have a reading disability,** with or without other disorders in other areas of learning. Early language problems can predict later learning disorders, even when language eventually develops normally. Many children experience combined problems with reading, mathematics, and written expression.

Learning disorders also often occur together with other axis I DSM-IV disorders. As many as **50% of children with learning problems also experience one or more definable psychiatric disorder** (Cantwell and Baker, 1987). The most common comorbid conditions are (a) attention-deficit disorder, (b) depression and anxiety disorders, (c) Tourette's syndrome and (d) conduct disorder. Conversely, it is generally to be expected that children with conduct disorder and, somewhat less so with attention-deficit/

hyperactivity disorder (AD/HD), will have a learning disorder. Many individuals are fortunate to have talents in areas other than those affected by their disability, providing compensatory opportunity for achievement and self-expression.

C. **Information processing model of learning.** A useful framework for conceptualizing learning is an information-processing model. In this model, the processes underlying learning are broken down into three primary areas (Table 15.1) in which difficulties can arise:

1. **Input:** the brain's ability to receive information from the environment
2. **Processing:** the interpretation, storage, organization, and integration of information received
3. **Output:** the expression of what is perceived and understood

1. **Input disorders** are the result of disturbed function at the level of central nervous system perception of sensory input.
2. **Processing disorders** are the result of interference with the organization and interpretation of sensory information. This involves a complex sequence of events. The primary sensory cortex interprets raw input, which must then be sorted or filtered from irrelevant stimuli. The sorted information must then be held in active working memory and meaning must be assigned. Relevant associations and memories related to previous knowledge must be retrieved from long-term memory and new combinations of information constructed. These must then be

Table 15.1.   Examples of learning disabilities in the information processing model

Input disabilities
    Visual perception disability
    Auditory perception disability
    Tactile dysfunction
    Vestibular dysfunction
    Kinesthetic dysfunction

Processing disabilities
    Short-term memory deficits
    Active working memory deficits
    Long-term memory storage deficits
    Abstraction deficits
    Executive function (organizational) deficits
    Planning deficits

Output disabilities
    Motor or Coordination deficits
    Speech and expressive language deficits

stored in long-term memory. Appropriate output must be planned, including gross and fine motor behavior, language, and kinesthetic and nonverbal communication. Dysfunction at any point in this sequence can result in a processing disability.

3. **Output disorders** result from dysfunction in systems of expression and include such problems as expressive language dysfunction and speech articulation problems.

The **ability to pay attention influences each of the steps in the process of learning.** Disorders and experiences limiting the capacity for sustained attention (e.g., AD/HD, anxiety disorders, depressive disorders) will affect the efficiency of learning.

D. **The major types of learning disorders.** The DSM-IV describes three types of learning disorders: reading disorder, disorder of written expression, and mathematics disorder.

1. **Reading disorder.** Professionals refer to this disorder using any of the following terms:
   - Learning disability in reading comprehension
   - Dyslexia
   - Developmental dyslexia
   - Learning disability in phonologic processing
   - Language or auditory-based learning disability
   - Specific reading disability

   Nuanced differences exist between these terms, but substantial overlap occurs. Because school is where reading is a required skill, these disorders are most often discovered after a child begins school. About **4%** of children experience reading disorders (Kavale and Forness, 1995).

   Most reading disorders are the result of problems with **phonologic awareness,** or the ability to decode word sounds rapidly and accurately, and can be thought of as coexisting with a phonologic language problem (see below). When these children misspell, one can usually not discern the meaning by sounding out the word. They either have the whole word learned (by rote memory) or they are at a loss. As they read aloud, they either recognize the word or stumble helplessly. If read to, however, it becomes apparent that **comprehension is intact** for these children.

   A few children experience reading and spelling problems related to an inability to visually recognize and decode groups of letters (i.e., whole words). Their phonologic skills are intact but they cannot see a word and rapidly decode it. To read, they must sound out groups of letters, which when heard aloud (or in their head) are decipherable to themselves. Hence, they can read slowly and haltingly by sounding out what they see. Similarly, they often have trouble spelling, although their misspellings are understandable (e.g., kat for cat).

Parents and educators often refer to reading problems as examples of **dyslexia.** The term "dyslexia" is problematic. Literally, the term describes some dysfunction associated with reading. However, various models of learning would assign the term dyslexia to very different neurologic processes. A popular misconception is that most reading problems are secondary to some form of difficulty with visual perception. According to this concept, dyslexia involves a child's inability to sort or retain visual cues, resulting in an inability to distinguish letters. This view has led to a fad treatment focused on optical retraining. On the other hand, whereas most reading problems are secondary to phonologic dysfunction, a tendency exists to overlook those problems related to the ability to recognize and recall complex visual signals. A few children with reading problems have difficulty with visual perception. They have difficulty developing a sight word vocabulary and may have persistence of letter reversal beyond a developmentally appropriate age. Thus, reading difficulties (dyslexia) are the result of many possible dysfunctional pathways, some of which are directly related to language processing (phonologic awareness) and some are not.

Although it is clear that **reading to young children** has a beneficial effect on the development of vocabulary and information about the world, the effect of this early experience on the **development of the ability to read is small.** No evidence indicates that early reading experiences will prevent or correct reading disorder. However, evidence suggests that **early training in phonologic processing** (i.e., practice in making the connection between the written letters and their associated sounds) can make a difference in long-term outcome for children with a phonologic disorder.

Appropriate **remedial intervention** depends on expert diagnosis of the type of reading and spelling problems present. Special attention can then be paid to teaching the child adaptive skills as well as challenging the disability with practice sessions to maximize the abilities that are present. Remedial approaches generally include a combination of phonetic practice, holistic comprehension instruction, and teaching of cognitive

learning strategies (self-monitoring, predicting, rehearsing by reviewing what is learned).
2. **Mathematics disorder.** Professionals refer to this disorder using any of the following terms:
   - Learning disability in mathematics
   - Dyscalculia or developmental dyscalculia
   - Nonverbal learning disability
   - Learning disability in sequential reasoning
   - Visual-perceptual learning disability

   Prevalence of mathematics disorder ranges from **1% to 6%,** with girls possibly slightly outnumbering boys (AACAP, 1998, 46S–62S). In first grade, children with this disorder demonstrate problems in retrieving basic arithmetic facts and using numbers. By the beginning of third grade, most children can count and put together numbers with groups of objects these numbers represent. They also can arrange numbers in the correct order and know which numbers are greater and smaller than others. Children with mathematics disorder have trouble retrieving facts and use inefficient strategies to solve the problems their peers solve with ease. Some know their mathematics facts but cannot manipulate numbers to answer questions about them or solve problems. Similarly, many children with this disorder have a hard time with spatial reasoning and with understanding mathematics concepts.

   The long-term effect of special education strategies for this disorder is not known. In general, the **course is life-long.** As with reading disorders, the strategies usually include a combination of teaching alternative skills (including the use of calculators and computers) and challenging the disability with remedial exercises to maximize the ability that is present.
3. **Disorder of written expression.** Of the disorders of learning, the least is known about disorders of written expression. Children with these difficulties have trouble **composing written texts.** Their written work appears to lack organization, with frequent grammatical and punctuation errors. Spelling errors and poor handwriting are common associated problems, but this diagnosis should not be given to those who have only these difficulties. This disorder should also be distinguished from fine motor coordination problems, which may not be associated with the organizational, "executive functioning" difficulties found in disorders of written expression. This disorder is commonly **found in association with reading disorder, mathematics disorder, or both.** The difficulties are usually

apparent by second grade. As children become older, difficulties taking notes becomes a prominent concern. This can be especially problematic in high school and college. Accommodations (e.g., using a computer or prepared lecture notes) are frequently helpful at that point. Little is known about its prognosis, although the **course is often lifelong.** Early intervention strategies generally involve repetitive, direct instruction following sequential, small steps.

E. **Another way to think about learning disorders.** School personnel and educational psychologists often talk about learning disabilities in terms of verbal and nonverbal skill deficits, related to testing results of standardized intelligence tests (Wechsler Intelligence Scale for Children [WISC-III], Wechsler Preschool and Primary Scale of Intelligence [WPPSI]).

1. **Verbal or language-based learning disorders.** Language disorders are included in the DSM-IV as one of five communication disorders. Prevalence rates depend largely on the definition of the type of language disorder studied, and range from **1% to 13%** of populations studied (Cantwell and Baker, 1991; Myers and Hammill, 1992).

Language is the medium through which most information is taught in schools. If a child has basic difficulties with language, it is expected that he or she will be at **great risk for specific learning disabilities.** Just as numerous types of language difficulties (e.g., phonologic or articulation, expressive, expressive-receptive and pragmatic) are seen, so can be seen numerous associated types of learning disability. It is helpful to think of language based-learning disabilities in a more descriptive way.

a. **Phonologic awareness** refers to the ability to discern the most basic sounds of a language, which blend together to make a word. In reading, this would correspond with the ability to assign sounds to symbols and blend those sounds into words. Children with good phonologic awareness usually have good receptive and expressive language ability. **Early indicators** that a child might have difficulty with phonologic awareness can include **difficulty with rhyming** (e.g., anticipating the next word in a nursery rhyme or Dr. Seuss-type book), persistence of **phonemic substitution and deletion** beyond developmentally appropriate age, and difficulty with **rapid naming** of pictures. During early elementary school, this may manifest as difficulty mastering sound and symbol relationships and developmentally inappropriate difficulty decoding words. As a child gets older, the decoding difficulty may interfere with comprehension and reading rate.

b. **Language-based learning disorder** would reflect a more pervasive problem with understanding language or formulating output. A child with this difficulty will have trouble understanding verbal instruction and with listening and reading comprehension. These children may also have difficulty with written expression. Children with **central auditory processing disorder** would be in this category. The PCP should monitor the academic progress of children with diagnosed speech and language delays.

c. **Pragmatic language delay** indicates that the child has excessive difficulty with the social and communicative function of language. Such children may have deferred eye contact and difficulty with social skills, monitoring the listener, and appreciating another's point of view. This combination of language problems and social difficulties must be differentiated from syndromes in the autistic spectrum (see Chapter 17).

2. **Nonverbal learning disorders.** Although language is typically thought to be predominantly a left hemispheric function, some learning disorders are associated with more traditional right hemispheric functions such as **spatial awareness, recognition of visual patterns, and coordination of motor patterns.** A child with a nonverbal learning disorder may show relative weakness in performance IQ cognitive testing. Such an individual may show any combination of difficulties in the following areas:

a. **Handwriting difficulties** can result from poor visual perception and spatial planning as well as from difficulty with fine motor execution. Handwriting samples may show inconsistent size and shape of letters and poor spacing between words. These children can have much difficulty copying from the blackboard. Mathematics problems requiring that digits be in the correct column can be problematic.

b. **Arithmetic difficulties** reflecting problems with understanding spatial concepts and relationships

c. Inability or difficulty in understanding information presented in a visual format, such as maps and graphs

   d.   Social skills deficits reflecting difficulty interpreting social space, body language, and nonverbal behavior of others

   Because of the combination of learning problems and social skills deficits, these disorders can be confused with autistic spectrum disorders. Indeed, some research has indicated considerable overlap between these syndromes. However, children with nonverbal learning disorders typically have solid interpersonal relationships and do not show the perseverative and obsessive behaviors commonly associated with autistic spectrum disorders.

F.   Etiology. For those children who have significant learning disorders, learning problems tend to have a **genetic or congenital origin.** Central nervous system insult (e.g., encephalitis or meningitis, fetal alcohol exposure, and traumatic brain injury) can also leave a residue of learning handicaps. For reading disorders, a familial risk exists among **first-degree relatives** of **35% to 45%** (Pennington, 1995). Twin studies have indicated a genetic factor in the cause of both reading and mathematics disorders. About 50% of siblings of children with identified mathematics disorder also experience this disorder (Shalev and Gross-Tsur, 2001).

G.   Natural history of learning and course of learning disorders. Patterns and rates of learning vary widely among normal children. Some children who have not developed two-word sentences by their second birthday will go on to experience significant language-based learning problems later in their development, whereas most others will soon thereafter explode into a barrage of language and show no problems with learning. Similarly, although some children who cannot read by the end of first grade will later experience significant learning disabilities, most will acquire a useful ability to use written language for learning. The learning process for every child involves a developmental interaction between the growing child's mind and brain, and environmental stimulation.

   Learning problems are usually **life long** with ongoing and changing need for adaptation as development proceeds. Other life skills beyond academic learning are often affected, especially those related to social relationships. Because school is such an important part of a child's life, learning disabilities often have a profound impact on self-esteem, which in turn interferes with the child's motivation to face and adapt to learning problems. Despite this, many individuals with learning disorders have had successful lives, by any measure.

A successful outcome depends on several factors:
1. Early recognition and intervention
2. High motivation in the family and the child
3. Appropriate understanding of the individual's strengths and limitations
4. Appropriate school programs to address special needs
5. Realistic matching of ability, achievement, and eventual career choice

H. Differential diagnosis. Many conditions and behaviors can influence the child's ability to learn. These must be considered when evaluating a child whose learning performance is below expectation. Factors to be considered in the differential diagnosis include:
1. Visual and hearing problems
2. Frequent school absence
3. Distraction based on stressful home or school environment
4. Overall low cognitive ability
5. Primary psychiatric disorder (Table 15.2)
6. Seizure disorder
7. Medication side effects
8. Traumatic brain injury

II. Practical office evaluation. The PCP does not need to be able to diagnose a specific learning disorder or create remedial education plans. However, the PCP is often in an excellent position to screen for possible learning problems.
   A. Presenting problems that may alert the PCP to the presence of a learning disorder are:
   - Early speech and language delays in a child with a family history of reading problems
   - History of nonacademic developmental delays in preschool
   - School-related somatic symptoms
   - Teacher questions of AD/HD
   - Frustration and externalizing behavior in school or related to school work
   - Increasing anxiety, especially related to school or academic work
   - Symptoms of depression
   - Dislike of school; school avoidance or refusal

Table 15.2. Primary psychiatric disorders interfering with learning

Attention deficit disorder
Mood disorders: Depression, cycling mood disorders
Anxiety disorders: Obsessive-compulsive disorder, separation anxiety disorder, generalized anxiety, posttraumatic stress disorder
Oppositional and conduct disorders
Psychotic disorders: Early onset schizophrenia (rare)

- Parental concern about child's learning
- Discrepancy in achievement among school subjects

General screening during well-child visits should include questions about school attendance, satisfaction, and sense of achievement. **Parental concerns** about school or academic performance should always be **taken seriously** and investigated further (Glascoe, 2000). **Review of a report card** from the past academic year would also be helpful. If the PCP has determined that problems with reading or mathematics exist, it may be useful to **ask the child to read aloud or perform simple arithmetic tasks** appropriate for age.

Once difficulties in school have been determined, consider and rule out conditions that can be contributing to learning problems. See above section on comorbid conditions and differential diagnosis.

B. **Beyond screening: specific questions**
  1. **For the child**
     a. What are your favorite parts of school?
     b. What are you really good at?
     c. What are your least favorite parts of school?
     d. Is there any part of school that is especially hard?
     e. When you have trouble finishing your work, what is going on for you—is the work too hard? Are you having trouble concentrating? Are you thinking about something else? Do you understand what you are supposed to do? Are you worrying about how well you will do? Are you worrying about something else?
     f. Who is your best friend at school? Who do you play with at recess? Who do you sit with at lunch? Do you get invited to other kids' houses? Do you get teased very much at school? About what?
     g. If one thing could change that would make school a lot better for you, what would it be?
  2. **For the parents**
     a. What do you think the problem is? Help the parent clarify whether the issues seem to be reading, reading comprehension, language comprehension and processing, graphomotor skills, mathematics skills, or other specific problems.
     b. How does homework go at your house? Ask questions about routines, who helps with homework; if a global problem with homework exists or if the problems are related to a specific task (e.g., reading or writing).
     c. Is the child showing school avoidance behaviors such as somatic complaints?

   d. Is the child's mood different on school days versus non-school days?
   e. Is there a family history of learning difficulties?
   f. Are there indications of problems with anxiety, attention, mood?

3. **Information from the school**
   a. Copies of school assessments of learning abilities and achievement. Children in most states are now required to take **standardized, group-administered tests of achievement,** results of which can supplement individual report cards and teacher comments (e.g., California Achievement Test, Stanford Achievement Test, and the Terranova tests).
   b. Copies of **individually administered tests of ability and achievement,** if they have been performed by the school. IQ and wide range achievement tests are used by school districts to determine the presence of learning disabilities and copies of these tests should be reviewed if they have been administered (see Chapter 7 for complete description of tests and their interpretation).
   c. Copies of **Individualized education plans (IEP)** or **504 plans** should be reviewed if the schools have already determined the presence of a learning disability and have an educational plan in place (see Chapter 7 for detailed description of these documents and their uses).
   d. **Narrative summaries by teachers** and other school personnel are useful for gaining an overall impression of the nature of the problems the child may be experiencing.
   e. **Standardized rating forms** completed by parents and teachers can be useful in screening for comorbid conditions including AD/HD or mood disorders. Broad screening instruments would include the Achenbach **Child Behavior Checklist** (there are separate forms for both parents and teachers) or the **Behavior Assessment System for Children.** Screening instruments specific for AD/HD include the Conners Teacher Rating Form, the Vanderbilt forms, ADDES (attention deficit disorders evaluation scale), and others (see Chapter 12).

C. **Physical examination and laboratory evaluations.** Although the physical examination is usually within normal limits, certain minor findings are more frequent in children with learning disabilities. At this time, **neuroimaging techniques are only used in**

research settings and are not indicated for clinical assessment or management. Therefore, the PCP should emphasize the following:

1. Is there a problem that can be treated?
   a. **Sensory abilities:** careful screening for visual acuity and hearing
   b. Evidence for **seizure** activity
   c. Signs of **thyroid disorder**
   d. Evidence of **medication side effects**
   e. Sleep apnea or **sleep disorder**
2. Are there physical findings consistent with a learning disorder?
   a. **Neurologic soft signs:** minor neurologic signs that persist beyond a developmentally appropriate age are frequently noted in children with learning disabilities, including synkinesia, motor overflow, motor clumsiness, and mixed dominance. These do not need further workup, and are **not diagnostic, but can increase clinical suspicion.**
   b. Markers of **perceptual difficulties:** poor right-left distinction, difficulty imitating finger movements or gestures, difficulty catching and throwing a ball
   c. **Dysmorphic features** that can suggest specific syndrome (e.g., fetal alcohol syndrome [FAS], fragile X syndrome, Williams syndrome)
3. Are there physical issues that may require accommodation or that may interfere with test performance?
   a. **Specific fine motor problems** that may need accommodation (e.g., tremor that interferes with writing)
   b. Attention to **abnormal movements:** tics, chorea, athetosis, tremor

      PCPs may want to become skilled at administering a specific **neurodevelopmental assessment instrument** such as the Pediatric Extended Examination at Three (PEET), Pediatric Examination of Educational Readiness (PEER), Pediatric Early Elementary Examination 2 (PEEX2), and Pediatric Examination Educational Readiness At Middle Childhood 2 (PEERAMID 2) developed by Levine. Some may also wish to have a battery of academic screening tests in the office (see *Suggested Readings*) (Table 15.3).

III. **Triage assessment and treatment planning.**
   A. **General treatment planning.** Establishing a **supportive treatment alliance** with the patient and family is especially important in the diagnosis and treatment of children with learning disabilities. Be-

Table 15.3.   Academic screening tests

Questionnaire	Where to Obtain
Global assessment instruments	
Child Behavior Checklist, parent form (CBCL) and Teacher Report Form (TRF)	TM Achenbach University of Vermont 1 South Prospect Street Burlington, Vermont 05401
Behavior Assessment System for Children (BASC)	American Guidance Service 4201 Woodland Road Circle Pines, Minnesota 55014-1796
AD/HD questionnaires	
Conners Parent Rating Scale-Revised Conners Teacher Rating Scale-Revised Conners Abbreviated Parent-Teacher Questionnaire	Multi-Health Systems 908 Niagara Falls Boulevard North Tonawanda, New York 14120
ADD-H Comprehensive Teacher's Rating Scale (ACTeRS)	Metri Tech 111 North Market Street Champlain, Illinois 61820
Neurodevelopmental assessment tests	
Pediatric Extended Examination at Three (PEET) Pediatric Examination of Educational Readiness (PEER) Pediatric Early Elementary Examination (PEEx 2) Pediatric Examination of Educational Readiness at Middle Childhood (PEERAMID 2)	Educators Publishing Service 31 Smith Place Cambridge, Massachusetts 02138-1000 www.eps.com

cause the problems are chronic and express themselves in such an important part of the child's daily life, **children and families can easily become discouraged** and need ongoing support and encouragement. Every school year will present a new challenge, because the understandings developed between teachers, students, and their families need to be redeveloped in each new classroom. **Transitions between schools,** especially as children move from elementary to middle and high schools, are particularly stressful because the subtle adaptations to learning disabilities do not easily translate from one school's approach to another. The PCP is in a unique position to provide continuity of support and understanding through these transitions.

B.   **Watching**
1.   **When to watch.** It is appropriate to wait and watch if parents, school personnel, or the child have raised questions about learning or school

performance, but a review of the child's report cards and an interview with the child indicate consistent and expected performance accompanied by a positive adaptation to school environment and expectations. Certain predisposing factors predictive of later school performance problems warrant **particular attention:**

    a. **Preschool** history of **language disorder**

    b. **Preschool** history of **AD/HD**

    c. School-aged child with **difficulty naming letters** of alphabet and associating sounds with letters

    d. Elementary school child reported as **"slow reader"**

    e. **Positive family history of learning disability or AD/HD**

    f. **Neurologic impairment** (e.g., traumatic brain injury)

2. **When watching**

    a. **Psychoeducation**

        (1) **Educate parents about normal variability in learning.** Advise parents about possible differences between the child's inherent abilities and parental expectation of performance. Most parents wish for outstanding achievement, but only a few children have outstanding ability.

        (2) **Address homework concerns.** Assist parents with ways to be involved with homework and school activities that are supportive and encouraging but not intrusive or demanding.

        (3) **Foster appropriate school contact.** Encourage parental involvement with teachers and other school personnel to reach consensus about the child's abilities, special talents, and achievements.

    b. **Advocacy.** Children sometimes encounter teachers whose expectations of behavior, compliance, or academic achievement exceed a normal child's abilities. A PCP can encourage parents to advocate for their children in such circumstances by seeking consultation with school administrators or guidance personnel. Direct PCP involvement may be necessary in the form of written documentation or suggestions to the school. A timely telephone call can also be of assistance in the resolution of **teacher–pupil mismatch.**

    c. **Psychotherapy** is not necessary while watching.

    d. Medication is not necessary while watching.

    e. Laboratory and other evaluations are not necessary beyond that indicated by physical signs and symptoms.

    f. Monitoring and follow-up planning. Establish a timetable to review and reassess the child's adaptation to school and learning. Report cards are typically issued every 10 to 12 weeks. If parents remain concerned despite reassurance, a review of the next 12-week assessment will provide further reassurance and assist in evaluating subtle learning problems that may have been missed in the initial assessment. A brief meeting with the child and parent at this time will allow a reassessment of the child's ongoing adaptation as well as a restatement of assurance and preventive counseling.

C. Intervening further

  1. When to intervene further. When the screening interview with the child and parents and a review of school performance from the teacher reveal evidence of learning problems, it is time to become more actively involved in further exploring the problem and providing assistance for the child and family. Sometimes, learning disorders present as behavior problems, the child acting out frustration about the learning difficulties. Specific examples of problems warranting further investigation and intervention are:

    a. Preschool history of moderate to severe language disorder

    b. School-aged child with teacher reports of **poor early academic achievement** in one or more areas

    c. School-aged child with **mild behavior problems**

    d. School-aged child **identified by school as learning disabled**

    e. Academic performance at school or when doing **homework produces stress and conflict for child, family, or both**

  2. When intervening further. The PCP is seldom in a position to treat learning problems directly. However, a careful investigation of contributory medical, social, and psychological factors is an important part of the treatment of learning disabilities. Furthermore, advocacy for children with learning disorders is important throughout their education and in planning for their occupational future.

a. **Psychoeducation**
   (1) **Educate about the Committee on Special Education (CSE) process.** When parents first encounter the need for special approaches to education for their child, they need clear and concise information about the processes by which their children's special needs will be met (see Chapter 7 for information about federal laws guaranteeing educational opportunities for all children and the processes by which parents and children gain access to them).
   (2) **Recognize the child's need for psychological support.** Children with learning disorders need extra support and encouragement in their approaches to school and learning. Parents must be helped to understand that the child's aversion to homework or school is not simply noncompliance or laziness, but a natural response to frustration and lack of efficacy. Parents can work together with teachers to develop approaches to homework and remedial work that are consistent with the child's ability and, therefore, more rewarding of the child's efforts.
   (3) **Address parental guilt.** Parents often feel guilty about any problem or perceived defect in their children. They must be helped to see that they did not "cause" this problem in their child.
   (4) **Encourage the parents' emotional neutrality with the child.** Many children with learning disorders have parents with the same or similar disabilities. These parents may feel shame, anxiety, or anger about their own educational experiences. As a result, they can have difficulty approaching their children's learning in an emotionally neutral way. Their emotional reactions can complicate the child's approach to learning. Supportive education in a nonjudgmental style can help the parents understand the differences between their own experiences and the opportunities they can give their child.

(5) Learning disorders are a **life-long problem.** Parents and children must be educated about the **patience and persistence** needed to achieve long-term goals. In addition, the PCP should have parents ascertain that a **transition plan** is included in the child's IEP beginning in early high school to ensure appropriate adaptation when the student leaves the secondary school system.

(6) Many **fad treatments** promising miraculous improvement in learning are available to parents and teachers through the internet and printed media. The PCP's familiarity with these fads and the scientific evidence for or against their efficacy can help families choose appropriate strategies to help their children (Silver, 1995). Examples of fad treatments lacking in scientific evidence for efficacy are:

- Optometric visual training
- Chiropractic applied kinesiology
- Megavitamins
- Food additive or preservative-restricting diets
- Allergy desensitization
- Patterning treatment ("Doman-Delacato" treatment)

b. Advocacy. Developing an effective approach to meeting the needs of children with learning disorders should be done by a **multidisciplinary team** including parents, the student, school psychologists, counselors, special education teachers, and administrators. Because of their long-term relationships with children and their families, PCPs can play an important advocacy role as members of this team. Specifically, the PCP's advocacy might include the following:

(1) Because schools are required to assess children's abilities and achievement in a timely manner, the PCP can assist parents who are meeting resistance from busy and sometimes overwhelmed school testing services by directly contacting special education school personnel to bring the needs of the child to their attention.

(2) By sending written documentation regarding the student, the PCP can assist teachers and administrators in their advocacy for increased services for children in their care.

(3) The PCP can refer parents to private clinicians and clinics specializing in assessment and educational planning and advocacy.

(4) The PCP can help the family access community agencies or support groups with specific expertise in learning disabilities.

c. **Psychotherapy**

(1) Many PCPs maintain **extended office visits** in their schedules to counsel children and their families. It is useful to have supportive contacts with parents to assist them with their understanding of the nature of learning problems and relieve feelings of guilt, grief, at the loss of the image of "the perfect child." Similarly, individual meetings with children are appropriate to assist them with their understanding of the nature of their problems in school and to encourage self-esteem and self-advocacy.

(2) Many **schools offer supportive individual and group counseling** to assist learning disabled children with approaches to learning and social skills.

(3) **Behavior modification** systems can be helpful to assist children with structuring their approaches to remedial homework that can be both arduous and emotionally taxing.

(4) Some children require further mental health intervention beyond the PCP's expertise and should be referred for collaborative care by mental health specialists (see section on referral).

d. **Medication.** No medications are specifically useful for learning problems. However, **many children have comorbid (AD/HD)** that complicates their adaptation to their learning difficulties. Stimulant medications can be helpful in these circumstances (see Chapter 12). Other comorbid conditions likely to interfere with adaptation to learning difficulties that respond to medications include depressive and other (bipolar) mood disorders, and anxiety disorders (see chapters 11 and 16, respectively, for more details about medications).

e. **Laboratory and other evaluations.** In those instances in which toxic exposure (e.g., lead exposure) or other medical problem has contributed to the learning problem, follow up with appropriate laboratory measures is indicated.

f. **Monitoring.** When a learning problem warranting intervention has been suspected or diagnosed, keep in close contact with the family at important points in the process, such as:

   (1) **After a CSE** or other school planning **meeting,** to help the family understand the conclusions of the meeting and to confirm the appropriateness of the plan

   (2) After a **new or updated IEP** is in place for an academic quarter to assess the progress of the student in response to the plan

   (3) At the **conclusion of an academic year** to assess the overall effectiveness of the strategy. Scheduling annual medical assessment at this time can make this assessment efficient and keep it in context of normal developmental assessment.

D. **Referring**

   1. **When to refer and transfer primary responsibility.** Several major circumstances warrant referral to specialists:

      a. Learning disability is **incidental to co-morbid psychiatric condition**

      b. Development of **school refusal** in child with learning disability

      c. **School and parents do not agree on the presence of a learning disability**

      d. **School and parents do not agree on needed services**

      e. Learning disability identified, but the child is making **unsatisfactory academic progress** despite intervention

      f. **Family is unable to accept learning disability diagnosis** and scapegoat child

      g. Major **concerns exist about transition to adulthood**

   2. **When referring.** Even when a referral to a mental health or learning disability specialist has been made, the PCP should remain a part of the assessment and planning team, providing continuity and an objective point of view.

a. **Psychoeducation**
   (1) **Destigmatize mental health re-ferral.** Children with learning dis-orders often experience a sense of stigma and social exclusion. Refer-ral to mental health specialists can add to this sense of being different and "crazy." Parents and children need supportive and reassuring edu-cation about the nature of contact with these specialists.
   (2) **Explain clearly to the family the reasons for referral.** Refer-ral should include a statement of the goals of the referral in rela-tion to the diagnosed learning dis-orders. Clear explanations of the interaction between learning and emotional and behavioral disorders can assist parents in the develop-ment of approaches to planning for their children.
b. **Advocacy**
   (1) Direct verbal and written contact with the professional or agency to which the family is referred is es-sential to clarify the goals and ex-pectations of the consultation and treatment.
   (2) When disagreement occurs with the school about the diagnosis or needed services it may be helpful to refer to a professional well versed in learning problems (e.g., develop-mental pediatricians, child psychol-ogists, or child neuropsychologists). These individuals generally have the greatest expertise in evaluating and advocating for children with learning disorders. When this still fails to bring resolution, parents may need to retain an attorney or education advocate to assist in set-tling the differences.
   (3) When the learning problems are com-plicated enough to require referral to specialists, parents and school usually need more than the usual encouragement to persist and remain engaged.
   (4) Some children and adolescents with learning disorders develop associated oppositional and conduct disorders. Families may need external support

to maintain discipline and can benefit from referral to family court (see
Chapter 9).

c. **Psychotherapy**
(1) Certain learning problems contribute
to problems with social skills development. Time-limited **social skills
groups** can be helpful and are often
available in school settings.
(2) If the child's learning problems have
become an unhealthy and inappropriate preoccupation for the family,
referral for **family-oriented therapy** is appropriate.
(3) **Individual supportive and dynamic therapies** can assist with the
development of self-advocacy, expression, and esteem.

d. **Medications.** As above, the approach to
prescription of medication is toward allevi-
ation of symptoms of comorbid conditions
that interfere with learning and general
adaptation.

e. **Laboratory and other evaluations.**
None necessary beyond those required for
comorbid medical conditions.

f. **Monitoring**
(1) When a referral to a specialist has
been made, follow-up with the family after the first visit to make sure
the consultation has occurred and is
proceeding as planned.
(2) Schedule a **review** of the success
of the program **after the plan has
been in place for enough time
to assess its effectiveness (8 to
12 weeks) and after an academic
year** has passed to reassess progress
(end of the school year).
(3) Just as the PCP appreciates a call or
written summary of the care of the
specialist, specialists appreciate a call
or written follow-up contact with the
referring doctor to maintain collaborative contact.

IV. **Practical use of medications.** No medications are specifically helpful in the treatment of learning disorders. As
noted, **comorbid conditions (e.g., AD/HD, depression)
can and should be treated** as outlined in the chapters
on those subjects. Some medications used for the treatment of other mental disorders can interfere with learning.
For example, nearly all the medications used as mood stabilizers can have side effects that interfere with various
learning functions. Similarly, antipsychotic medications

can also affect learning efficiency (refer to Medication Appendices at the end of the book).

V. **Summary.** Learning disorders are neurologically based differences in the way an individual's brain processes information These disorders are really life problems, often affecting social skills, performance in extracurricular activities, and adaptation as an adult. The role of the PCP is to recognize the need for further evaluation, to advocate for the child, and to support the child and family over the course of time. Because the terminology associated with learning disorders is not standard across disciplines, this advocacy includes education and explanation for children, families, and educators. The long-term relationship PCPs enjoy with their patients is an important context for developing and maintaining enthusiastic and creative approaches to these lifelong challenges.

SUGGESTED READINGS

American Academy of Child and Adolescent Psychiatry. Practice parameters for the assessment and treatment of children and adolescents with language and learning disorders. *J Am Acad Child Adolesc Psychiatry* 1998;37(suppl. 10):46S–62S.

American Academy of Pediatrics and American Academy of Ophthalmology. Learning disabilities, dyslexia, and vision: a subject review. *Pediatrics* 1998;102(5):1217–1219.

Beitchman J, Young A. Learning disorders with a special emphasis on reading disorders: a review of the past 10 years. *J Am Acad Child Adolesc Psychiatry* 1997;36(8):1020–1032.

Cantwell DP, Baker L. *Developmental speech and language disorders.* New York: Guilford Press, 1987.

Glascoe F. Early detection of developmental and behavioral problems. *Pediatr Rev* 2000;21(8):272–280.

Kavale KA, Forness SR. *The nature of learning disabilities: critical elements in diagnosis and classification.* Mahwah, NJ: Lawrence Erlbaum, 1995.

Myers PI, Hammill DD. *Learning disabilities: basic concepts, associated practices, and instructional strategies,* 4th ed. Austin, TX: PRO-ED, 1992.

Pennington BF. Genetics of learning disabilities. *J Child Neurol* 1995;10(suppl. 1):S69–S77.

Shalev R, Gross-Tsur V. Developmental dyscalculia. *Pediatr Neurol* 2001;24(5):337–342.

Shapiro B. Specific reading disability: a multiplanar view. *Mental Retardation and Developmental Disabilities Research Reviews* 2001; 7(1):13–20.

Shaywitz S. Current concepts: dyslexia. *N Engl J Med* 1998;338(5): 307–312.

Silver L. Controversial therapies. *J Child Neurol* 1995;10(suppl. 1): S96–S100.

Toppelberg C, Shapiro T. Language disorders: a 10 year research update review. *J Am Acad Child Adolesc Psychiatry* 2000;39(2):143–152.

US Department of Education. *Seventeenth Annual Report to Congress on the Implementation of the Individuals with Disabilities Education Act.* Washington, DC: US Office of Special Education Program, 1995.

For Parents

Silver L. *The misunderstood child. Understanding and coping with your child's learning disabilities,* 3rd ed. New York: New York Times Books, 1998.

Smith C, Strick L. *Learning disabilities: A to Z.* New York: The Free Press, 1997.

Web Sites

LDOnline, a nonprofit site affiliated with WETA Public Broadcasting Co., has much advocacy and educational information for parents and teachers about learning disorders. Especially well-done site has extensive list of links. Available at www.ldonline.org. Accessed on 6/29/02.

Learning Disabilities Association is a nonprofit self-help organization that sponsors an educational and advocacy web site for families with learning-disordered individuals. Available at www.ldanatl.org. Accessed on 6/29/02.

National Association for the Education of African American Children with Learning Disabilities. An advocacy site for the promotion of quality education for African–American children. Available at www.charityadvantage.com/aacld/homepage.asp. Accessed on 6/29/02.

National Center for Learning Disabilities sponsors an advocacy and educational website primarily for parents about learning disabilities. Available at www.ld.org. Accessed on 6/29/02.

Schwablearning.org provides educational information for parents and teens about learning disabilities. Includes excellent and practical information for parents about how to help their child. Available at www.schwablearning.org. Accessed on 6/29/02.

16 ♣ Mood Disorders

Anna C. Muriel, Jeffrey Q. Bostic,
and Jeanne M. Dolan

I. **Background.** Mood disorders refer to **unpleasant moods** that are **sustained (i.e., most of the day) and persistent (i.e., every day or almost every day, for weeks to months), and accompanied** by distressing neurovegetative symptoms that have a negative impact on a child's functioning. As primary care physicians (PCPs) follow children through developmental transitions, they are well positioned to identify when a child's mood state crosses from a normal variation to an impairing disorder. Normal "developmental" mood fluctuations are usually mild and time-limited and do not interfere significantly with a child's functioning. However, persistent, intense mood states can **impair functioning** at:
- **Home (strained family relationships)**
- With **peers (withdrawal or alienation)**
- At **daycare or school (drop in grades or school absences)**

Most importantly, significant mortality is associated with juvenile mood disorders. **Mood disorders** are the **most important risk factor for youth suicide,** the third leading cause of death in adolescents. When symptoms lead to functional impairment or suicide risk, intervention is warranted.

Unlike adults who present to their physicians complaining of feeling "down" or "depressed," children and adolescents with mood disorders are typically brought by their parents to the PCP with **presenting complaints** of:
- **Irritability** or anger
- **Decline in school performance**
- **Oppositional or defiant** behavior ("a bad attitude")
- **Withdrawal** from age-appropriate activities
- **Somatic complaints** (e.g., headaches, stomachaches, or fatigue)

Therefore, the PCP must be alert to signs and symptoms of mood disorders and be prepared to treat or refer patients appropriately.

A. **Epidemiology.** Depressive disorders increase throughout childhood and adolescence. **Major depressive disorder** occurs in approximately **2% of children and up to 5% of adolescents, and dysthymia in 2% of children and 4% of adolescents.** Girls and boys are equally likely to suffer depression in childhood; by adolescence, however, girls are twice as likely to become depressed. Cause is considered multifactorial, with some evidence for genetic as well as environmental risk. Although controversy exists about biological markers for depression, genetically mediated vulnerability to depression likely involves dysregulation of central neurotransmitter functions. **Bipolar disorder** occurs in approximately 1% of both female and male adolescents. With the onset of puberty occurring earlier in the United States, earlier onset of mood disorders has also been identified in the past 10 years. Accompanying this earlier age of onset is an increase in the severity and duration of symptoms, comorbidity with other psychiatric disorders, and poorer response to treatment.

The *Diagnostic and Statistical Manual of Mental Disorders,* Fourth Edition, Text Revision (DSM-IV-TR) provides diagnostic criteria to identify mood disorders. However, these criteria were developed for adults, and are often difficult to apply to children and adolescents. Thus, the American Academy of Child and Adolescent Psychiatry and the American Academy of Pediatrics developed the DSM-Primary Care—Child and Adolescent version in 1996. Primary mood disorders, which are summarized in Table 16.1, include (a) major depressive disorder, (b) dysthymia, and (c) bipolar disorder. A high degree of overlap exists between major depressive disorder and dysthymia, with many patients having both conditions either at the time of presentation or on follow-up (e.g., dysthymic patients are subsequently at high risk for a major depression).

B. **Developmental differences in presentation of mood disorders.** Although depressive disorders can occur in **infancy,** they are difficult to diagnose. However, depressed infants can be particularly worrisome, because symptoms can threaten their physical and emotional development and attachment formation. These infants may have feeding difficulties and sleep disturbances; reject eye contact or appear either irritable or apathetic. Depressed **preschoolers** may exhibit more behavioral problems, aggression toward peers, irritability, and regression. Any of these signs should alert the PCP to a possible mood disorder that will require family assessment and psychosocial intervention to prevent problems with the child's future growth and development.

Latency age children with depression can display sad, irritable, or depressed mood; crying spells and lack of pleasure in activities. They complain that "nobody likes me" or that they have "no friends." They can also exhibit high levels of "externalizing behaviors" (e.g., aggressive outbursts, biting, kicking, throwing things, or prolonged tantrums). Their condition can be misdiagnosed as oppositional defiant disorder or attention-deficit/hyperactivity disorder (AD/HD) because of the defiant and impulsive nature of their actions. Clues to the diagnosis of depression can be found by investigating the child's feelings of self-worth, thoughts of dying, and parental

Table 16.1. Primary mood disorders

Major Depression[a]	Dysthymia[a]	Bipolar Disorder[b]
Depressed or irritable mood or diminished interest or pleasure, associated with significant distress or impairment in function, that represents a change from previous functioning and is accompanied by at least 5 of the following criteria nearly everyday for at least 2 weeks Insomnia or hypersomnia Weight loss or gain Fatigue, decreased energy Decreased ability to concentrate Feelings of guilt or worthlessness Psychomotor retardation or agitation Recurrent thoughts of death and suicide	May be less severe or disabling, but more persistent than major depression Depressed or irritable mood most of the day, for more days than not, for at least 1 year, associated with at least 2 of the following: Insomnia or hypersomnia Decreased or increased appetite Fatigue, low energy Poor concentration or decision-making ability Feelings of hopelessness Individuals with dysthymia are at greater risk for episodes of major depression	Elevated, expansive, or irritable mood lasting at least 1 week, accompanied by at least 3 of the following: Inflated self-esteem or grandiosity Decreased need for sleep Flight of ideas or racing thoughts Distractibility Increase in goal-directed activity or psycho motor agitation Excessive involvement in pleasurable activities that have a high potential for painful consequences (e.g., buying sprees, promiscuity) Juveniles appear less likely to have distinct "episodes," frequent (up to multiple times daily) "episodes" or mixed states are more commonly described in younger patients

[a] *Diagnostic and Statistical Manual of Mental Disorders—Primary Care-Child and Adolescent version.*
[b] *Diagnostic and Statistical Manual of Mental Disorders, Fourth Edition.*

observations of sleep and appetite changes or with-drawal from previously enjoyable activities. Younger children may be less likely than adolescents or adults to have classic neurovegetative signs. A crucial consideration in school-aged children with depression, however, is the high incidence of somatic complaints, the development of phobias, or onset of nightmares and sleep disruption. Somatic complaints, which most frequently take the form of stomachaches or head-aches, can interfere with school attendance. These children **can be precariously suicidal** and this needs to be seriously considered even though the statistical risk is small. The possibility of comorbid anxiety disorders or obsessive-compulsive disorder (OCD) must also be assessed in this population.

As the child reaches **adolescence,** clinical symptoms more resemble those of adults and are distinct from adolescent development. As teenagers seek an identity separate from the family, mood shifts, questioning of authority, and changing family relationships are considered normal. A depressed adolescent, however, can have feelings of sadness, hopelessness, and self-hatred, fearing isolation from all peer groups. This adolescent may also describe neurovegetative symptoms (e.g., decreased sleep, appetite, and concentration) or "atypical" depressive symptoms (e.g., hyperphagia, hypersomnia, and excessive fatigue). Comorbid dysthymia, substance use, and conduct and anxiety disorders are also common in adolescents. Suicide risk must always be considered in teenagers with mood disorders. Suicide has increased markedly in recent decades with **5% to 10% of high school students making suicide attempts each year.** Access to various means of suicide warrants assessment, because completed youth suicide most commonly occurs with firearms (see Chapter 23).

Whenever assessing for mood disorder, also be aware of the possibility of the child having **bipolar disorder.** Although the diagnosis of bipolar disorder in young children remains controversial, severe irritability and extreme explosive behavior; unpremeditated aggression; tantrums lasting hours; or mixed euphoria, giddiness, and agitation should alert the PCP to this diagnostic possibility. Switching from depression to mania occurs in up to **one-third of juveniles initially exhibiting depressive symptoms,** and appears unrelated to antidepressant exposure. Predictors of switching include family history of bipolarity, psychomotor retardation, psychosis, and rapid onset of depression. In particular, prepubertal children and young adolescents are more likely to present with initial depressive episodes, or with rapid cycling, mixed, or non-episodic mood states. Also, **high comorbidity with AD/HD** is seen, which further complicates diagnosis. Older adolescents may have more adultlike presentations, with more easily identifiable mania and discrete mood onset and offset. Among adolescents with bipolar disorder, comorbid substance use is common, and must also be addressed.

C. **Course.** With appropriate treatment, gradual improvements (i.e., over a period of months) in mood and function usually occur. However, because approximately 40% of individuals who have a depressive episode during childhood will have another episode within 2 years (72% recurrence within 5 years), clinicians should follow-up with these patients every 2 to 4 months for at least 8 to 12 months after treatment is discontinued. In addition, patients and their families should identify the symptom progression (e.g., stopped eating, became irritable, could not sleep, then stopped practicing musical instrument) so that recurrent episodes can be more rapidly treated.

II. **Practical office evaluation.** Assessment of childhood mood disorders requires integration of information from **multiple sources,** as well as an awareness of baseline temperament, developmental phase, and psychosocial stressors. Children tend to report internalizing or subjective symptoms, whereas parents or other adults are often more reliable reporters of external indicators. Children and adults, therefore, should be interviewed independently, as both parties may be more candid in the absence of the other. PCPs can also consider using a **screening questionnaire such as the Children's Depression Inventory** (Kovacs, 1985), which is a 27-item, symptom-oriented scale designed for children and adolescents. Whereas the specificity of this instrument is only fair, it is the most widely used tool available for juvenile depression. Other questionnaires for parents (e.g., the Pediatric Symptom Checklist see Chapter 5 [Jellinek, 1998]) include items for depression, but screen more generally for psychosocial dysfunction.

A. **Questions for the child**
   1. **Mood.** Have you been feeling sad, blue, down, or irritable and grouchy most of the day, more days than not? Do you find yourself crying a lot? Do you get into more hassles or arguments with others?
   2. **Anhedonia.** Are you unable to enjoy things you used to enjoy? Do you have less interest in doing fun things? Do you feel "bored" or "tired" a lot?
   3. **Guilty feelings or negative self-image.** Do you feel badly about yourself? Or feel badly about things you have done? Do you feel not worthwhile as a person? Do you have any friends? (Depressed children will report they do not, even when others say that they do.) Do other kids like you? (Again, depressed children will report that others do not.)

4. **Neurovegetative signs.** Have you noticed changes in your sleep pattern? For example, do you have difficulty falling asleep or staying asleep, sleeping too much? Are you having trouble concentrating in school? Have you had any changes in appetite? Increased? Decreased?

5. **Somatic symptoms.** Do you have headaches? Stomachaches? How often? How severe? How is your energy level?

6. **Suicidal ideation.** Do you ever wish you were dead? Wish you would not wake up in the morning? Think that it would be all right to get hit by a car? Do you think about death, or make plans for how to kill yourself? Have you ever tried to hurt yourself?

7. **Substance use.** What kinds of drugs or alcohol are you using? How much? How often? Is this a recent change?

B. **Questions for the parents**

1. **Mood/affect.** Have you noticed a change in your child's mood? Does he or her seem sad? Does the child cry a lot? Seem irritable? Does the child argue a lot or have anger outbursts?

2. **Neurovegetative signs.** Have you noticed changes in your child's sleep pattern (e.g., difficulty falling asleep or staying asleep, sleeping too much)? Have you noticed changes in your child's appetite or energy level? Increased? Decreased? Has the child's weight changed recently?

3. **Suicidal ideation.** Has your child voiced any thoughts about wishing he or she was dead? Has the child done anything to hurt self? Are you worried that the child might hurt self? Does the child seem preoccupied with death or morbid writings, music, or movies?

4. **Impaired school or peer functioning.** Have your child's grades declined? Is your child showing less interest in social or after-school activities? Has the child missed much school? Is he or she spending less time with peers? Or has the peer group changed significantly? Any signs of substance use?

C. **Physical examination and laboratory.** Perform a complete physical examination and consider screening laboratory tests (thyroid function tests [TFTs], complete blood count [CBC], toxicology screen) if the child demonstrates signs or symptoms of a medical condition associated with depressed mood. Also, gather a thorough history of substance use or other medications (e.g., steroids, thyroid supplements, megavitamins) that might be contributing to mood changes. Medical disorders that can mimic or cause mood disorders are listed in Table 16.2, although physical examination will usually clarify the likelihood of these disorders.

Table 16.2. **Medical conditions that can present as or cause mood disorders**

Depression	Mania
Anemia	Steroid use
Vitamin B_{12} deficiency	Asthma medications
Cushing's syndrome	Hyperthyroidism
Connective tissue disorders	
Juvenile rheumatoid arthritis	
Systemic lupus erythematosus	
Diabetes mellitus	
Chronic fatigue syndrome	
Fibromyalgia	
Hypothyroidism	
Infections	
Mononucleosis	
Hepatitis	
Human immunodeficiency virus (HIV)	
Inflammatory bowel disease	
Multiple sclerosis	
Seizure disorder	
Tumors	
Medications	
Benzodiazepines	
Beta-blockers	
Clonidine	
Corticosteroids	
Isotretinoin (Accutane)	
Oral contraceptives	
Substance abuse or withdrawal	
(alcohol, cocaine, amphetamine, opiates)	

III. **Triage assessment and treatment planning**
  A. **Watching**
    1. **When to watch**
      a. Child has specific stressors or losses associated with mood changes
      b. Symptoms are mild and not sustained
      c. No psychiatric comorbidity and little or no suicidal ideation seen
      d. Peer and academic functioning is adequate
      e. Family functioning appears good or improving
      f. The child demonstrates the ability to discuss stressors with parents, peers, or nonparental adults.
      g. Family history of mood disorder
    2. **When watching**

a. **Psychoeducation**
   (1) **Review the circumstances.** In age-appropriate language, clarify stressors or losses contributing to mood changes.
   (2) **Clarify coping strategies** that have been tried, or that have been successful in the past. Support the child's capacity to discuss his or her feelings with parents, other adults, and peers.
   (3) **Destigmatize the acknowledgment of emotional difficulties.** Note that it is a sign of health to recognize when one is struggling and to be open to help.
   (4) **Normalize developmental struggles** (i.e. "Many kids your age . . .") This may help connect the child to peers or allow the child to consider how others have coped with similar distressing circumstances.
   (5) **Identify self-esteem enhancing activities, skills, or strengths** that parents and other adults can cultivate. Camps, school-based programs, and community recreational and parks programs that can bolster self-esteem should be aggressively sought. Summer vacation is an especially good time to find these opportunities. Advise parents to think about these programs and discuss them with their child in the winter, if not before, to assure availability.
   (6) **Reinforce good self-care habits.** In addition to learning to talk about one's feelings, it is important for one's mental health to establish regular eating, sleeping, and exercise habits.
   (7) **Rule out maltreatment** as a contributing factor.
   (8) **Educate child and family about signs of increasing depression.** Describe specific symptoms (e.g., sleep disturbance, change in appetite, school problems, argumentativeness). If noted, the family should call the PCP for a follow-up appointment.
b. **Advocacy** is usually not needed in cases of transient depressed mood, although if school functioning is beginning to be affected, consider school accommodations as described below in the intervention section. Consider opportunities for prevention (e.g.,

recommending additional activities as described above). In addition, be alert for signs of abuse or neglect that might require the involvement of Children's Protective Services.

c. **Psychotherapy** is generally not needed in the mildest cases, although it might be considered even at this stage if signs indicate that the child's coping strategies are inflexible or likely to lead to greater difficulty in the future. However, youth at this stage should not be "forced" into psychotherapy, as this will sometimes be counterproductive. Nonetheless, vulnerable young people will benefit from relationships with supportive, interested adults in their school and community settings.

d. **Medications** are not indicated in the setting of transient, mild mood symptoms.

e. **Laboratory and other evaluations** are not indicated unless reason exists to suspect an underlying medical condition.

f. **Monitoring.** The family should call to report on the child's progress in 4 to 6 weeks. Follow-up appointments can be made in 2 to 3 months to track the progress of symptoms and to reinforce continued mental health hygiene practices.

B. **Intervening further**
  1. **When to intervene further**
     a. The child is persistently sad or irritable more days than not, over a period of weeks, with moods interfering with day-to-day activities.
     b. Peer or academic functioning beginning to deteriorate.
     c. Significant sleep, appetite, or energy changes are noted.
     d. Mild to moderate family disturbance occurs, but parents are allied in best interest of child.
     e. More than fleeting suicidal ideation exists, without any specific plan or intent, and the PCP is comfortable with the parents' capacities to assess and protect the child.
  2. **When intervening further**
     a. **Psychoeducation**
        (1) **Educate** children and parents **about depression** being a biologically based illness that can be treated with a range of modalities. It often bears emphasizing that clinical depression is fundamentally real, and that the symptoms are not feigned

or under the child's conscious control. Parental misconceptions about depression being willful or the result of moral weakness must be explored and dispelled to allow the child to receive appropriate treatment.

(2) **Destigmatize treatment** by recognizing it as a sign of strength and health (just as going to a doctor for treatment of diabetes is considered a sign of health; refusing to go is a sign of avoidance and "weakness"). Many well-known rock stars, movie stars, politicians, and others in the public eye have had clinical depressions. Being familiar with current events and letting the child or adolescent know about this can help these patients address their own situation without feeling ashamed.

(3) Regularly **assess suicidal ideation** and thoughts of self-harm. Investigate all self-harm comments or behaviors and create a safety plan to address any potential suicidal ideation (see Chapter 23). The child should actively identify a hierarchy of others to contact (e.g., parent, then other parent, then particular relative, then friend) and alternatives to self-harm (e.g., attempting distracting activities, exercise, writing) if thoughts of self-harm emerge. In addition to reviewing this plan with the child, the safety plan with parents must include eliminating the child's access to means of self-harm (e.g., removing firearms from the home).

(4) **Look for underlying psychological issues or life concerns.** Explore developmental issues, family conflict, peers, and medical illness in the child or parent. Young people wrestling with sexual preference are at particular risk of depression and suicide. Inquiring about romantic feelings, dreams, or interests rather than about "having boyfriends or girlfriends" may facilitate discussion of this topic.

(5) **Employ cognitive techniques.** While acknowledging and validating feelings, address unrealistic or dis-

torted thoughts about self-esteem, social issues, and so forth. Depressed young people may selectively emphasize one negative event to conclude they are inept, while dismissing positive events or activities. It is helpful if the PCP can genuinely reassure them or place their concern into a more positive frame. Encourage the child or adolescent to learn his or her own strategies for countering this negative self-talk.

(6) As with other disorders, younger patients sometimes benefit from **"objectifying" the disorder** (i.e., distinguishing it from the person) so that the family, the patient, and PCP can ally in their efforts to "fight" the disorder. For example, clinicians might clarify how much time today (or the last week) the patient spent "with depression" (children may generate their own names for the disorder). They can also be engaged in discussions of how their life has changed since depression entered it or how they can "talk back" to depression or find other ways to "rebel" so that it takes up less energy and they can attend to more positive peer interactions and activities.

(7) Support the continued use of family, school, and community resources as above.

(8) Reinforce good self-care and **mental health hygiene**.

b. **Advocacy**

(1) **School accommodations and modifications.** (Chapter 18 addresses prominent school absenteeism.) It is important to maintain frequent communication between school, home, and the PCP. Frequently revising (e.g., weekly) any intervention plan with child, family, and school staff may be necessary.

In the setting of a major mood disorder, it is legitimate to consider the following modifications:

(a) **Alter the school day** (abbreviating or starting with classes or teachers where likelihood of success is greatest).

> > > **(b)** Diminish stress by reducing academic workload or by frequent check-ins with teachers.
> > > **(c)** Address school environment issues that prevent attendance (e.g., bullying, courses where failure is likely).
> > > **(d)** Structure opportunities for sanctuary and reassurance (e.g., guidance or nurse's office).
> > **(2)** **Assess for maltreatment.** Assure the child's safety and the parents' capacities to monitor and protect the child. Involve the Department of Social Services for any question of abuse, neglect, or parental conflict that works against the best interest of the child (including refusal of parents to secure and protect the child from lethal means when child has made a credible suicide threat).
>
> c. **Psychotherapy** is indicated for the treatment of depression. Referral should be made to a qualified child mental health specialist for individual cognitive-behavioral, interpersonal, or psychodynamic therapy. These therapies should generally occur on a weekly basis. Family therapy, often a crucial part of the treatment plan, is done in conjunction with the individual work.
> d. **Medications** should be considered after psychosocial interventions have been tried for 2 to 3 months without success, or if symptoms are particularly severe. For specific medications see *Practical Use of Medications* below.
> e. **Laboratory and other evaluations.** Screening laboratory tests including a CBC and TFTs should be considered if a child meets criteria for major depression. Further testing is done if any additional underlying medical condition is suspected.
> f. **Monitoring.** Follow-up should occur in 1 month to assure that the family has followed through with obtaining mental health treatment. If medications have been prescribed, these can be followed up at that time as well.

C. **Referring**
  1. **When to refer and transfer primary responsibility**
     a. Any evidence of dangerous behavior (e.g., assaultiveness, suicide gestures or attempts)

b. Evidence of another significant psychiatric disorder (e.g. anxiety disorder, OCD, psychosis, conduct disorder, substance abuse)

c. Moderate to severe interference in academic functioning

d. Evidence of serious family disturbance, including parental mental illness or substance abuse, physical or sexual abuse, neglect or social chaos

e. Failure of two medication trials

f. Bipolar disorder is suspected because of rapid cycling or mixed moods that may or may not be episodic. Extreme explosive behavior, unpremeditated aggression, or tantrums lasting hours also raise suspicion. In rare cases, the PCP may lack access to other providers more familiar with bipolar disorder and, thus, be required to treat this disorder. **However, referral is always recommended for juveniles suspected of having bipolar disorder.**

g. **Hospitalization** is necessary for depressed children and adolescents in cases of significant suicide risk. Depending on community resources, innovative, intensive outpatient programs or partial hospitalization programs may be available as alternatives to acute inpatient hospitalization. Initial episodes of mania usually require hospitalization to stabilize symptoms.

2. **When referring**
   a. **Psychoeducation**
      (1) **Support continuity in mental health treatment.** Mental health treatment should generally continue for a minimum of 6 months. Termination before this can represent minimization or avoidance of the problem. Encourage the family to remain in treatment until a satisfactory conclusion is reached. If necessary, caution the parents that recurrence is common and that suicide can be a serious risk without definitive treatment. Destigmatizing treatment, as noted, also helps to maintain the patient in treatment.
      (2) **Reinforce education regarding depression as an illness** (i.e., the symptoms, nature, and cause).
      (3) Encourage continued use of **family and extra-family supports.**
      (4) Reinforce self-care and **mental health hygiene.**

       (5) **Continue to monitor for signs of maltreatment.**

       (6) Continue to carefully **monitor for suicide risk through the recovery period.** Be aware that patients may be at *higher* suicide risk when they appear to be recovering. This may be because they then have enough energy and motivation to act, or it may be that their mood has lifted because they have found a way out of their psychic pain (i.e., they decided to kill themselves).

  b. **Advocacy.** The mental health clinician generally will interface with the school or social services. PCP referral for mental health visits is required by many insurance companies and managed healthcare organizations. Intensive treatment efforts beyond standard outpatient care (see below) may require PCP support and advocacy with managed care companies to ensure reimbursement for services.

  c. **Psychotherapy** will most likely be a cornerstone of treatment. The child can benefit from both individual and family therapy by a qualified child mental health specialist. Treatment generally should last a minimum of 6 months, and often longer. In more severe cases, treatment needs to be carried out more than once per week.

  d. **Medications** will be indicated under these circumstances. Generally, a child and adolescent psychiatrist will manage them.

  e. **Laboratory and other evaluations.** None indicated, unless suggested by ongoing physical signs and symptoms.

  f. **Monitoring** should occur as a face-to-face contact every few months initially, including evaluating general physiologic status.

IV. **Practical use of medications.** Medications are often helpful in the treatment of mood disorders in children and adolescents. For children or adolescents with major depression, psychotherapy can be tried first before medications are started. If the child remains depressed despite a reasonable trial of psychosocial interventions (i.e., 2 to 3 months) or if symptoms are severe and persistent, medications warrant consideration. At this time **selective serotonin reuptake inhibitors (SSRI)** (Appendix N) are considered the **first-line treatment** for pediatric depression. Although none of the SSRI currently have US Food and Drug Administration (FDA)-approved indications for pediatric depression, controlled trials support the use of fluoxetine, paroxetine, and citalopram for children and adolescents with depression. Open trials also support the use of citalopram, fluoxetine, paroxetine, sertraline, and fluvoxamine for juvenile depression. Current information about psychopharmacologic treatment of pediatric mood disorders is available at the Texas Children's Medication Algorithm web site (see *Web Sites* in *Suggested Readings*).

A. **Depression**
   1. **"Start low and go slow"** with respect to dosing. See Table 16.3 for dosing guidelines. SSRI are given once per day. Dosing can be increased every 5 to 7 days until a target dose is reached. Dosage should be held for 4 to 6 weeks before further increases are made.
   2. Patients are more likely to adhere to treatment if **side effects** are described when giving the initial prescription and plans are made for addressing any that emerge. Patients should be made aware of the risks of **serotonin syndrome,** and be forewarned about the possibility of agitation or restlessness; apathy or amotivational syndrome; gastrointestinal upset or diarrhea, headaches, insomnia; and, in adolescents, sexual side effects.
   3. SSRI appear to have equivalent benefits. The differences are in side effect profile, half-life (Table 16.3) and effects on the P450 cytochrome system. Citalopram and paroxetine are thought to cause the least activation or agitation; fluoxetine the most. Paroxetine and fluvoxamine are thought to cause the most sedation. Although it is generally not a major problem (as it is with the atypical antipsychotics), paroxetine is most associated with weight gain; the others are less likely to do so. With respect to P450 effects, Table 16.4 summarizes the differences between SSRI. Table A.5 in Appendix lists specific P450 substrates.
   4. If intolerable side effects emerge or a maximal dosage is reached without improvement after 8 to 12 weeks, then an alternative SSRI should be cross-tapered and substituted.
   5. If a second SSRI trial is unsuccessful, then atypical antidepressants (e.g., bupropion, venlafaxine, and mirtazapine) can be tried. Fewer data are available for use of these agents in juveniles. **Bupropion** (Appendix F) has stimulant-like properties and has been helpful in some cases of depression and AD/HD. It has been associated with an increased risk of seizures and should not be used in patients with eating disorders or substance abuse histories. **Venlafaxine** (Appendix R) has been helpful for adolescents with depression and anxiety disorders. It causes blood pressure elevations in

Table 16.3. SSRI dosing in depression

Medication	Trade Name	Half-life ($T\frac{1}{2}$)[a] and Dosing Interval	Initial Dose	Maintenance Dose[b]	Maximal Dose[c]
Citalopram	Celexa	24 h (no active metabolite); q.d.	Ch: 2.5–5 mg Adols: 5–10 mg	Ch: 10–20 mg Adols: 20–40 mg	Ch: 40 mg Adols: 60 mg
Fluoxetine	Prozac	1–3 d (active metabolite 7–9 d); q.d.	Ch: 2.5–5 mg Adols: 5–10 mg	Ch: 10–20 mg Adols: 20 mg	Ch: 40 mg Adols 60–80 mg
Fluvoxamine	Luvox	14–18 h (no active metabolite); q.d.	Ch: 12.5–25 mg Adols: 25–50 mg	Ch: 50–150 mg Adols: 50–200 mg	Ch: 200 mg Adols: 300 mg
Paroxetine	Paxil	20–25 h (no active metabolite); q.d.	Ch: 5–10 mg Adols: 10–20 mg	Ch: 10–20 mg Adols: 20–40 mg	Ch: 40 mg Adols: 60 mg
Sertraline	Zoloft	20–28 h (active metabolite 60–70 h); q.d.	Ch: 12.5–25 mg Adols: 25–50 mg	Ch: 50–100 mg Adols: 50–200 mg	Ch: 150 mg Adols: 250 mg

[a] Based on adult studies
[b] Once level of maintenance dose reached, hold for 4 to 6 weeks to check response before further increases.
[c] Unusual to need doses in this range for depression.
SSRI, serotonin reuptake inhibitor; q.d., everyday; Ch, children; Adols, adolescents.

Table 16.4. Relative effects of SSRI inhibition on P-450 isoenzymes

CYP-450 Isoenzyme	Citalopram	Fluoxetine	Fluvoxamine	Paroxetine	Sertraline
1A2	Unlikely	Unlikely	++	Unlikely	Unlikely
2C9/10	No data	Contradictory	Contradictory	None	None
2C19	No data	++	+++	No data	None
2D6	+	+++	None	+++	+
3A4/5	Unlikely	+	++	Unlikely	Unlikely

SSRI, serotonin reuptake inhibitor.
Based on table in Preskon S. Clinically relevant pharmacology of SSRIs. *Clin Pharmacokinet* 1997;32 (suppl. 1):1–21.

5% to 7%, which must be monitored. **Mirtaza-pine** (Appendix K) has not been used widely in juveniles, but is available for use. It is highly sedating and, rarely, is associated with agranulocytosis. **Nefazodone** (Appendix L), another atypical antidepressant, has recently received a "black box" warning regarding hepatotoxicity, and should be used cautiously.

6. Because of their narrow therapeutic margin of safety, and their lack of benefit in 12 controlled studies with juveniles, the **tricyclic antidepressants** are not currently supported as first-line agents for juvenile depression.

7. Be vigilant for signs of switching into mania (e.g., increased activity, irritability, aggression, euphoria, giddiness, decreased sleep) and be prepared to stop antidepressant treatment. This can occur with any of the antidepressants in predisposed individuals.

8. Patients and family members must be reminded that antidepressants often **take 2 to 4 weeks to alleviate symptoms,** and once symptoms improve, the medication should be **continued for 6 to 12 months.** Children should be stable and symptom free for at least 3 months before the drug is slowly tapered down. A gradual taper prevents withdrawal syndromes (paroxetine is the most problematic) and allows for rapid retitration if depressive symptoms recur.

B. **Bipolar disorder**

1. If **bipolar disorder** is suspected, antidepressants alone may exacerbate manic symptoms. Although mood stabilizers (e.g., lithium, valproic acid, carbamazepine) have been the mainstay of treatment, **atypical antipsychotics** (e.g., risperidone [Risperdal], olanzapine [Zyprexa], quetiapine [Seroquel], and ziprasidone [Geodon]) are increasingly used as **first-line agents** for juvenile bipolar disorder. These mood stabilizers and atypical antipsychotics **should be used by clinicians familiar with their use in psychiatric disorders or with appropriate consultation.**

2. **Atypical antipsychotics** (Appendix D). Risperidone, olanzapine, or quetiapine have the most support for use in this age group. Common **side effects** include sedation, weight gain and hyperglycemia (most with olanzapine and risperidone, less with quetiapine, least with ziprasidone), constipation, and hyperprolactinemia (most with risperidone, least with quetiapine). QT prolongation can be an issue with risperidone and the newer medication ziprasidone, so electrocardiographic monitoring is

recommended. Risperidone can be started at 0.25 to 0.5 mg every day and titrated as tolerated up to a maximum of 6 mg/day in divided (usually twice daily) doses. Olanzapine is usually initiated at 2.5 mg every bedtime and increased to a maximum of 20 mg/day in juveniles; weight gain should be carefully monitored and diet and exercise addressed. Quetiapine is usually initiated at 25 mg/day and titrated up in divided doses up to 800 mg/day in older juveniles. Ziprasidone is a newer agent, but may have less appetite-stimulation than the other atypical agents; dosage parameters have not yet been clearly established in children.

3. **Lithium** (Appendix J) can be started at 150 mg/day for children and 300 mg for adolescents and titrated up every 3 to 5 days to achieve serum levels between 0.8 to 1.2 mEq/L for acute mania, and decreased to achieve serum levels between 0.6 and 0.9 after acute symptoms have abated. Routine monitoring of lithium levels, thyroid function, and renal function must be maintained, and families must be warned of the risks and signs of toxicity.

4. **Valproic acid** (Appendix Q) can be started at 125 to 250 mg/day in children (250 mg twice daily in adolescents), and titrated to achieve serum levels of 75 to 125 mEq/L, which is higher than what is used for seizure control. Monitoring of serum levels and liver function tests should be done at least every 3 months, and families should be warned about the risks of weight gain and counseled about nutrition and exercise for their child. Hair loss and gastrointestinal distress are other common side effects. Although concerns of polycystic ovaries were reported in young women taking valproate, this may have been related to weight gain, so careful monitoring is necessary. Of major concern, hepatotoxicity, pancreatitis, and agranulocytosis can occur with this medication.

5. **Carbamazepine** (Appendix H) should be used in consultation with someone familiar with its use for juvenile bipolar disorder, because of rare but serious risks of agranulocytosis or Stevens-Johnson syndrome.

6. Child and adolescent psychiatrists also may use newer anticonvulsants (e.g., **gabapentin, oxcarbazepine, topiramate, lamotrigine**) in the management of bipolar disorder.

V. **Summary.** Mood disorders such as major depression and bipolar disorder are a significant cause of psychosocial dysfunction and distress among children and adolescents, and they carry a risk of suicide and self-harm. As PCPs follow patients through developmental stages, they are well positioned to assess, treat, and appropriately refer these patients. The keys to detection are being alert to the varying presentations of mood disorders, attentive to signs of mood disorders, and ask children and parents about symptoms. Effective treatments now available present the PCP with crucial opportunities to help their pediatric patients.

SUGGESTED READINGS

American Academy of Child and Adolescent Psychiatry. Practice Parameters for the Assessment and Treatment of Children and Adolescents with Depressive Disorders. *J Am Acad Child Adolesc Psychiatry* 1998;37(suppl. 10):63S–83S.

Birmaher B, Ryan ND, Williamson DE, et al. Childhood and adolescent depression: a review of the past 10 years. Part I. *J Am Acad Child Adolesc Psychiatry* 1996;35(11): 1427–1439.

Birmaher B, Ryan ND, Williamson DE, et al. Childhood and adolescent depression: a review of the past 10 years. Part II. *J Am Acad Child Adolesc Psychiatry* 1996;35(12): 1575–1583.

Bostic J, Wilens T, Spencer T, et al. Juvenile mood disorders and office psychopharmacology. *Pediatr Clin North Am* 1997;44(6): 1487–1503.

Carlson GA, Meyer SE. Bipolar disorder in youth. *Current Psychiatry Rep* 2000;2(2):90–94.

Geller B, Luby J. Child and adolescent bipolar disorder: a review of the past 10 years. *J Am Acad Child Adolesc Psychiatry* 1997;36:9.

Jellinek M, Snyder J. Depression and suicide in children and adolescents. *Pediatr Rev* 1998;19(8):255–264.

Kovacs M. The children's depression inventory. *Psychopharmacol Bull* 1985;21(4):995–998. Available at http://assessments.ncspearson. com. Accessed on 6/29/02.

Shoaf T, Emslie G, Mayes T. Childhood depression: diagnosis and treatment strategies in general pediatrics. *Pediatr Ann* 2001;30(3): 130–137.

For Families

Cobain B, Verdick E. *When nothing matters: a survival guide for depressed teens.* Minneapolis: Free Spirit Publishing, 1998.

Dubuque S. *Survival guide to childhood depression.* Plainview, NY: Childswork/Childsplay 1996.

Fassler D, Dumas L. *Help me, I'm sad: recognizing, treating, and preventing childhood and adolescent depression.* New York: Viking Penguin, 1998.

Greene R. *The explosive child: a new approach for understanding and parenting easily frustrated, "chronically inflexible" children.* New York: HarperCollins. 1998.

Lynn G. *Survival strategies for parenting children with bipolar disorder: innovative parenting and counseling techniques for helping children with bipolar disorder and the conditions that may occur with it.* London: Jessica Kingsley Publishing, 2000.

Miller J. *The childhood depression sourcebook.* New York: McGraw Hill, 1999.

Papolos D, Papolos P. *The bipolar child.* New York: Broadway Books, 1999.

Seligman M, Reivich K, Jaycox L, et al. *The optimistic child.* New York: Harper Trade, 1996.

Swedo S, Leonard H. *Is it just a phase? How to tell common childhood phases from serious problems.* New York: Bantam Books, 1999.

Web Sites

Child and Adolescent Bipolar Foundation. Available at www.cabf.org. Accessed on 6/29/02.

NAMI (National Alliance for the Mentally Ill). Available at www.nami.org. Accessed on 6/29/02.

NDMDA (National Depressive and Manic-Depressive Association). Available at www.ndmda.org. Accessed on 6/29/02.

Parents of Bipolar Children. Available at www.bpparent.org. Accessed on 6/29/02.

Texas Children's Medication Algorithm Project is a site that contains updated medication practices for mood disorders, including in children. Available at www.mhmr.state.tx.us/centraloffice/medicaldirector/CMAP.html. Accessed on 6/29/02.

The Bipolar Child. Available at www.bipolarchild.com. Accessed on 6/29/02.

17 ♣ Pervasive Developmental Disorders

David L. Kaye

I. **Background.** Pervasive developmental disorders (PDD) are a group of severe problems that reflect disturbances in **multiple areas of a child's life (hence, "pervasive").** They present **from the first years of life (hence, "developmental").** The core disability that characterizes all PDD is a **social communication deficit** consisting of difficulty:

- Reading and responding to social and emotional cues **(affective reciprocity)**
- Establishing **joint attention** (i.e., the ability to share attention with another person as in pointing or showing)
- Developing a **"theory of mind"** (i.e., intuitively and fluidly understanding others' thoughts and feelings, a prerequisite for pretend play)

Children with milder forms of PDD might be described as having little "common sense," whereas those with more severe PDD may appear to be "in a world of their own." Children with the most severe form (autism) show no apparent interest in social relationships. When children with PDD do show interest, their disability usually precludes the establishment of mutual friendships. They show **deficits in "social knowledge"** (e.g., how to start a conversation, chose a topic, take turns, read others' nonverbal cues).

A second key feature of PDD (especially autism, disintegrative disorder, Rett syndrome, but not Asperger's) is **disturbance of speech and language** in which deficits or delays in expressive, receptive, or pragmatic language occur.

Rigid and stereotyped behavior patterns are common and are required for the diagnosis of autism. Associated features include attentional problems and symptoms like attention-deficit/hyperactivity disorder (AD/HD) and anxiety symptoms (especially with obsessive-compulsive features). Overall cognitive limitations (i.e., **mental retardation**) are present in more severe forms of the disorders, especially autism. Unlike mental retardation, the PDD do **not** represent **"delays"** of development but **rather are deviations** (i.e., the features are not found in normally developing children).

   A. **Prevalence** for autism is 5/10,000 and for the broader PDD group (excluding autism) 15/10,000. Although higher prevalence rates have been reported over the past decade, the most likely explanation for this is use of broader and less stringent inclusion criteria in the studies. No credible scientific reason (including the purported effects of immunizations) exists for this apparent increase. The American Academy of Pediatrics (2001) recommends that the primary care physician (PCP) "should continue to promote immunizations for all children."

B. **Gender.** Of children with PDD, 75% to 80% are **boys.** The exception to this is Rett syndrome, which is seen only in girls.

C. **Etiology** is unknown but the disorder is presumed to be neurologically based. Family studies strongly support a **genetic** factor in the development of autism and autistic-like disorders. Many first-degree relatives show similar social deficits, although usually not as severe. **Siblings have an elevated risk of 3% to 7%.** Also, an over-representation of **major depression and social phobia** is seen in the first-degree relatives of persons with autism. This appears to predate the birth of the autistic child. Current research is demonstrating the influence of specific gene sequences that act early in intrauterine life to influence the development of autistic spectrum disorders. **No evidence** indicates that particular styles of **parenting** or other adverse psychosocial events play a role in the etiology of autism.

D. **Associated medical conditions.** A substantial percentage (33%) of autistic individuals develop a **seizure disorder** by adolescence. Otherwise, most are entirely healthy. In the unusual case (generally in the severely retarded group), autism has been associated with tuberous sclerosis, congenital rubella infection, Angelman's syndrome, and **fragile-X** syndrome. Despite earlier reports to the contrary, the latter syndrome accounts for a small percentage (**2% to 5%**) of autistic individuals. Rarely, PDD co-occurs with Williams syndrome and neurofibromatosis. Because of their social deficits children with PDD are at risk for **pica** and consequent **lead poisoning.**

E. **Neuropathology.** The many attempts that have been made to localize the affected areas of the brain have largely been unsuccessful. The only consistent findings are:
   1. Up to 30% of autistic persons have an **increase in head circumference** that develops in early to middle childhood.
   2. **Decreased Purkinje** cell counts

F. **Course** is **lifelong,** with the more severely affected individuals entirely unable to live or function outside of supervised settings. Most require lifelong supports, structured and sheltered work activities, and supervised living situations (e.g., group homes). In milder situations, independent functioning is more feasible, although significant social deficits interfere with satisfactory functioning at work and with peers. It is only the unusual situation (in some cases of Asperger's syndrome) in which the individual is able to live independently, work in a competitive job, and have intimate peer relationships (e.g., marry).

Although the *Diagnostic and Statistical Manual of Mental Disorders,* Fourth Edition, Text Revision (DSM-IV-TR) lists five categories of PDD, many experts refer to all PDD as "autistic spectrum disorders," with the core social deficits common to all and the differences being ones of severity. Although this dimensional view is increasingly accepted, the traditional categories remain widely used as well. These categories are as follows:

1. **Autism,** the most well recognized of the conditions, presents with typical social skills deficits, stereotyped and rigid motor and behavioral patterns, and speech and language difficulties (50% are entirely mute); 75% are also mentally retarded. Generally, they are attractive physically and do not appear dysmorphic, although a small percentage does have an underlying medical disorder (e.g., fragile X syndrome, tuberous sclerosis). Symptoms typically appear in the first 18 months and must be present before 30 months to meet diagnostic criteria. Development of useful speech by age 5 is the best predictor of future functioning and prognosis.

2. **Asperger's syndrome,** a disorder first written about in the 1940s, was not included in DSM until DSM-IV. Controversy exists about whether this should be thought of as a separate disorder or whether it merely represents the "high functioning autistic" individuals (i.e., those with normal IQ). These children have normal early speech and language development and usually, although not always, show milder social deficits than seen in autism. Their IQ subtest scores reveal poorer performance (i.e., nonverbal tasks) versus verbal scores. Neuropsychologists have described similar individuals as having **nonverbal learning disabilities.** These children are often not identified until well into elementary school or even later (many are probably never identified and are just seen as "odd" or unusual adults), as they often achieve adequately in school and are not typically behavioral problems. They may come to attention because of symptoms of anxiety or depression. At that time, others may note a history of teasing, lack of friends, and characteristic social disability. These children often have circumscribed interests that dominate their conversations (e.g., geology, astronomy and space, maps).

3. **Pervasive developmental disorder not otherwise specified (PDD NOS).** This category, also termed "atypical autism," represents the largest number of those with a diagnosis of PDD. It is used for children who have some autis-

tic features but not others (e.g., lack the rigid and stereotyped patterns of behaviors and interests); age of onset is after 30 months; or features lack sufficient severity (i.e., have some ability to relate but clearly not at a normal level). Whether these children have mild autism or another disorder is unclear at this point.

4. **Disintegrative disorder** is a rare condition (incidence much lower than autism) that has its onset after 2 to 4 years of normal development. Often acutely or subacutely (i.e., over 3 to 6 months), the child becomes dramatically different. Onset may be heralded by innocuous appearing events, including viral infections, chicken pox, and so forth. Speech is lost, cognitive abilities decline, and many of these children appear as classically autistic. Some have a presentation that appears psychotic, with agitation, apparent hallucinations, and disrupted sleep. Mental retardation is the rule. Seizures occur in most and prognosis is poor. Although this has been associated with a number of neurologic disorders (e.g., metachromatic leukodystrophy), in most cases no other medical condition is identified.

4. **Rett syndrome** is a rare, X-linked dominant condition that develops in girls after a period of normal development (usually 6 months to 4 years). The defect is presumably fatal for male fetuses. Whereas social skills deficits become prominent after the onset, the disorder usually begins with deceleration in head circumference. This is followed by loss of use of hands, with characteristic hand wringing movements, speech and language regression, ataxia, and breathing dysfunctions.

II. **Practical office evaluation.** The evaluation of **social relatedness** is the central issue. Secondarily, **speech and language functioning** and **general cognitive abilities** must be assessed. Current research demonstrates that **parents are highly accurate reporters** of early developmental concerns. **Attentive listening** to these concerns is **essential in the early recognition** of autistic spectrum disorders and other developmental or behavioral problems. In addition to listening to parents, it is critical for the PCP to **ask** the parents questions and then to **observe** the child themselves.

Developmental prescreening, including for social-emotional milestones, should occur at all well-child visits from infancy through school age. A number of excellent general developmental prescreening tools are available (*Parents' Evaluations of Developmental Status, Ages and Stages Questionnaire,* BRIGANCE screens, and the *Child Development Inventories);* the traditional and revised Denver screens are *no longer* recommended because of poor sensitivity and specificity (see Chapter 5 for references to these instruments). PCPs should routinely use one of these recommended tools. If suspicion warrants more specific screening, the **Checklist for Autism in Toddlers (CHAT;** Baird et al., 2000) is a standardized screening tool that can be used by the PCP. It has excellent specificity, although sensitivity is only fair. This can be used at 18 months, although revisions have improved the sensitivity if used at 24 months. This instrument continues to evolve, but now consists of both **questions for the parents and observations made by the PCP** or other healthcare worker. Key items are those that measure joint attention and pretend play (Table 17.1).

Children who are **screen positive** are **rescreened 1 month later.** Children who fail a second screen should be referred for comprehensive evaluation, as almost all of these children will have a PDD. Use of this screening strategy has yielded false-negative findings for many children with PDD, often because of parent over-reporting of early skills that on closer examination are not present. Questionnaire **screens for Asperger's syndrome** or high functioning autism in older children have recently been developed as well, although are not as well standardized. One such screen has been developed by **Ehlers**

Table 17.1.   Five Key Items on the CHAT[a]

A. Parent questions
   1. Does your child ever *pretend,* for example, to make a cup of tea using a toy cup and teapot, or pretend other things?
   2. Does your child ever use his or her index finger to point, to indicate *interest* in something?

B. Practitioner observation
   1. Get child's attention, then point across the room at an interesting object and say, "Oh, look! There's a (name of toy)!" Watch child's face. Does the child look across to see what you are pointing at?
   2. Get the child's attention, then give child a miniature toy cup and teapot and say, "Can you make a cup of tea?" Does the child pretend to pour out tea, drink it, and so on?
   3. Say to the child, "Where's the light?", or "Show me the light." Does the child *point* his or her index finger at the light? To record "Yes" on this item, the child must have looked up at your face around the time of pointing.

CHAT, checklist for autism in toddlers.
[a] *High risk* children fail all five items; *moderate risk* fail A1 and B3.
From Baird G, Charman T, Cox A, et al. Current topic: screening and surveillance autism and pervasive developmental disorders. *Arch Dis Child* 2001;84:468–475, with permission.

and Gillberg (1999) and another is the **Australian Scale for Asperger's syndrome** (Attwood, 1998), available as a download from the Online Asperger Syndrome Information and Support web site (see *Web Sites* in *Suggested Readings*).

A. **Further screening for social relatedness**

1. In the **infant,** look for the following:

    a. Has the baby developed a social smile?

    b. Does the baby make good eye contact with the caregiver?

    c. Does the baby appear to enjoy being held or cuddled?

    d. Does the baby show signs of playful reciprocity (i.e., visibly enjoyable back-and-forth interacting with others as in peek-a-boo, bye-bye, pat-a-cake)?

    e. Does the baby show signs of initiating the establishment of joint attention (e.g., pointing, vocalizations, showing)?

2. For **preschool-age** children, questions might include:

    a. Does the child show interest in other children, babies?

    b. Does the child show ability for playing games with others?

    c. Does the child play symbolically (i.e., does child appear to be playing out an organized "story" versus stacking objects, lining up, or using objects to produce sight or sound)?

    d. Does the child initiate joint attention in activities?

    e. Can the child have a conversation (i.e., back-and-forth verbalizations) about a topic?

3. For **older children,** screening questions might include:

    a. Does the child show interest in other children (this is usually true for children with Asperger's syndrome)?

    b. Does the child have at least one friend (i.e., someone the child wants to be with and who wants to be with that child (rare, even in Asperger's syndrome)?

    c. What does the child do with this friend? Play dates? Sleepovers? Talk on phone? (These are all unusual in children with PDD, including those with Asperger's syndrome.)

    d. Do other children pursue relationships with this child? (Typically no, but depends on the other children also.)

    e. Does the child get teased frequently? If so, why? (Many reasons exist for why children are teased but one is the social awkwardness of PDD; i.e., they "don't know how to make friends.")

B. Screening for speech and language deficits
1. For the infant:
   a. Does the infant babble in the first year?
   b. Does the infant appear to hear adequately?
   c. Does the baby orient (i.e., turn, look, or show other sign of recognition) to the parent's calling their name?
   d. Does the infant communicate needs clearly? If so, how?
   e. Does the infant point, wave, or grunt to establish joint attention?
2. For the older child:
   a. Does the child use toys appropriately to play?
   b. Does the child draw? If so, does it represent something to the child or is it merely a scribble?
   c. Does the child use full sentences that are entirely understandable to the PCP by age 4?
   d. Does the child have conversations with others? (Autistic children will have no ability for this; children with Asperger's syndrome will but conversations will be narrow and perseverative, often relating back to the child's circumscribed interest.)
   e. Does the child use speech to request material needs only (e.g., a cookie, bathroom)? Or, does child seek contact for social ends?
   f. Does the child respond appropriately to who, what, when, where questions?
   g. Does the child use pronouns properly or does he or she "reverse pronouns"?
   h. Does the child understand and use age-appropriate idioms?

C. Physical examination and laboratory. Although typically normal, a thorough physical examination is appropriate to reassure the parents that the child is otherwise healthy and to rule out neurologic conditions. **Audiologic evaluation** is indicated for any child with developmental delay in social or language areas. In cases of a child having an abrupt loss of language and socialization abilities, an electroencephalogram (EEG) can assist with the diagnosis of the rare Landau-Kleffner syndrome. The usual onset of this syndrome is between 3 and 7 years of age in an otherwise normally developing child; diagnosis is generally made by sleep EEG, which shows epileptiform pattern in the temporal regions. Other specific **laboratory or neuroimaging studies are unnecessary** unless indicated by the physical examination or symptoms of seizures or other neurologic symptoms are present (Table 17.2). Inadequate evidence supports testing for trace elements, allergies (e.g., food

Table 17.2. Indications for laboratory
investigation in autistic spectrum disorders

Test	Indications
Audiologic evaluation	All children with social or language delay
Electroencephalogram (EEG)	Symptoms suggest seizure, or history of regression in social, motor, language skills
Genetic testing	Dysmorphic features, family history of fragile x syndrome or tuberous sclerosis, MR with undetermined etiology
Lead screening	Pica
Metabolic consultation or testing	Dysmorphic, MR, early seizures
Neuroimaging	Focal neurologic signs or symptoms, seizures

MR, mental retardation

allergy for gluten, candida), vitamin levels, or immunologic abnormalities. Megalencephaly is present in 25% of patients, but is not a reason in and of itself for further testing.

III. **Triage assessment and treatment planning.**
   A.   **General issues.** The goals of assessment are to establish the diagnosis of PDD **early in the child's life** (i.e., before 3 years of age) and to initiate a treatment plan. Useful practice parameters on this topic, prepared by the American Academy of Neurology and Child Neurology Society and American Academy of Pediatrics, have been recently published (Filipek et al., 2000; American Academy of Pediatrics, 2001). Because these parameters already exist, this chapter follows closely their recommendations. Filipek et al. (2000) have distinguished between the:
   Level I investigation: routine developmental surveillance and screening specifically for autism.
   Level II investigation: diagnosis and evaluation of autism.
      It is generally accepted that early intervention substantially improves social, language, and emotional functioning. An example of such an intervention is the applied behavioral analysis regimen that has become the standard of care in some communities. **Treatment goals** generally involve **maximizing the child's potential,** as opposed to remediating the core social deficit. Despite periodic "miracle" cures in the media, no current treatment effectively alleviates this core deficit. The needs of the child and family are lifelong, requiring persistent support, advocacy, and

guidance. General management addresses the following areas:

1. **Psychoeducation of patient and family.** Initially, it is helpful to provide a **diagnosis,** information about the **nature and cause** of these disorders (i.e., neurologically based and not due to inadequate parenting), and **what can be done** at this time (i.e., a treatment plan). As with the presentation of any chronic and serious illness, the PCP should recognize that families need to be **educated in stages,** according to their ability to assimilate new information. The PCP should not expect that all information will be taken in and understood at the first discussion. Many discussions may ensue over a period of years. Being **given a diagnosis** is often a **crisis** for the family and initiates a **grieving process** that unfolds over months to years. Coming to terms with this reality is not easy for any parent and with each life milestone (e.g., birthdays, graduations, marriages, births) often comes further grieving reactions as they are met with unrealized hopes for their child. Understanding this process and supporting the child and family through this can be enormously helpful to them.

2. **Advocacy regarding schools** and assuring optimal educational placement and services for the child is critical. Being situated in an environment that recognizes and responds to the needs of children with PDD is crucial to the development and well-being of the child and to relieving family stress. A child in an unsuitable school environment is disastrous for both the child and the family! In the best of circumstances, the child's teacher is familiar with PDD; **academic, social, and behavioral programming** are in place; and the school administration (e.g., principal, school psychologist) will approach the situation flexibly and with a positive problem-solving attitude. Families should be encouraged to work together with the school in the best interests of the child. At times this can be extremely frustrating for the families, especially in the face of the current pressures on schools to limit expenditures. Controversy exists whether these children do best in "inclusion" classes or in "self-contained" (i.e., smaller numbers of children, often with other disabilities). This must be decided on a case-by-case basis, taking into account the particular child's needs, the teacher's strengths, and the resources available in the school (especially the availability of extra support in the classroom if the child is in an "inclusion" setting).

3. **A life span perspective** should be taken to prepare the child for independent living as he or she becomes older. Further **education or vocational training** and **life skills development** should begin to be addressed by mid-adolescence. Schools and developmental disabilities advocates are most helpful in identifying relevant programs. Parents may need to consider filing for **guardianship** (see Chapter 9) as their child approaches the age of majority. This is necessary to maintain the right to manage a child's finances and to maintain involvement with, and the right to consent for, decisions regarding treatment, vocational training and placements, or residential arrangements.

B. **Watching**
1. **When to be concerned about a PDD**
    a. Parental concern of social skills deficit (e.g., poor eye contact, does not enjoy being held, no playful reciprocity) in infant
    b. Failure to meet any of the following early language milestones:
        a. No babbling by 12 months
        b. No gesturing (pointing, waving bye) by 12 months
        c. Any **loss** of language or social skills at any age
    c. Failure to meet the following, if concerns also present for receptive language and pragmatics:
        a. No single words by 16 months
        b. No two-word sentences by 24 months
    d. Sibling with autistic spectrum disorder
    e. Positive family history of tuberous sclerosis or fragile X syndrome
2. **What to do when concerned (i.e., Level I investigation)**
    a. **Formal audiology evaluation,** including electrophysiologic procedures, behavioral audiometric measures, and assessment of middle ear function
    b. **Speech and language evaluation**
    c. **Lead level for children at risk who put "everything" in mouth**
    d. **CHAT**
    e. If problem identified, **referral to an early intervention program (<3 years of age) or local preschool committee on special education** (>3 years of age) for intervention services
    f. **Medications.** No medications are indicated for the at-risk child, as none are effective in preventing the development of PDD.

    g. **Monitoring.** CHAT should be repeated in 1 month for children who initially screen positive, which can be done by telephone in many situations. If positive 1 month later, child should be referred for diagnostic evaluation (see below). For children who screen negative but show some signs of social deficit, follow-up appointment for the child should be made in 2 to 4 months.

C. Intervening further

  1. When to evaluate and intervene further

    a. Screen positive on CHAT

    b. Screen negative on CHAT, but concerns persist at next visit

    c. Preschool child who regresses in social, language, or motor skills

    d. School-aged child with history of never having made a friend

    e. School-aged child, or older, with circumscribed and unusual interests

  2. What to do when evaluating and intervening further (level II investigation)

    a. **Further screening,** if desired, can be obtained by using an instrument such as the **Childhood Autism Rating Scale** (Schopler et al., 1988). This 15-item questionnaire has good psychometric properties and could be incorporated into PCP practice, although it does require training to use. **Refer to clinician (i.e., developmental pediatrician, child and adolescent psychiatrist, or child psychologist) or clinic (i.e., PDD or autism spectrum disorder clinic) with expertise in developmental problems for definitive diagnosis.** Although diagnosis is generally made using DSM-IV criteria, a number of standardized evaluation tools are available for clinical use. These take much time and, therefore, are not appropriate for general primary care use. The best tools available at this time are the **Autism Diagnostic Interview-Revised** (ADI-R; Lord et al., 1994), a parent-interview instrument, and the **Autism Diagnostic Observation Schedule** (ADOS; Lord et al., 1989), based on clinician observation.

    b. If a clinic is not available, it is important that a **multidisciplinary team** be involved in evaluating these children. This team should include a developmental pediatrician (or one with experience with PDD), clinical psychologist, social worker, speech and language pathologist, and occupational therapist. Consultants in genetics, neurology, and child and adolescent psychiatry are often helpful as well. In addition to PDD-specific diagnostic tools, the comprehensive evaluation should include:

(1) **Psychological testing** (i.e., *Wechsler Intelligence Scale for Children* [WISC] or other appropriate IQ testing; see Chapter 8.)

(2) **Adaptive functioning evaluation** is generally also done by a psychologist. The Vineland Adaptive Behavior Scales is the most widely used instrument for this.

(3) **Educational testing** to measure the child's academic readiness or skill levels.

(4) **Speech and language evaluation**

(5) **Family assessment** of resources, psychological strengths, stressors, and approach to behavior management can be done by a child mental health specialist (e.g., psychologist, social worker).

(6) **Behavioral assessment** is important in that many children with PDD have additional behavioral problems. General screening instruments such as the Child Behavior Checklist can be helpful starting points. Referral to a psychologist or child and adolescent psychiatrist is often helpful here.

c. **Further medical evaluation** should follow from the specific signs and symptoms (Table 17.2). No further medical evaluation is generally indicated for the child whose physical examination is otherwise normal (including appearance) and has no symptoms of neurologic disorders (e.g., seizures).

d. **Educate families about the condition, especially etiology (i.e., not due to parenting), and treatment.** In particular, the issue of fad treatments should be discussed. Every few years a new "miracle cure" emerges for autistic spectrum disorders that begins to circulate. With the advent of the internet, this trend is likely to escalate and parents may come in with questions about or, at times, insistence on receiving new unproved treatments. Although it is understandable that parents hold out hope, much time and money can be wasted on these treatments. Perhaps most damaging is the pursuit of these "miracles" while other modestly effective treatments are not received or the child becomes embroiled in the parents' avoidance of coming to terms with the diagnosis. This can become explosive fuel for behavioral problems in these children. The following **fad treatments** for the core deficits of PDD are **lacking in scientific evidence for efficacy** (Hyman and Levy, 2000; Tanguay, 2000):

(1) **Auditory integration training,** which is generally delivered by "therapists" trained in this procedure, involves training the child to decrease auditory hyper-responsiveness.

(2) **Desensitization for "cerebral allergy"**

(3) **Elimination diets** (e.g., dairy, wheat, gluten, sugar, additives). Anecdotally, the associated problems of some children (e.g., hyperactivity, difficulty falling asleep) have reportedly improved from these diets, although the results are often unimpressive when viewed by objective observers.

(4) **Facilitated communication,** which involves a trained "facilitator" guiding the child's hand and fingers to type on a keyboard, which is then used to communicate. Research has demonstrated that the communications are those of the "facilitator" and not the child.

(5) **Higashi daily life therapy**

(6) **Kaufman's "options" programs**

(7) **Megavitamin and magnesium treatments**

(8) **Secretin.** Despite much recent, initial excitement, controlled studies have failed to document efficacy (Osley et al., 2001), at least for single-dose treatment.

(9) **Steroids** can be helpful in the rare epilepsy condition, Landau-Kleffner syndrome, but are not effective for PDD.

(10) **Systemic candidiasis therapy**

e. **Referral to early intervention program or the committee for preschool special education** at the local school district. It is critical for parents to be linked with these programs as early as possible because these programs provide for the child's educational needs and also generally know the resources available in a community for evaluation, support, and treatment.

f. **Psychotherapy** may be indicated for associated family problems or difficulty managing the child. With higher functioning children and adolescents, individual or group therapy can be helpful as well.

g. **Medications** can be helpful for the associated problems (see below), although no medications have documented efficacy for the core deficits.

h. **Support groups** are available in many communities and are of enormous help to many families in providing support, education, and resources for daily living needs for children and adults with PDD. Some are specialized autistic spectrum support groups and others part of, or available through, a generic learning disabilities support group.

i. **The mental retardation/developmental disabilities (MR/DD)** system often offers case managers and other support services (e.g., respite services, recreational programs, vocational or work programs) to families. Children and adults with PDD are generally eligible for services in this system. These services are outside the mental health and education systems and, therefore, it is best to contact the MR/DD agencies directly to explore available services.

j. **Monitoring.** The child who has been diagnosed with a PDD and is receiving appropriate services should be seen for follow-up no less than every 6 months. This allows the PCP to provide sufficient support, education, and linkage with needed services.

D. **Referring**
   1. **When to refer to child and adolescent psychiatrist or developmental-behavioral pediatrician**
      a. Confirmed autistic spectrum disorder with comorbid:
         - Self-injurious behavior
         - Aggression
         - Severe oppositional behaviors
         - Depression
         - Severe sleep disorder
      b. Consider referral if autistic spectrum disorder with comorbid:
         - AD/HD-like symptoms
         - Anxiety disorder

2. **When referring.** Subspecialty clinics often are available for evaluation, consultation, and annual reviews. Ongoing management and support of the child and family often falls to the PCP. These children frequently have behavioral or emotional problems that require attention. At times, these problems can be managed in the PCP office. At others, a referral is indicated. All of the considerations mentioned above remain relevant to the situation when the child has been referred for a complicating psychiatric concern. The child and adolescent psychiatrist or developmental pediatrician typically can be expected to carry out some or all of the above functions.

   a. **Psychotherapy** is generally helpful in these situations and referral should be made to a child mental health professional with specialized experience with PDD. With younger children or those with externalizing behavior problems, **family therapy** often focuses on behavior management issues. In the older child or adolescent, **individual or group psychotherapy** can be useful in addressing social skills issues. **Cognitive behavioral** approaches can also be beneficial to some higher functioning older children or adolescents who have depressive or anxiety disorders. **Psychodynamic** approaches are helpful in selected higher functioning individuals to develop social skills, but this is more the exception and should not be routinely recommended.

   b. **Medications** are often used in these situations. They frequently are a critical part of the treatment plan, allowing the child or adolescent to benefit from the other programming and treatments they are receiving in addition to relieving symptoms.

   c. **Monitoring** for the child who has been referred for ongoing treatment should follow the guidelines above, in "when evaluating and intervening further."

IV. **Practical use of medications.** Medications have been sought to treat the core deficits in PDD but have been unsuccessful to date. Recently, excitement was generated about anecdotal reports of improvement with **secretin** in the amelioration of these core symptoms, but controlled trials of single doses have not confirmed its efficacy. Nevertheless, medications do have a prominent place in the management of many individuals with autistic spectrum disorders. These medications are targeted at the frequently associated behavioral and emotional symptom clusters that co-occur with PDD. Although virtually every type of psychotropic medication has been tried in this population, few controlled studies have been conducted. The recommendations that follow are based on the literature and clinical experience. Because data are so limited, it is recommended that the **PCP obtain consultation when prescribing in this population.** In using any medications with children with PDD, or other neurologic impairments, it is best to **start low and go slow** with dosing. Common symptom clusters and clinical treatment recommendations include:

A. **Aggression-agitation-tantrums cluster** is a common set of problems in these children. It often is related to rigidity, poor affect modulation, poor impulse control, and limited frustration tolerance, although mood disorders can contribute as well. The medications that have the best evidence for efficacy are the selective serotonin reuptake inhibitors (SSRI) and the atypical antipsychotics. Some evidence also supports the use of clonidine.

   1. The **SSRI** (Appendix N) are used in doses similar to those used in depressive disorders (see Chapter 15 for more details). No specific SSRI has established better efficacy than any of the others. SSRI can be activating (especially fluoxetine) and this can cause an increase in agitation, hyperactivity, or insomnia.

   2. The **atypical antipsychotics** (appendix D) have been widely used for this and other problems in autistic spectrum disorders. Risperidone has the most support and is commonly prescribed. Usual starting doses are 0.25 mg/day for children, and 0.5 mg for adolescents. Increased appetite, weight gain, hyperglycemia, and sedation are the most common side effects. Electrocardiographic (ECG) and liver function tests should be monitored. Olanzapine, quetiapine, and ziprasidone have also been used, although research support for them is even more limited. These also cause weight gain (less so with quetiapine and ziprasidone). Other side effects for this group of medications include galactorrhea (less with quetiapine) and anticholinergic effects for some (primarily olanzapine). These agents have virtually replaced the use of older antipsychotics (i.e., haloperidol, thioridazine, chlorpromazine), although these older agents may still be used in unusual circumstances by child and adolescent psychiatrists. The reason for this change is the relative infrequency of extrapyramidal side effects with the atypical agents. Although dystonias, Parkinson-like symptoms, akathisia, and tardive dyskinesia occur much less frequently than with the older agents, they can occur and any child on an atypical anti-

psychotic needs to be monitored for the development of these movement disorders. Neuroleptic malignant syndrome, another scourge of the older agents, occurs less frequently with the newer agents. In this syndrome, an acute onset of muscle rigidity occurs, followed by fever and autonomic instability. Treatment is supportive to prevent excess muscle breakdown, renal failure, and death (10%). Bromocriptine and dantrolene have been effective in some cases.

3. **Alpha adrenergic agonists** (clonidine, guanfacine, Appendix A) can be useful for these symptoms. These agents can cause hypotension, and require blood pressure monitoring. Families should be instructed not to miss doses or stop suddenly as this can cause rebound hypertension. Clonidine, but not guanfacine, is highly sedating. At times, this may be a desirable effect (see Chapter 12 for further details on prescribing).

4. When the aggression is minor and caused by poor impulse control (often in the context of AD/HD-like symptom picture), **stimulants** (Appendix O) have been helpful. Children with PDD often respond better to **low to moderate doses** (methylphenidate 1 mg/kg/day), whereas higher doses can cause withdrawn behavior, dysphoria, or increases in stereotyped patterns, including self-picking. Children with a lesser degree of mental retardation may show better responses to stimulants. Other side effects include tics, decreased appetite, anxiety, and irritability (see Chapter 12 for further details about using stimulants).

5. **Tricyclics** (Appendix P) have been used as second-line agents with this cluster of symptoms. PCPs are reminded of the cardiac effects, especially for desipramine, and the need for ECG monitoring. These agents also can lower seizure threshold, which may be especially relevant in this population because of the high incidence of seizures. Imipramine or desipramine have been started at doses of 1 mg/kg, gradually increasing to a maximum of 5 mg/kg which, in the higher ranges, is often given in divided doses to minimize side effects (e.g., cardiac, sedation, and anticholinergic effects). The dangers of overdose need to be fully reviewed with the family and patient.

6. **Naltrexone** has been modestly helpful in some cases of hyperactivity and aggression but is not a first-line treatment.

7. In cases of more severe aggression **mood stabilizers** have been used. Valproate (Appendix Q),

carbamazepine (Appendix H), and lithium (Appendix J) have all been helpful in selected cases, but should be reserved for use by child and adolescent psychiatrists or others experienced with this population. Use can be limited by the need for blood monitoring, which can be difficult in this population.

8. **Propranolol** (Appendix M) has been helpful as an adjunctive medication (usually with an antipsychotic agent) in moderate to severe aggression. Use in this population should be restricted to child and adolescent psychiatrists or other experts in this area.

B. **Self-injurious behavior (SIB).** This common problem (usually biting or hitting self, or head banging) can run from mild to severe, including serious injuries such as detached retinas and fractured skulls.

1. **SSRIs** have been helpful in some cases, in dosing similar to that used for depressive disorders.

2. **Naltrexone** had early reports of success but these have not held up.

3. Frequently, when symptoms are severe, SIB requires treatment with **atypical antipsychotics.** Low dose risperidone is commonly used for treating this problem.

C. **Hyperactivity-inattention-impulsivity cluster.** Although this cluster of symptoms is common in PDD, by convention these individuals are not given an additional diagnosis of AD/HD, despite that by every other measure they would meet criteria for the diagnosis. Treatment of this set of symptoms in the context of PDD is similar to that for AD/HD (see Chapter 12).

1. **Stimulants** are often used, although they generally are not as effective as in typically developing children with AD/HD. Side effects (i.e., irritability, dysphoria, and insomnia) are common. Stimulants can be more effective when used in lower doses and in combination with other medications (often atypical antipsychotics).

2. **Alpha agonists** also have support as treatment for hyperactivity.

3. Low dose **atypical antipsychotics** are frequently used for these symptoms. Because of the side effects cited, older antipsychotics are generally no longer used.

4. **Naltrexone** has been helpful in some cases, and might be tried when other agents have failed.

5. **Buspirone,** in doses of 5 to 10 mg twice or three times daily, has decreased hyperactivity in some children, although it is unclear if this results from its antianxiety effects.

D. **Stereotyped-perseverative-anxious cluster.** Narrow and repetitive rituals or interests may become a focus of treatment. They can have an "obsessive-compulsive" flavor with repeated worrying or perseverative statements dominating the symptom picture (e.g., Are you coming home? Is the bus coming?). This can lead to states of agitation that are problematic for families.

1. **SSRIs,** in doses used in depressive disorders, are first-line treatment for this cluster.
2. **Buspirone** may have a role in selected cases, although clinical experience has not been impressive.
3. **Atypical antipsychotics** are often helpful in low doses, but are generally utilized cautiously due to their side effect profile.
4. **Benzodiazepines** have been noted to increase hyperactivity and aggression in autistic children and, therefore, should be used only with caution.

E. **Mood disorder cluster.** Mood disorders or prominent irritability are frequent problems in this population. They are generally treated as in normally developing children and adolescents (see Chapter 16).

1. **SSRIs** are first-line treatment for these symptoms and are used in typical doses.
2. **Newer antidepressants** (e.g., venlafaxine, bupropion, mirtazapine) can also be helpful, although little or no data exist regarding their use in this population.

V. **Summary.** The pervasive developmental disorders are a group of serious, lifelong conditions that have an impact on all areas of the child's and family's life. Early recognition and prompt referral for appropriate educational, medical, psychological, and psychiatric treatment are paramount. The PCP is pivotal in initiating treatment and remains critical in the lives of the family members who look to them over many years for support, understanding, and guidance through a difficult path. As with other chronic conditions, optimal outcomes are achieved by early recognition, prompt treatment, family support, and lifelong interventions.

SUGGESTED READINGS

For the Physician

American Academy of Child and Adolescent Psychiatry. Practice parameters for the assessment and treatment of children, adolescents, and adults with autism and other pervasive developmental disorders. *J Am Acad Child Adolesc Psychiatry* 1999;38 (suppl.):32S–54S.

American Academy of Pediatrics Committee on Children with Disabilities. The pediatrician's role in the diagnosis and management of autistic spectrum disorder in children. *Pediatrics* 2001;107(5): 1221–1226.

Attwood T. *Asperger's syndrome: a guide for parents and professionals.* London: Jessica Kingsley Publishers, 1998:16–20.

Baird G, Charman T, Baron-Cohen S, et al. A screening instrument for autism at 18 months of age: a 6-year follow-up study. *J Am Acad Child Adolesc Psychiatry* 2000;39(6):694–702.

Baird G, Charman T, Cox A, et al. Current topic: screening and surveillance for autism and pervasive developmental disorders. *Arch Dis Child* 2001;84:468–475.

Buitelaar J, Willemsen-Swinkels S. Medication treatment in subjects with autistic spectrum disorders. *Eur Child Adolesc Psychiatry* 2000;9(suppl. 1):I85–I97.

Ehlers S, Gillberg C, Wing L. A screening questionnaire for Asperger's syndrome and other high-functioning autism spectrum disorders in school age children. *J Autism Dev Disord* 1999;29:129–141.

Filipek P, Accardo P, Ashwal S, et al. Practice parameter: screening and diagnosis of autism: report of the Quality Standards Subcommittee of the American Academy of Neurology and Child Neurology Society. *Neurology* 2000;55(4):468–479.

Filipek P, Accardo P, Baranek G, et al. The screening and diagnosis of autistic spectrum disorders. *J Autism Dev Disord* 1999;29(6): 439–484.

Halsey N, Hyman S. Measles-mumps-rubella vaccination and autistic spectrum disorder: report from New Challenges in Childhood Immunization Conference Convened in Oak Brook, Illinois June 12, 2000. *Pediatrics* 2001;107(5): E84.

Hyman S, Levy S. Autistic spectrum disorders: when traditional medicine is not enough. *Contemporary Pediatrics* 2000;17:101–116.

Kormaz B. Infantile autism: adult outcome. *Seminars in Clinical Neuropsychiatry* 2000;5(3):164–170.

Lord C, Rutter M, Goode S, et al. Autism diagnostic observation schedule: a standardized observation of communicative and social behavior. *J Autism Dev Disord* 1989;19:185–212.

Lord C, Rutter M, LeCouteur A. Autism diagnostic interview-revised: a revised version of a diagnostic interview for caregivers of individuals with possible pervasive developmental disorder. *J Autism Dev Disord* 1994;24: 659–685.

New York State Department of Health. Clinical practice guideline for autism/pervasive developmental disorders: assessment and intervention for young children (age 0–3 years), 1999. Available by calling the NYS Department of Health, Early Intervention Program (518-473-7016) or available on the web at www.health.state.ny.us/nysdoh/eip/menu.htm. Accessed on 6/29/02.

Osley T, McMahon W, Cook E, et al. Multisite, double blind, placebo controlled trial of porcine secretin in autism. *J Am Acad Child Adolesc Psychiatry* 2001;40(11): 293–1299.

Schopler E, Reichler R, Renner B. *The childhood autism rating scale.* Los Angeles: Western Psychological Services, 1988.

Tanguay P. Pervasive developmental disorders: a 10-year review. *J Am Acad Child Adolesc Psychiatry* 2000;39(9):1079–1095.

For Parents

Attwood T. *Asperger's syndrome: a guide for parents and professionals.* London: Jessica Kingsley Publishers, 1998.

Grandin T. *Talking in pictures and other reports from my life with autism.* New York: Random House, 1996.

Ives M, Munro N. *Caring for a child with autism.* London: Jessica Kingsley Publishers, 2001.

Jessica Kingsley Publishers, London, publishes widely for parents and professionals on autistic spectrum disorders. 1-800-634-7064. Available at www.jkp.com. Accessed on 6/29/02.

Myles B, Southwick J. *Asperger's syndrome and difficult moments: practical solutions for tantrums, rage and meltdowns.* Shawnee Mission, KS: Autism Asperger Publishing, 1999.

Willey L. *Pretending to be normal: living with Asperger's syndrome.* London: Jessica Kingsley Publishers, 1999.

Web Sites

Many web sites are dedicated to autism and related disorders. Parents should be advised that the quality of these sites is variable. In particular, parents should be cautioned about the possibility of misinformation, especially regarding the association of autism with immunizations and "miracle cures."

Asperger Syndrome Coalition of the United States is a private nonprofit organization providing information and advocacy for individuals with the syndrome. Available at www.asperger.org. Accessed on 6/29/02.

Autism Society of America is a private nonprofit organization dedicated to education and advocacy for individuals with autism. Available at www.autism-society.org. Accessed on 6/29/02.

Developmental Disabilities: Resources for Health Care Providers is a state of California initiative to educate primary care physicians and other healthcare providers about a wide variety of developmental disabilities and their treatment. Available at www.ddhealthinfo.org. Accessed on 6/29/02.

Division TEACCH (Treatment and Education of Autistic and Related Communication Handicapped Children) of the University of North Carolina is dedicated to research, cutting edge service delivery, and disseminating this information nationally and internationally. Extensive information from an academic program for parents and professionals. Has a list of summer programs, special schools, and college programs. Available at www.unc.edu/depts/teacch. Accessed on 6/29/02.

Online Asperger Syndrome Information and Support is a parent support website with extensive information, including downloads for the Australian Scale for Asperger's syndrome and the CHAT. Available at www.udel.edu/bkirby/asperger. Accessed on 6/29/02.

18 ♣ School Refusal

Jeffrey Q. Bostic and Harwood S. Egan

I. **Background. School refusal** is defined as **persistently** missing school despite being physically able to attend and having access to school. Approximately **1% to 3%** of schoolchildren refuse to attend school **each school year,** and 8% of all students will refuse at some point in their school careers. School refusal shows **peaks of onset at ages 7, 11, and 14,** consistent with **transitioning to elementary, middle, and high school.** For every day a child misses school, it becomes more difficult to return, with long-term risks including increased social difficulties, employment problems, later psychiatric illness, and lowered educational attainment.

When a child resists school, the primary care physician (PCP) must determine **what has made school less attractive than staying at home.** To best gauge the situation, the PCP must determine what is being avoided at school as well as what is gained by the child being at home. In addition, the PCP should consider what parents or schools may similarly be avoiding or gaining when the child is refusing school because their investment in the child's return to school will ultimately prove important in treatment planning. Multiple factors (see below) are typically involved, but three different patterns most commonly emerge:

1. The child wishes to attend school but **cannot successfully attend** (e.g., separation anxiety, "school phobia," depression, family illness).
2. The child wishes to remain at home to **avoid school** (e.g., unsafe school milieu, bullies, learning issues).
3. The child avoids school to **pursue more attractive activities** (e.g., conduct disorder, substance abuse).

The first pattern is most common for younger children, whereas the other two patterns are more common in adolescents. "School phobia" has been discarded as most cases are better captured by the *Diagnostic and Statistical Manual of Mental Disorders,* Fourth Edition term separation anxiety disorder. Typically, the child refuses to go to school for more than a week; or, over a number of months repeatedly complains of stomachaches, headaches, fatigue, or dizziness; and "can't" go to school. Over time, adult reactions turn to irritability or anger at feeling manipulated. This problem is especially likely to occur at the **beginning of school years or after school breaks or vacations.** Of children who experience one episode of school refusal, **one third will experience an additional episode.**

A. **Factors involved in school refusal.** Table 18.1 provides a framework for clinicians to identify factors relevant to school refusal. A number of factors should be considered in each child's refusal to attend school:

Table 18.1.   Factors in school refusing children and adolescents

	Child Onset	Adolescent Onset
Individual factors	1. Temperament 2. Physical illness 3. Psychiatric disorder 4. Loss (separation, divorce, death)	1. Psychiatric illness (psychosis, depression) 2. Conduct disorder 3. Substance abuse
Family factors	1. Parent(s) with separation sensitivity or anxiety disorder 2. Disabled parents unable to care for selves 3. Parents fearful of violence, other dangers 4. Psychotic parents incorporating children into delusions	1. Limited or poor supervision and monitoring 2. Parental substance abuse
School factors	1. Learning problems (learning disabled, MR, or borderline intellectual functioning especially when unrecognized) 2. Unsupportive or mismatched teaching environment (yelling, harshness, criticism) 3. Unsafe school milieu (fighting, neighborhood violence) 4. Peer stress (bullies, teasing) 5. Situational demands (oral presentation for shy children)	1. Academic failure 2. Failure to provide adequate academic support or special education services 3. Social ostracism

1. **Acute situational stress.** School failure or academic deterioration; fear of humiliation by a teacher or peer; bullying by another student; loss (divorce or death); problems at home, which either the child fears will be detected at school (e.g., physical or sexual abuse) or which make the child fear leaving the parent alone (e.g., substance abuse, chronic illness) can deter school attendance. If acutely stressful factors are identified and modifications are made (e.g., changes

in a class, alternative to showering with others, bullying stopped) but the school refusal persists, other underlying issues must be explored. As students mature, sexual orientation issues can become overwhelmingly stressful for students. A particularly difficult, and too common, problem in urban settings is that the school milieu may not be safe. Frequent fighting, neighborhood violence, and general unruly behavior can interfere with school attendance for many children.

2. **Internalizing emotional disorders.** Most commonly, children resist school because of internalizing disorders, such as anxiety, depression, and somatoform disorders. These disorders interfere with motivation, persistence, and ability to stay on task. **Up to 75% of school-refusing children exhibit anxiety disorders,** usually separation anxiety in elementary students and agoraphobia or social phobia in older students. The older the student, the more likely depressive disorders are present.

3. **Externalizing emotional disorders.** Students may avoid school because of externalizing disorders such as conduct disorder.

4. **Emerging psychiatric disorders.** Schizophrenia, bipolar disorder, obsessive-compulsive disorder, or major depression with psychotic features often emerges during the school years. Substance abuse must also be considered in adolescent-onset school refusal.

5. **Physical health.** Medications, asthma, seizures, cystic fibrosis, diabetes, chronic fatigue syndrome, anemia, hypothyroidism, and chronic illness can have an impact on school effort.

6. **Learning disabilities.** Students with no previous school refusal who suddenly complain that academics are "just too hard" may be embarrassed about an underlying learning disability.

7. **Temperament.** "Bad fits" between the temperament of the child and that of the teacher can culminate in school refusal. This is especially true in younger children who may be highly reactive to teachers who are stern or are perceived as frightening.

II. **Practical office evaluation.** Assessment of the school-refusing child requires the clinician to appraise the relative contributions of the factors noted above. It is preferable to begin the interview with a parent, but at some point attempts should be made to interview the patient alone. If the child cannot tolerate the parent leaving, or if the parent cannot tolerate the child being alone with the PCP, this often reveals separation anxiety. Physical illnesses (e.g., infection, anemia, hypothyroidism, chronic illness) can lower a child's ability to cope with the demands of a school day. Although these conditions can increase lost school days, excessive absenteeism more often suggests an emotional component. The PCP should pursue a workup to a point at which he or she can allay patient and family fears that symptoms (i.e., stomachaches, headaches, fatigue) might be attributable to a physical illness. The PCP should perform a **complete physical examination** along with screening laboratory tests (e.g., complete blood count, liver function tests, thyroid stimulating hormone, electrocardiogram [ECG], as appropriate) to identify physical illnesses suspected to contribute to school refusal. The PCP should be mindful that extensive medical workups may only reinforce parental fears of organic illness, and should make an effort to balance the child's fears of needles or laboratory procedures with perceived benefits from proposed procedures.

A. **For the child**
   1. **Absences.** How many days has the child missed? Which days? Has this ever happened in other grades? A psychiatric disorder is suggested when symptoms diminish at home (i.e., on weekends or over the summer), but increase the day before returning to school each week, the month before school starts, after vacations/holidays.
   2. **Feelings.** How does the child feel about missing school? Children who deny the existence of a problem more often have a psychiatric disorder.
   3. **Trauma or loss.** Has the child experienced anything traumatic? Any evidence of physical or sexual abuse? Any recent losses (including separation, divorce, or death)?
   4. **Child response.** What does the child *do* when not in school? Who stays with child? How does the child respond to the situation? Children who stay home and participate in enjoyable activities (e.g., TV, shopping) with the parent(s) are likely to have an anxiety disorder.
   5. **Family response.** What does the mother do to encourage the child to go to school? The father? Other important adults? Is the family in some way reinforcing the child's absences?
   6. **Child's stated reasons for absence.** Why is the child missing school? Is there evidence of an anxiety disorder (e.g., separation fears, panic attacks, agoraphobia)? Any problems with a teacher? With other students (bullies)? With the school milieu and climate? Academically? On the bus?
   7. **Somatic symptoms.** Does the child have trouble with headaches, stomachaches, or fatigue? Somatic symptoms that do not point to a medical cause may signify an anxiety disorder or depression. Typically, somatic symptoms in anxiety disorders evaporate once the child knows he or she can stay home for the day.

B. **For adolescents (in addition to questions above)**
   1. What does the youth **do when not in school?** Does he or she want to do something else (e.g., go to the mall, get high, hang out, make money)?
   2. Any evidence of **substance abuse?**
   3. Any evidence of a broader **conduct disorder** (stealing, fighting, lying, other criminal behavior)? Note: this is usually better asked of the parent(s).
   4. Is the **educational programming** for the adolescent appropriate? Should the youth be oriented more into a vocational track versus an academic track?
   5. Is the adolescent **avoiding** something at school? Academically? Socially (e.g., broken romantic relations, bullies)?

C. **For the parents**
   1. **School performance.** How is the child performing in school? On homework? Any evidence for a learning disability or other cognitive difficulties? Other problems in school? With teachers? With peers? If so, is the school responsive to the needs of the child?
   2. Does the child have a history of **conduct-disordered behavior?** Substance abuse?
   3. Does the parent(s) want the child to **remain at home?** If so, why? Is there domestic violence, community violence, physical illness, or psychosis in parent?
   4. Any evidence for **trauma or loss?**
   5. Are **both parents actively involved** in trying to solve the problem? When this is not the case, evidence is often seen for a separation anxiety difficulty.

D. **For the school**
   1. Remember that **parental consent is required** for communication with schools.
   2. Does the school have concerns about the child's functioning? **The Teacher Report Form** is an efficient way to obtain information about the child's academic, social, and emotional functioning in the school setting. We recommend using this routinely.
   3. Has the school adequately evaluated the child? Is it advocating for the child's school needs?
   4. Does the school agree with the **current educational placement** of this student?
   5. Are different or additional school-based services recommended? How have the **parents responded to the school's recommendations?**

III. **Triage assessment and treatment planning**
   A. **General issues.** The main goal of treatment is to **return the child to the school setting as quickly as possible.** This requires an understanding of the

factors involved in the child's school refusal as well as a deft handling of parents, child, and school personnel. A **firm but gentle approach,** with clear expectations that it is best for the child to return to school, generally provokes the least counter-resistance. Overly authoritarian directives to return to school or to return for longer periods than the child is able are counterproductive. Often it is best that the child **return to school in a graded manner,** starting with partial return and working up over a few weeks to full return. It is also critical **to involve the child actively** in collaboratively planning and problem-solving to avoid the child feeling that this is one more thing adults are "forcing" him or her to do. It is far preferable for children to see that the adults are merely trying to help them do what is in their best interest. Most of these situations are handled with an outpatient treatment plan. **Hospitalization** is rarely employed for the school-refusing child. It is often traumatic for the child with separation fears to be placed in an unfamiliar "locked" place where parental contact is limited. Accordingly, hospitalization is indicated only (a) when the child exhibits symptoms suggestive of an underlying medical disorder, which can be expeditiously determined in the hospital; (b) when the child is psychotic or suicidal; or (c) if home factors (e.g., abuse allegations) necessitate the child being in a safe environment to disentangle factors contributing to the school refusal.

B. **Watching**
   1. **When to watch**
      a. Child has missed minimal school
      b. No associated psychiatric condition is present
      c. Academic functioning is adequate
      d. Family functioning appears good or improving
   2. **When watching**
      a. **Psychoeducation**
         (1) **Review evaluation** with parents and child. It is recommended that **both parents be present** to discuss the findings of the PCP and to review the various factors thought to be relevant to the child's absences. For the child who has somatic complaints, the PCP can allay the family's fears by stating that the child "does not have a serious or life-threatening medical condition" causing the symptoms. Instead, the symptoms appear to be the child's way of communicating a feeling of being stressed.
         (2) **Encourage the child's return to school.** At this point, parents and

child can be encouraged to return to school with a firm message that it is medically safe for the child to attend school. It is not helpful for parents to reason or bargain with the child about going to school, to allay their own anxiety by telling the child the school or PCP is imposing this plan, or to entice the child with stories of how much fun school is. Instead, parents should present the plan to the child in **a neutral, matter of fact** way.

(3) **Provide a rationale for school return.** Frame interventions in the **child's best interest.** Although parents may complain that a teacher, class, peer, or other is traumatizing the child, usually parents can recognize that staying home and being deprived of other peers and opportunities for activities at school does not prepare the child for the future. If parents complain that the current school situation is intolerable, it sometimes helps for parents to realize their child's life cannot be "put on hold" to wait for another class, new teachers or aides to be found, and so on. As noted, it is important to emphasize to the child that the reasons to return are to help him or her feel better about self (i.e., children who don't go to school usually feel worse about themselves); to feel less anxious (e.g., the longer a child stays home the more anxious the child feels about returning, the more work to catch up, the more explanations needed to others); and to get in the habit of "facing your fears" rather than avoiding them. It is best for the PCP to resist strenuously asserting adult authority with the child ("You **will** go to school by Wednesday!"), which likely promotes a counterproductive power struggle. Usually the parents have already tried this strategy without success.

(4) **Reassurance of child and parents.** Parents usually report better success when empathizing with the child's fear, making appropriate contact available during the school day, and reassuring the child that they will see the child at a certain time

(e.g., pick up the child at 2:45 p.m.). Similarly, parents often need reassurance that it will not damage their child psychologically to return to school and cry, feel anxious, have stomachaches, and so on. Often attending to the parents' fears, allowing them to ventilate, and providing reassurance to them are sufficient to resolve mild or insidious difficulties.

(5) **Problem-solve with child and family regarding return to school.** Give the child some say in returning to school, but toward successful reintegration. Asking the child to agree to return to school by a certain date is rarely successful and further frustrates school and treatment personnel. Rather, asking which school person the child prefers to have meet him or her at school or what time and with whom he or she wants to read a note from home during the school day better empowers the child. Compromises occur around **how** the child will resume school, never about **whether** the child should resume school. Children who avoid school learn to isolate themselves when confronted with difficulties in later life circumstances (e.g., work).

(6) **Reinforce success.** Reward **any** successes (e.g., getting to the school building, staying for 10 minutes) rather than punish for not succeeding throughout the entire school day. Suggest opportunities for parents to demonstrate support (e.g., letters from them in lunch-box, phone calls at designated time).

b. **Advocacy** by the PCP with the school is generally not necessary in these mild situations. Parents generally manage satisfactorily by discussing the situation with the child's teachers or school administrator. Occasionally situations arise in which the parents decide that the main problem is a mismatch with the teacher or school. Changes in classroom or school may ensue, often with resolution of the school refusal. The PCP may not know whether to support these complex decisions. In most situations what the parents need is help in thinking through their decision (versus being told what is best to do). If parents proceed with a decision that the PCP feels is not in the child's long-term best interest, this issue can be raised while recognizing that the parents are the "experts" when it comes to their child and that they bear responsibility for them.

c. **Psychotherapy** is not necessary in these situations unless clear comorbid psychiatric conditions exist.

d. **Medication** is rarely indicated in these cases, unless sleep disturbances or specific, overwhelming fears (e.g., getting onto the bus) are present.

e. **Laboratory and other evaluations** are not necessary beyond the examination already completed during the course of the initial evaluation. Any new or different symptoms that emerge should receive standard pediatric attention.

f. **Monitoring.** Parents can be asked to call in 1 to 2 weeks and verify that the child has indeed returned to school. The child should be brought back for an office visit in 4 to 6 weeks for follow-up. Scheduling an appointment regardless of symptomatology (versus on "an as needed" basis) prevents the fostering of symptoms caused by the child "needing" to be ill to receive attention.

C. **Intervening further**
 1. **When to intervene further**
  a. Child has missed more than 1 week of school since the beginning of the school year
  b. Academic functioning shows mild drop
  c. Appearance of inadequate school support or placement
  d. Mild to moderate family disturbance, but parents allied in best interest of child
 2. **When intervening further**
  a. **Psychoeducation**
   (1) **Encourage return to school, reinforce rationale, provide reassurance, problem-solve, and promote rewarding success as above.**
   (2) **Promote realistic goals.** Help parents and child appreciate that full return to school and activities may take more time than they hoped or thought it "should" take. The main idea is to "keep moving in the right direction" and "putting one foot in front of the next."
   (3) **Recognize treatable psychiatric conditions.** Look for signs of anxiety

or depressive disorders that are frequently present in school refusers. Watch for signs of substance abuse in adolescents.

(4) **Support and reassure parents** that separating is not "scarring" the child. It may be helpful for the parents to call the school an hour after the child has arrived to reassure themselves that the child has made a satisfactory transition into the classroom setting. For younger children, parents can unobtrusively observe the child after he or she is dropped off at school to see the child's capacity to regroup. If a child is consistently unable to regroup, a referral for mental health treatment is indicated.

b. **Advocacy.** Direct involvement with the school is usually needed at this point. First, the PCP must make sure that the child's **academic skills and school needs** have been adequately **assessed.** It is often helpful to have the **parents observe the child at school** to obtain direct information about the school environment, the responsiveness of the staff, and the congruence of the school's assessment of the child. This can clarify the contribution of school-based factors and inform a decision whether the child would be best served by a change in schools or classes. Although moving a child should not be the first consideration, at times it is clearly the most appropriate. The following are clues that the placement may need alteration:

1. Persistent harshness by the classroom teacher toward the child
2. Teacher's or administrator's assessment of the child that is more negative and seriously at odds with parental perceptions
3. Teacher or administrator unable to discuss the child's needs productively, leaving parents frustrated and not "heard"

(1) Assuming that a change in placement is not indicated, the next major consideration is the establishment of a **"safety net"** for if and when the child needs to leave class. A key ingredient to success here is designating someone at school (e.g., guidance counselor, social worker, psychologist)

whom the child can contact on an as needed basis in the course of the school day.

(2) A second issue is establishing a **nursing plan** for evaluating somatic symptoms at school to which both parents and school personnel agree. Typically, an arrangement will be made with the school nurse to evaluate the child if symptoms develop. If the child does not appear ill and is afebrile, the child can stay in the nurse's office for a few minutes and then is encouraged to return to class. Parents should not be contacted unless the nurse feels this is medically necessary (e.g., child appears ill or has a temperature >100°F).

(3) Other school issues that need to be practically addressed can be accomplished by the family in conjunction with the school. At other times, these details require a third party to come to agreement. Some communities have **educational advocates** available to parents for this purpose. Common considerations are:

1. **Altering the school day** (abbreviating, or starting with classes or teachers where likelihood of success is greater)
2. Diminishing stress by **reducing academic workload,** particularly redundant work
3. Addressing school environment issues that prevent attendance
4. Allaying the child's fears by structuring opportunities for **sanctuary** and reassurance. Identify places of sanctuary (e.g., library, counselor's office) and "safe" peers with whom the student can readily affix when entering school, going to lunch, waiting for or riding the bus.
5. Revise frequently (e.g., weekly until stabilized) any intervention plan with child, family, and school staff.
6. Maintain frequent communication among school, home, and the PCP.
7. Identify small steps toward feared or avoided school activities.

8. **Home tutoring is usually best avoided,** as it slows the child's return to school, making future efforts to get the child back into school more difficult. Follow-up of students treated with home tutoring revealed these students more often experienced further educational, social, and psychiatric problems.

9. In rare cases, the child will not return to school. If modifications are made but the student makes little effort or if the parents cannot comply with the intervention program, the school may be required to report the case to **Child Protective Services** or commensurate agencies. Follow through is important and can actually avail the student, family, and school of additional resources to conquer school refusal. Helping the school to recognize that it only "keeps score" of absences may help school personnel act appropriately and with less emotion. Accordingly, as the plan is devised it should be made clear what expectations are (usually 50% to 75% attendance if the child has been attending <25%), how revisions will occur, and at what point the school will be required to report what to whom (e.g., "If child misses 12 days over next school quarter we are obligated to report to. . . .").

c. **Psychotherapy.** Cognitive behavioral strategies are often helpful at this stage. The PCP can use the following principles effectively:

   (1) Establish a **fear hierarchy.** What does the child fear? Discern a hierarchy from most fear to least fear and begin efforts with the least fears. These can be determined during a walk-through at the school, if they cannot be described outside school.

   (2) **Clarify antecedents and consequences** or rewards the child obtains by missing school. Strategies based on this analysis provide **intervention targets** to address antecedents

(e.g., child is afraid when dropped off for school that others will speak meanly to him) or consequences (child remaining at home gets to watch television).

(3) Strategies beneficial for the school-refusing child usually include **desensitization** to anxiety-provoking circumstances and **graded exposure,** whereby the student gradually is exposed to larger parts of the distressing situation. **Desensitization** involves identifying concrete steps for the student to take to diminish particular fears surrounding school attendance. This might include visiting the school building before the year starts, showing up early to connect with a teacher or staff person, and so on. **Graded exposure** involves establishing "steps" to more regular participation in school. If the child fears humiliation, devise steps to allow the student to initiate responses to teachers, then respond to teacher questions he or she knows (raise right hand if >80% sure of answer), and then to be called on randomly.

(4) **Relaxation or visual imagery.** Help the child relax through deep breathing or **emotive imagery.** Have the child identify and practice having images of superhero friends accompany him or her into distressing situations. Or, decide on "transitional objects" (e.g., plastic superhero figures, pictures or cards of powerful others or conventional objects, e.g., a piece of cloth) to keep in a pocket or inside a notebook, which can accompany the child from home to school.

(5) Identify **distraction techniques** (when anxious, internally repeating an encouraging word such as "brave" or phrase such as "I can make it.")

(6) Adolescents sometimes benefit from imagining how other **role models** would contend with similar circumstances.

   If none of the above strategies is sufficient, referral to a qualified child mental health may be necessary.

      d. Medication is usually unnecessary at this point. If psychoeducational and psychotherapeutic approaches have not been successful, use of short-term benzodiazepines (alprazolam, clonazepam, or lorazepam) may be helpful. Medications may also be considered if an anxiety or depressive disorder is identified.

      e. Laboratory and other evaluation. Unless new somatic symptoms arise, no additional laboratory test or examination is necessary.

      f. Monitoring. When symptoms are more disabling, follow-up should occur every 2 to 4 weeks. Telephone calls are helpful between appointments to update the PCP, reinforce gains, and clarify approaches.

D. Referring

  1. When to refer and transfer primary responsibility

      a. Child has missed more than 2 weeks of school (not necessarily consecutively)

      b. Evidence of another significant psychiatric disorder (e.g., separation anxiety disorder, depression, psychosis, conduct disorder, substance abuse)

      c. Moderate to severe interference in academic functioning

      d. Evidence is seen of severe family disturbance, including physical or sexual abuse, substance abuse, chaos; in some cases, separation or divorce is also accompanied by temporary and severe decrements in parental functioning.

      e. Any evidence of dangerous behavior (e.g., assaultiveness, suicidality)

  2. When referring

      a. Psychoeducation. Continued application of principles discussed above. Primary objective at this stage is to **continue support and encouragement** of parents and child, especially if progress is going slowly. Recognizing that "Rome wasn't built in a day" and that "sometimes we need to take one step back to make two steps forward" can be helpful in providing a much-needed perspective and in containing anxiety. Supporting the effort toward continued psychotherapeutic treatment is also critical to prevent the family from prematurely stopping treatment.

      b. Advocacy. At this point, the child and family may need assistance in procuring intensive treatment resources from the school, social services, or mental health systems.

    c. **Psychotherapy** is critical at this point and may include individual, group, and family components. More intensive psychotherapeutic programs may be necessary (e.g., day treatment, specialized schools, intensive support programs). Qualified child mental health professionals should be familiar with local programs and resources. They should take the lead in accessing these higher levels of services.

    d. **Medication** is generally indicated at this stage (see section below on *Psychotropic Medication Management*).

    e. **Laboratory and other evaluation.** Unless new somatic symptoms arise no additional laboratory test or examination is necessary.

    f. **Monitoring.** Until the child is comfortably back in school, follow-up appointments should occur every month to monitor progress and assure that a comprehensive treatment plan is being carried out.

IV. Psychotropic medication management. If the child is not able to attend school **after a psychosocial intervention plan** has been implemented, medications warrant consideration. Treatment should be directed at an underlying disorder (e.g., separation anxiety, depression). Although no medications are available specifically for conduct-disordered children who avoid school, some may be helpful for associated conditions (e.g., attention-deficit/hyperactivity disorder, depression). Children who have missed school with significant substance abuse histories should not be prescribed medications before having adequate psychosocial treatment for the substance abuse.

    A. Open trials support the use of **selective serotonin reuptake inhibitors (SSRIs)** (Appendix N) such as citalopram, fluoxetine, paroxetine, sertraline, and fluvoxamine as first-line treatment for juvenile anxiety and depression. Citalopram, fluoxetine, paroxetine, and sertraline are available in liquid formulations for patients unable to tolerate pills.

    B. Citalopram, fluoxetine, or paroxetine 5 to 10 mg every day, and titrated up to 20 mg after 1 week or sertraline (12.5 to 25 mg and titrated up weekly to 50 to 100 mg every day) is usually sufficient. Citalopram and sertraline have medium half-lives (~35 hours in juveniles), so that missing a dose does not usually lead to immediate withdrawal symptoms.

    C. SSRIs are often started in conjunction with **benzodiazepines** (Appendix D), with the benzodiazepine gradually reduced to "as needed" (p.r.n.) or tapered after approximately 4 weeks on the SSRI. The PCP can initiate a short-acting benzodiazepine, both at night when anxiety escalates about expectations for the next day and in the morning before going to school. Alprazolam (Xanax) is the most rapid acting of the commonly used benzodiazepines; it can be dosed 0.5 mg p.r.n. severe anxiety every 4 hours. Lorazepam 0.5 to 1 mg p.r.n. every 4 hours or clonazepam 0.25 to 0.5 mg every 6 hours may also allay sudden overwhelming anxiety or panic attacks.

  D. If the above are ineffective, the **tricyclic antidepressant (TCA) imipramine** (Appendix P), 50 to 150 mg about 1 hour before bedtime, may be helpful. TCAs require obtaining baseline and final dose ECGs. Clarifying that this is to detect any pre-existing heart conduction disturbance may be important to ensure patients and parents do not interpret this as a sign that the child has heart problems and become more anxious.

 V. **Summary.** School refusal is not a diagnosis, but rather a symptom resulting from a confluence of numerous factors. The understanding of the many factors involved in each case allows for a comprehensive approach to treatment. In most situations, the PCP is the key player in orchestrating the child's return to school. Most cases resolve satisfactorily, although recurrence is not uncommon.

SUGGESTED READINGS

Berg I, Nursten J, eds. *Unwillingly to school,* 4th ed. Washington, DC: American Psychiatric Press, 1996.

King NJ, Bernstein GA. School refusal in children and adolescents: a review of the past 10 years. *J Am Acad Child Adolesc Psychiatry* 2001;40(2):197–205.

Kleckner K, Engel RE. A child begins school: relieving anxiety with books. *Young Children* 1988;43(5):14–18. Presents an annotated bibliography of children's books, which parents and teachers can use to help young children deal with separation anxiety and other feelings associated with the beginning of school.

Velosa JF, Riddle MA. Pharmacologic treatment of anxiety disorders in children and adolescents. *Child Adolesc Psychiatr Clin N Am,* 2000;9:119–133.

Williams T, Hodgman C. Medication for the management of anxiety disorders in children and adolescents. *Pediatr Ann* 2001;30(3):146–153.

Web Sites

American Academy of Child and Adolescent Psychiatry. Click on Facts for Families and search for School Refusal. This is a one-page concise review for parents. Available at www.aacap.org. Accessed on 6/20/02.

National Association of School Psychologists. Search for "school refusal." A two- to three-page summary for parents available in English and Spanish. Available at www.naspcenter.org/index2.html. Accessed on 6/20/02.

19 ♣ Sexuality

William N. Friedrich and William J. Barbaresi

I. **Background.** Sexual behavior in children is often a concern in the pediatric office practice. However, the physician has only a scant body of literature to refer to regarding the management of behaviors such as compulsive masturbation in a 4-year-old or precocious sexual interest. Problematic sexual behavior (e.g., "has forced someone into sexual activity") is one of fifteen criteria for conduct disorder in children, and when evident, is of considerable concern. However, a range of less severe behaviors is more commonly seen. It is not surprising that many of these behaviors can be both troubling and puzzling to parents and professionals.

According to research questioning parents about their children, developmentally related sexual behaviors occur in at least 20% of children at given age levels (Table 19.1).

In addition, other sexual behavior that can be initially concerning to a parent may fall into a category of **normal sex play,** similar to other types of role-playing observed in children. In younger children, this can include pretend weddings, having a "boyfriend or girlfriend," being "married," and "playing doctor." Conversations about genitalia or reproduction or the use of dirty words with peers or similar age siblings should also be considered normal. Preadolescents may play "truth or dare" or similar games that fall into the normal range as well. Adolescents normally show an interest in erotica, have sexually explicit conversations with peers, and learn to flirt. Private masturbation should also be considered normative. Although individual families or cultural or religious groups restrict or prohibit it, sexual activity with a partner should also be considered normal unless problematic features are present.*

Sexual orientation also unfolds during adolescence. Parents or teenagers may come in with concerns related to homosexual thoughts, feelings, or behaviors. Sexual experimentation, including same-sex activities during childhood and adolescence, is common in childhood and adolescence and does not predict future sexual orientation. The origins of homosexuality are not clear, and consensus is that particular parenting practices do **not** determine sexual orientation. Further, no credible evidence suggests that parents (or others, including psychotherapists) can alter an adolescent's sexual orientation once formed. From a psychiatric perspective, gay or lesbian orientation is part of the continuum of sexual expression and is not considered a psychiatric disorder. It should not be seen as a "choice" that individuals willfully and consciously decide. Nevertheless,

---

*For both males and females, about half of high school students, and nearly two-thirds of 12th graders, have had sexual intercourse at least once (CDC data). Nearly 10% have been sexually active before age 13. All rates are substantially higher for African–American youth, with Hispanic and then white rates lower.

Table 19.1.   Developmentally related sexual behaviors

Boys 2–5 yr
    Stands too close to people
    Touches sex parts when in public places
    Touches or tries to touch their mother's or other women's breasts
    Touches sex parts when at home, and tries to look at people when
       they are nude or undressing

Girls 2–5 yr
    Stands too close to people
    Touches or tries to touch their mother's or other women's breasts
    Touches sex parts when at home
    Tries to look at people when they are nude or undressing.

Boys 6–9 yr
    Touches sex parts when at home
    Tries to look at people when they are nude or are undressing

Girls 6–9 yr
    Touches sex parts at home
    Tries to look at people when they are nude or are undressing

Boys 10–12 yr
    Very interested in the opposite sex

Girls 10–12 yr
    Very interested in the opposite sex

---

many families find homosexuality very disturbing. This often results in gay or lesbian youth who find themselves isolated within their families as they struggle with their sexual orientation. For this reason, as well as limited acceptance with peers and the wider community, these youth are vulnerable to a variety of mental health problems. Most important are the **substantial risks** of:

1. **Suicidal behavior and suicide**
2. **Depression**
3. **Substance abuse**
4. Stress, trauma, or physical injury caused by **violence and victimization** at school or in the community

The attentive primary care physician (PCP) can be of critical importance to gay and lesbian youth in providing psychological support and, at times, advocating for them through the major risk period of adolescence and the "coming out" phase. Community-based support groups (e.g., P-FLAG, see *Web Sites* in *Suggested Readings*) can literally save lives. The PCP should be familiar with these resources and assist in referral.

Given that much of sexual behavior and interest is developmentally normative, comorbid behavior problems are not expected. When other behavior problems are described along with the sexual behavior, the management decision becomes more complex. Problematic sexual behavior for both children and teenagers is significantly associated with a range of symptom clusters, including anxiety, bipolar disorder, posttraumatic stress, aggression, social skills deficits, delinquent-spectrum behaviors, and developmental disorders.

In general, the child's caretakers determine whether a young child's sexual behavior is identified as a problem. A 4-year-old girl who daily grabs her crotch in one day-care setting can legitimately be seen as normal, whereas a single instance of prolonged genital auto-exploration in another 4-year-old girl will prompt a referral that may not turn up anything inappropriate.

In determining whether a given sexual behavior is problematic, consider the following:

1. **Frequency.** Higher frequency brings forth more concern.
2. **Compulsiveness.** More compulsive behavior arouses greater concern.
3. **Context.** Some behaviors are acceptable in private (e.g., masturbation), but not in public.
4. **Physical safety.** Behaviors that put self or others at risk are problematic.
5. **Mutual consent.** Lack of consent in behaviors involving others is problematic and requires adult intervention.
6. **Equality.** Lack of equality (i.e., age, cognitively) between the two (child or adolescent) requires adult intervention.
7. **Coercion.** Physical or psychological threats require adult intervention.

   Keypoints to keep in mind include:
1. Most children and nearly all adolescents will exhibit sexual behavior, interest, or both.
2. Problematic levels of sexual behavior more often than not are associated with other behavior problems.
3. Referral of children and teens is often subjective and can reflect beliefs and values of the individual caregiver.
4. Consideration of child maltreatment or other psychosocial problems is advisable, but may not be present in the child you are seeing.
5. When sexual behavior problems are present, without other behavior problems, their management can be relatively straightforward.
6. Family violence is related to increased sexual behavior problems in children.
7. Children's sexual behavior is influenced by the family's attitudes and behavior about sexuality, including open nudity, safe touch, and many other issues.

II. **Practical office evaluation.** Physicians can be reluctant to manage these behaviors for several reasons. The first may reflect a lack of comfort talking about sexuality with parents and children. A second is fear that the case may become entangled in the legal or social service systems.

It is important to become comfortable asking questions about sexuality. With a matter-of-fact approach, the typically more anxious parents will follow the lead. In addition, the first report of sexual behavior problems may occur at a distressing time in the child's life (e.g., marital separation). Medical professionals may then opt to find out less about the behavior rather than more and, thus, lose a chance to educate the parents and defuse a situation that more often than not is benign.

Questions to ask. The questions found to be most useful in handling sexual behavior problems in children fall into eight categories. These are:

1. A description of the behavior
2. Where, when, and with whom the behavior occurs
3. Parental expectations about sexual behavior
4. Presence of stressful events in the child's life
5. Sexual climate of the family
6. Existence of other behavior problems
7. Steps the parent has taken to manage the behavior
8. Parents' capacity to monitor their child

A. **Description of the behavior**
   1. What exactly does your child do that is concerning?
   2. Does he or she do anything else that appears sexual?
   3. Describe that for me.

   When parents "pathologize" the child's behavior, help educate them about the frequency with which preschoolers touch themselves sexually and the fact that many types of behaviors are relatively normative.

B. **Where, when, and with whom**
   1. When did you first notice this behavior?
   2. At its most intense, how often does it occur per day?
   3. Does this occur every day or are there days where the child does not engage in this behavior?
   4. Do you have any ideas why it varies like this?
   5. Does this behavior occur only at home? Other places?
   6. Have other adults reported seeing your child do this?
   7. Who else has noticed these behaviors?
   8. Does your child involve other children in this?
   9. Who are these children?
   10. How does your child know them?
   11. If someone walked into your child's room, would the behavior stop?

   Behaviors that occur across settings are often more persistent, less related to situational variables, and may require the involvement of two or more caregivers to eliminate the behavior.

C. **Parental expectations.** The parent's view of the behavior will drive the referral of the child. Possible questions for parents of preschoolers could include the following:

1. What is your theory about why your child does this?
2. Do you think that sexual behavior in children can be a natural occurrence?
3. Would you be surprised to hear of two preschool children who were caught playing "doctor"?
4. Would you expect those children to be disturbed?

D.   Stress in the child's life

1. Has anything upsetting happened in your child's life recently?
2. Has there been any major change in caregiver arrangements?
3. Are there any concerning children at daycare?
4. Any new adults or teens living in the home?

E.   Family sexuality. Because the following are very personal questions, we have found it helpful to preface these questions with the following: "I am going to ask some questions about things that happen in families that may stir up children to act in some unusual ways. Research has shown that these things are related to sexual behavior in young children."

1. How would you describe your family's attitudes toward sexuality?
2. How about nudity in front of the children? Bathing with them?
3. What types of sexual behaviors has your child seen within your home?
4. Has he or she observed you having sex?
5. Is pornography in the home?
6. Does your child ever hear loud conflict between you and your spouse?
7. Is there any pushing or shoving going on between the grown-ups at home? The kids?
8. How do you feel when you see him or her doing this?

F.   Comorbid behavior problems

1. Is your child's teacher reporting any behavior problems in school?
2. Does your child tend to be more active and impulsive than other same-age children?
3. Is your child more aggressive with other children than you expected?

G.   Previous attempts to manage the behavior

1. How good is he or she at minding you?
2. What steps have you used to reduce the frequency of this behavior?
3. Were these steps effective?
4. Has the behavior decreased, increased, or remained the same?

H.   Parental monitoring

1. When at home, are you typically within eyeshot of your child?

2. Given how busy you are, does your child spend much time unsupervised?
3. How many children are in the daycare? How many staff?
4. Are you aware of any children at daycare who are aggressive or provocative?

A decision can be made about the severity of the child's sexual behavior problem by taking into consideration the fact that a number of behaviors are not unusual, particularly in younger children (Table 19.1).

Questionnaires. The only published questionnaire to help the office pediatrician standardize their formal assessment of sexual behavior in children is the *Child Sexual Behavior Inventory* (CSBI; Friedrich, 1997). The PCP may find this instrument useful. It is a 38-item measure completed by the parent about the frequency of different sexual behaviors in the prior 6 months. The normative frequency of each of these behaviors has been determined and several subscale scores can help the PCP to determine whether or not the behavior is more developmentally related, or possibly related to other negative events in the child's life, including sexual abuse. The questionnaire is available from Psychological Assessment Resources (www.parinc.com).

III. **Triage assessment and treatment planning.** Identifying when a sexual behavior is problematic can be confusing. Many situations are unclear, it is difficult to find out specifically what happened, and the data informing professionals on normal behavior are limited. Using the guidelines in the previous section can help with these triage situations. A major consideration: make sure that the child has not been sexually abused or is in no danger of such. Although sexual abuse is statistically unlikely, it is a problem that can ill afford to be missed. When children exhibit problematic sexual behavior, intervention typically consists of:
1. Education of the parent and child about normal sexual behavior
2. Increased monitoring of the child
3. Use of standard behavior management strategies, when necessary

With adolescents, the situation can be more complicated and the PCP may need to involve other systems (e.g., the schools, social services, legal system). Particularly problematic for PCPs is the situation in which a parent describes an occurrence at home that is clearly of concern, but is unsure if Child Protective Services or commensurate authority should be contacted. For example, a 13-year-old boy has had inappropriate sexual contact with a 5-year-old sibling or cousin. In such a situation, the central **clinical** issue is to assure referral for evaluation and treatment of the children involved. The central issue from a **legal** standpoint is whether a child is in danger because of maltreatment or neglect by the responsible adult. In these cases the question is: Are the parents neglecting their duties to supervise their child such that a danger exists to that child (or another)? If the PCP concludes that the adults have failed to adequately supervise and protect the child, this situation must be reported to the authorities as a case of neglect. On the other hand, if the PCP concludes that the adults were not derelict in their duties, then contact with Child Protective Services may not be required. Although pregnancy, sexually transmitted diseases (STD), the human immunodeficiency virus (HIV) and acquired immunodeficiency syndrome (AIDS), and contraception are of critical importance in adolescent healthcare, they will not be addressed in this chapter.

A. **Watching**
   1. **When to watch**
      a. **Sexual behaviors are occasional.** Examples, according to Ryan (2000), include:
         (1) Preoccupation with sexual themes
         (2) Sexual graffiti
         (3) Sexual teasing or embarrassment of others
         (4) Precocious sexual knowledge
         (5) Single incident of peeping or exposing
         (6) Single incident of pornographic interest or rubbing against other (if prepubescent)
         (7) Attempting to expose other's genitals (if prepubescent less concerning)
         (8) Simulating foreplay with dolls or peers with clothing on (i.e., kissing, petting in prepubescent children)
         (9) Mooning and other obscene gestures
      b. No comorbid conditions
      c. No interference with peer relations
      d. No interference with parent–child relationship
      e. Observed only in one setting
      f. Recent onset
   2. **When watching**
      a. **Psychoeducation**
         (1) **Take an emotionally neutral attitude.** Sexual issues stir up a lot of emotion in adults. Taking a neutral tone can be more effective in decreasing the family's anxiety, which is typically counterproductive in these situations. The goal of "sex education" is to promote a healthy appreciation for sexual impulses as well as a recognition of the need for responsible and appropriate expression of them.
         (2) **Education and normalization**
             (a) Provide information about the relative ubiquity **and nor-**

malcy of some sexual behaviors (e.g., touching genitals in preschoolers).

(b) Explain how parental attitudes and anxiety about child sexuality can foster conflict and increase the likelihood of harsh parenting and persisting problems that are more a function of the parent–child relationship than they are about sexual behavior

(c) Explain how family stressors can effect behavior

(d) Teach parents how to praise their child when he or she is behaving appropriately

(3) **Discuss directly what is problematic.** Instruct parents to discuss with the child specifically what is problematic. Is it the behavior itself, its context, or its frequency? Because of adult anxiety, the issue may be addressed only vaguely, which can send the message that "this is dangerous and bad," and shut down future communication between parent and child.

(4) **Encourage discussion between parent and child.** Having an exchange with the child is more effective than authoritarian, "just say no" approaches. Understanding the child's point of view, what prompted the behavior, and how the child felt during and after are important in addressing concerns. Maintaining an open line of communication between parent and child is, in the long run, the most important factor in preventing sexual acting out and other problem behaviors.

(5) **Parental monitoring.** Evidence indicates that simple monitoring, by itself, is actually a low-level and appropriate intervention. Parents are expected to track the daily frequency of the concerning behavior. These data will inform the PCP about the scope of the problem and whether the behavior is increasing, remaining the same, or decreasing in frequency.

(6) **Distraction or ignoring** can be encouraged with younger children,

especially when behaviors are not dangerous (e.g., touching their genitals).

  b. **Advocacy.** It is also useful for the parent to keep in touch with other adults (e.g., at school) in the child's life to determine whether this behavior is being seen in other settings. If the behavior is more generalized, and particularly if it is beginning to interfere with adult–child relationships or peer–peer relationships, moving to a treatment mode is recommended. If the child has been the victim of maltreatment, then the PCP must call Child Protective Services or the appropriate authority.

  c. **Psychotherapy** is not indicated at this stage.

  d. **Medications** are not indicated for problems at this stage. The PCP should resist any effort by the parents to medicate children for these types of concerns. If parents persist in this effort to medicate, it is an indication of the need for specialist mental health referral.

  e. **Laboratory and other evaluations** are indicated only to investigate specific health complications that may be suggested by the behaviors (e.g., masturbation) and history of physical complaints (e.g., urinary tract infection symptoms).

  f. **Monitoring.** A follow-up appointment should be made within 2 to 4 months to monitor the situation and the child's progress.

B. **Intervening further**
  1. **When to intervene further**
    a. Some interference with peer relations
    b. Interfering with parent–child relationships
    c. Persistent behavior (i.e., has occurred more than once) that has not diminished despite reasonable interventions by parents. Examples, based on Ryan, include:
      (1) Peeping or exposing self
      (2) Mooning or other obscenities
      (3) Pornographic interest or rubbing against other with clothes on
      (4) Compulsive masturbation or interrupts tasks
      (5) Simulating intercourse with dolls, peers, or animals with clothing on (i.e., humping)
      (6) Adolescent promiscuity
    d. Behaviors that involve lack of consent or age inequality, based on Ryan:

(1)   Touching other's genitals without permission
(2)   Degradation or humiliation of self or others with sexual themes
(3)   Sexually explicit proposals or threats, including written notes
(4)   Violation of other's body space (e.g., pulling skirts up, pants down)
(5)   Sexually explicit conversation between adolescent and prepubescent child
(6)   Touching other's genitals without permission (i.e., goosing, grabbing)

2.   **When intervening further**
   a.   **Psychoeducation**
      (1)   **Take an emotionally neutral tone** in discussing the issues with the parents and child. Condemning or shaming approaches are ineffective and promote the movement of the problem "underground," so that the behaviors persist while the child becomes more secretive.
      (2)   **Affirm that the child or adolescent has not been the victim of maltreatment.** When behaviors persist or are more serious, the chances of sexual or other abuse are greater.
      (3)   **Encourage explicit and direct discussion** of the problems between the parents and child. If they are unable to do so, it is reason to refer the family for specialist mental health treatment.
      (4)   **Develop a plan for monitoring** the child's behavior. The parents must be able to obtain the data necessary to know whether the child is continuing with the behavior. Reinforcing that the parents know the "4 Ws" (i.e., **w**ho they are with, **w**here they are going, **w**hen will they be back, **w**hat are they doing) with adolescents is especially important. Optimally, the child participates in this, recognizing that the parents are attempting to help. When the child cannot or will not recognize this, the case should be referred for specialist mental health treatment.
      (5)   **Parents should be cautious about ignoring behavior at this level of concern.** Instead, they should generally be monitoring the child and

setting limits on the behaviors in question.

(6) **Limit setting** (see Chapter 3 for more about behavior management). Mild limit setting can be effective and not harmful to the child. Brief **time-outs** with the child visually monitored by a parent can be helpful for younger children (e.g., compulsive masturbation in a 4-year-old.)

(7) **Establishing rules regarding sexual behaviors and a mild consequence** when a rule is violated is also important. Some children have actually benefited from being sent briefly to their room for scheduled "masturbation sessions." These are children who prefer to be involved with peers, watching a favorite TV program, and so on, and the "session" is scheduled at the time of a favorite program. The parent must maintain a neutral stance and say, "You seem to need to touch yourself. Since it is important to you, I think you need a special time. Each day, you are to spend 10 minutes, between 3:50 and 4:00 p.m. in your room. If you need to touch yourself, that is the time to use." For the adolescent, consequences generally are greater and need to match the severity of the problem. Grounding, loss of privileges (e.g., ability to attend events, use of TV, computer, car) and early curfew are some of the common responses parents can make. The important thing is for parents or other adults responsible to:

(a) Monitor the behaviors

(b) Work together to establish consequences for **future** behavior

(c) Apply and follow through with consequences

b. **Advocacy** is often important at this phase. Contact with the school may be necessary to assure appropriate (i.e., not too harsh or punitive, not too minimizing or lenient) responses to behaviors occurring at school. Arranging for additional psychosocial support (e.g., a school social worker) to be available to the child or adolescent, either on a regular or an as-needed basis, may help prevent future problems. If problems continue to escalate, the parents should be made aware of persons in need of supervision (see Chapter 9) or similar petitions available through the family court to monitor and supervise the youth. If the child has been the victim of maltreatment, the PCP must call Child Protective Services or the appropriate authority.

c. **Psychotherapy** is often indicated at this point. Family therapy directed at parent management issues must be a central part of treatment. Individual therapy with a cognitive behavioral approach is also often helpful. Group treatment, if available, can be especially helpful for these children. Although child mental health specialists who have particular expertise and experience working with these situations may be available, from a national perspective this is more the exception than the rule. If these subspecialists are not available in the community, the PCP must be sure that the mental health professional has specific expertise working with children, adolescents, and their families.

For example, a 7-year-old boy who grabbed at his mother's breasts and exposed himself to his mother and older sister, was also a child who was frequently sent to the school principal's office for fighting and making provocative comments to teachers and peers. Given the coercive nature of the mother-son relationship, any corrective response by her would have been followed by an escalating response in the boy. What was most successful for them was to spend four sessions over the course of 5 weeks with a therapist skilled in parent–child interaction therapy. These sessions afforded the mother a chance to work hard to repair the relationship with her son. His oppositionality began to decrease at home following the second week, and by the third week, his teacher had noted that he was less angry and impulsive as well. Although his sexual behavior problems had been nearly eliminated by this time, he still was exposing himself to his sister. Because the mother had introduced some positives into her relationship with her son, she was much more effective at using time-out with him the next several times that he exposed himself at home, which effectively eliminated the behavior.

      d. Medications are indicated only for comorbid conditions. No medications should be used to target sexual behavior problems.

      e. Laboratory and other evaluations are indicated when signs and symptoms exist for a medical disorder or the youth is felt to be at risk for such (e.g., the promiscuous adolescent who may require HIV, pregnancy testing)

      f. Monitoring. The patient and family should be seen in follow-up within 1 to 2 months. This allows the PCP to monitor the situation, confirm follow through with treatment referrals, and communicate that the problem should not be ignored.

C. Referring

  1. When to refer and transfer primary responsibility

    a. Sexual behavior appears related to sexual abuse.

    b. Preoccupation with sexually aggressive pornography, literature, web sites

    c. Sexual behavior that includes the sexual touching (or threat) of other children. Examples, based on Ryan:

      (1) Oral, vaginal, or anal penetration of dolls, children, or animals

      (2) Simulating intercourse with peers with clothing off

      (3) Exposing other's genitals

      (4) Sexually explicit threats

      (5) Adolescent touching another's genitals without permission

    d. Sexual behavior has resulted in legal action:

      (1) Obscene phone calls

      (2) Voyeurism, exhibitionism

      (3) Sexual harassment

      (4) Forced sexual contact

      (5) Forced penetration

      (6) Sexual contact with animals

      (7) Genital injury to others

    e. Less severe sexual behavior problems exist in context of a family that is unable or unwilling to implement parenting changes.

  2. When referring

    a. Psychoeducation

      (1) Continue to take a steady, neutral approach to the child and family. It is expected that the PCP will have strong feelings about these situations. The neutral approach is taken in the interest of helping the child, and recognizing that these children or adolescents do not just disappear from our society but continue to be a risk for serious behavior problems into adulthood. The PCP can convey disapproval of the **behavior,** but not of the **child.**

(2) **Reinforce the need for ongoing treatment.** This includes challenging the family that withdraws from treatment prematurely and without satisfactory completion.

(3) Reinforce the importance of **parental monitoring, working together, and follow through** with consequences.

(4) Monitor for signs of **sexual exploitation of other children** in the home (i.e., other siblings) or community **by the youth.**

(5) Continue to monitor for signs of **maltreatment of the child or adolescent** by the caretaker.

b. **Advocacy** is best left to the treating mental health professional. The PCP, however, may be required to report cases of maltreatment to the proper authorities.

c. **Psychotherapy** must occur at this stage. Many children or adolescents at this stage may be under the jurisdiction of court supervision. Younger children at this stage can be treated on an outpatient basis, although many adolescents will require an inpatient or residential setting initially. Regardless of the setting, treatment must be aimed at the sexual behavior problems themselves. Treatment can also include addressing other mental health issues (e.g., attention-deficit/hyperactivity disorder [AD/HD], depression) but must not be done *in lieu* of addressing the sexual problems. Programs for "sexual perpetrators" may exist in a given community, including outpatient and inpatient approaches. Psychotherapeutic treatment often uses a cognitive behavioral method. Both individual and group treatments are typically included. Family therapy is an essential part of treatment as well.

d. **Medications** should not be used to target the sexual behaviors themselves unless they are considered a symptom of another disorder (e.g., sexual promiscuity when a patient with bipolar disorder is manic). In these cases, the overarching condition should be treated. Other comorbid conditions should be similarly addressed pharmacologically.

    e. **Laboratory and other evaluations** are indicated only to rule out medical conditions for which the youth is felt to be at risk (e.g., HIV, pregnancy, STD).

    f. **Monitoring** will generally be done by the treating mental health professional. The PCP should see the youth for follow-up in 6 to 12 months. This conveys that the PCP has not "given up" on the youth and remains interested in the child's health and well-being.

IV. Practical use of medications. No literature exists on the use of medications in the management of sexual behavior problems in children or adolescents. When these problems are incidental to another psychiatric condition, treatment of that condition is indicated. For example, cases were reported on children whose sexual behavior problems were part of the impulsive symptoms of AD/HD or bipolar disorder and whose behaviors were eliminated once the child responded to appropriate medication.

At times, the question has arisen whether the compulsive masturbatory behavior of a child or a teenagers' apparent compulsion to use internet pornography falls within the category of an obsessive-compulsive disorder. Currently, no evidence supports that children with compulsive sexual behavior problems have other obsessive-compulsive features. Consequently, the use of a specific medication has not been tried. However, that does not rule out the possibility of medication use in the future.

V. Summary. It is expected that physicians will increasingly be asked to evaluate children and adolescents who have some difficulty related to sexual behavior. With younger children, the difficulty is typically related to a parent's perception that the child's behavior is inappropriate. In fact, parent and caregiver perceptions are likely to be critical in determining whether the child has a problem. Educating the caregiver about the normative aspects of a preschooler's sexual behavior can go far in diffusing these problems and allowing development to take its course. Sexual behavior problems are usually short-lived, particularly when no comorbid behavior problems exist, family stress is minimal, and no other negative life events have occurred in the child's life.

Teenagers with sexual behavior problems present a greater challenge. It is more often appropriate to refer for therapy—individual, family-based, or both. However, that does not preclude that some combinations of education, monitoring, and appropriate limit setting can be useful in helping parents manage children's behaviors and, in so doing, feel more successful as a parent. Interventions of this type are certainly part of being the physician to the "whole child."

SUGGESTED READINGS

For the Physician

Davies SL, Glaser D, Kossoff R. Children's sexual play and behavior in preschool settings: staff's perceptions, reports, and responses. *Child Abuse Negl* 2000;24:1329–1343.

Friedrich WN, Fisher J, Broughton D, et al. Normative sexual behavior in children: a contemporary sample. *Pediatrics* 1998;101(4):E9.

Friedrich WN, Grambsch P, Broughton D, et al. Normative sexual behavior in children. *Pediatrics* 1991;88(3):456–464.

Friedrich WN. *Child sexual behavior inventory.* Odessa, FL: Psychological Assessment Resources, 1997. Available at www.parinc.com. Accessed on.

Gordon BN, Schroeder CS. *Sexuality: a developmental approach to problems.* New York: Plenum, 1995.

Hembree-Kigin T, McNeil C. *Parent–child interaction therapy.* New York: Plenum, 1995.

Remafedi G. Suicide and sexual orientation: nearing the end of controversy. *Arch Gen Psychiatry* 1999;56(10):885–886.

Ryan G. Childhood sexuality: a decade of study. Part II. Dissemination and future directions. *Child Abuse Negl* 2000;24(1):49–61.

Ryan G. Childhood sexuality: a decade of study. Part I. Research and curriculum development. *Child Abuse Negl* 2000;24(1):33–48.

Stronski Huwiler S, Remafedi G. Adolescent homosexuality. *Adv Pediatr* 1998;45:107–144.

For Parents

Johnson TC. *Understanding your child's sexual behaviors: what's natural and healthy.* Oakland, CA: New Harbinger, 1999.

Web Sites

Centers for Disease Control Youth Risk Behavior Survey. Report and data available on a large cohort of high schoolers' sexual behaviors. Available at www.cdc.gov/nccdphp/dash/yrbs/index.htm. Accessed on 6/29/02.

OutProud. Well-done and extensive education and support web site for gay and lesbian youth. www.outproud.org. Accessed on 6/29/02.

Parents, Families, and Friends of Lesbians and Gays (P-FLAG) is an international support, advocacy, and education organization with many local chapters and an excellent website. Available at www.pflag.org. Accessed on 6/29/02.

20 Somatoform Disorders and Functional Syndromes

Caroly S. Pataki and David L. Kaye

I. **Background.** Children and adolescents frequently present to their primary care physicians (PCP) with physical symptoms that do not fully fit into traditional medical categories of disorder. These types of symptoms have historically been referred to as "psychosomatic," but in the current psychiatric nomenclature are grouped together as "somatoform disorders." Typically **parents and the child believe that an unidentified medical diagnosis is present.** Although it is evident that the symptoms cause significant distress and impairment to the child and the family, no medical condition can be found that fully accounts for the physical symptoms. In **contrast to "factitious disorders" or "malingering,"** in which symptoms are intentionally produced or feigned, the symptoms in somatoform disorders are not planned. They **are not under voluntary control** and **serve no overt purpose to the patient** (e.g., to avoid school, diminish social interactions, to gain medical attention, or obtain financial benefits).

Associated features likely to be present in children and adolescents with somatoform disorders are:

1. **Temperamental characteristic of "somatosensory amplification."** Individuals susceptible to these conditions often have a neurobiologically mediated, longstanding, and pronounced attention and sensitivity to bodily sensations and changes, even when not painful or unpleasant. They may interpret them as dangerous and react fearfully to these changes.
2. **Difficulty connecting life events to feelings, and verbalizing these feelings**
3. Symptoms often begin after a **specific stressful life event** (e.g., child abuse, loss, death).
4. **School refusal** is a frequent complication.
5. **Anxiety and depressive disorders are frequently comorbid conditions.**
6. **Sleep** is often **disrupted** (usually difficulty falling asleep).
7. The symptom becomes more prominent in situations when the child is observed.
8. A family member may have a similar condition.

The five primary somatoform disorders grouped together in the *Diagnostic and Statistical Manual of Mental Disorders,* Fourth Edition (DSM-IV) are pain disorder, conversion disorder, body dysmorphic disorder, hypochondriasis, and somatization disorder. An additional category, undifferentiated somatoform disorder, is common in pediatric primary care and subsumes conditions such as chronic fatigue syndrome (CFS), fibromyalgia (FM), and multiple chemical sensitivity (MCS) syndrome.

A. **Pain disorder** is the most frequently encountered problem. It consists of persistent or recurrent pain (e.g., **recurrent abdominal pain, headaches**) for which an adequate general medical explanation is not found and which is refractory to usual medical treatments. The pain causes significant distress, along with a marked change in the child's or adolescent's functioning, usually resulting in inability to attend school on a regular basis, frequent trips to the doctor, and an inability to participate in usual family and peer activities. Prevalence rates for this disorder are estimated to be 10% to 15% at a given time.

B. **Conversion disorder** consists of motor, sensory, or visceral symptoms typically suggesting neurologic disease that cause dysfunction and cannot be adequately explained by physiologic findings. Prevalence rate estimates vary widely, from 1/10,000 to 5/1000. It is more common in females. As with the other somatoform disorders, patients have no conscious voluntary ability to produce or stop their symptoms.

   1. Common **motor symptoms** are:
      a. **Psychogenic nonepileptic seizures.** Historically termed **"pseudoseizures,"** a more neutral and preferred description is "nonepileptic seizures" or "stress-related events." These are sudden and dramatic episodes of falling down or paroxysms of flailing movements of arms, legs, and trunk resembling a seizure, but have no:
         1. Postictal paralysis or incontinence
         2. History of injury following the event(s)
         3. Electroencephalographic evidence of seizure activity
         4. Elevated serum prolactin after the episode

         Typically, these events last much longer (i.e., usually 15 minutes or longer, even hours) than the 2 to 3 minutes expected for electrical seizures. Patients may also respond verbally to questions during the episode. These often occur in patients who have confirmed epilepsy, so the clinical picture can be complex and confusing.
      b. **Paralysis** of one or more extremity, typically leading to inability to walk
      c. **Involuntary movements** that do not conform to a known movement disorder
      d. **Astasia-abasia:** a staggering gait along with jerking movements in the upper extremities, sometimes preventing standing or walking without help
   2. **Sensory symptoms** can include:
      a. **Lack of sensation** in extremities that does not conform to underlying nerve distribu-

tion (e.g., "glove or stocking" distribution of anesthesia)

b. **Blindness,** although pupils are reactive to light and visual field deficits are not consistent with known patterns of physiology. Patients usually do not harm themselves bumping into objects even when they cannot "see" them.

3. **Visceral symptoms**

a. **Cyclic vomiting** (i.e., vomiting in cycles or repeatedly without evidence of explanatory medical condition)

b. **"Globus hystericus"**—repeated episodes of feeling as if choking, as if the throat is closing, without demonstrable medical disorder to explain it

C. **Body dysmorphic disorder** is characterized by **severe distress** and preoccupation with a **perceived defect in appearance,** often of the skin or face (e.g., acne, facial features, or hair). The defect can be imagined or be insignificant compared with the excessive concern and feelings of repulsiveness that the patient develops. This preoccupation with personal "ugliness" often leads to social avoidance and extreme self-consciousness. It causes significant impairment in the child or adolescent's social life, school life, or family life. Body dysmorphic disorder has been viewed as a variant of obsessive-compulsive disorder (OCD). Individuals with body dysmorphic disorder have higher than expected rates of mood disorders and OCD in their family histories. The disorder generally begins in adolescence, and less frequently in childhood. The pediatric prevalence is unknown in the community, but is frequently seen in dermatologic practices.

D. **Hypochondriasis** consists of bodily preoccupation for at least 6 months. Patients believe that bodily symptoms represent serious or life-threatening illnesses. A child or adolescent with hypochondriasis might be convinced that feeling his or her own heartbeat was an indicator of a heart attack. A minor injury (e.g., a scrape) would elicit an overwhelming fear that an infection would ensue and the entire limb would be lost. Even vague sensations (e.g., mild fatigue) are interpreted as signs of serious illness. Children, adolescents, and adults with hypochondriasis tend to seek a great deal of medical care, but are not relieved even when medical reassurance is given. Often it is the **parents** who are preoccupied with the child's physical complaints. Separating out the parent's anxiety from the child's can be challenging.

E. **Somatization disorder** also termed "Briquet's syndrome" after Pierre Briquet who believed the disorder resulted from a dysfunction in the central nervous system. Prevalence of this disorder is estimated to be between 0.2% and 2% among females and less than 0.2% in males. Because of stringent diagnostic criteria this disorder is unusual among youth. Core features of this disorder include:

1. At least a **2-year history** of **multiple physical complaints** that cannot be explained by any detectable medical conditions.
2. Diagnostic criteria require **six or more symptoms** that occur in at least two different organ systems among the following: gastrointestinal, cardiovascular, genitourinary, or skin and pain symptoms.
3. Preoccupation with the symptoms causing significant distress, and a persistent inability to accept medical reassurance that no serious medical condition is present.

F. **Other somatoform disorders.** DSM-IV-TR has other broad categories (i.e., **"undifferentiated somatoform disorder"** and **"somatoform disorder not otherwise specified"**) that encompass conditions commonly encountered in pediatric practice. The most important of these are **CFS, MCS, and FM.** Although CFS is described in some major pediatric textbooks, the other two conditions are rarely mentioned at all. The most controversial is MCS, for which no consensus in diagnostic criteria exists, and prominent medical organizations have proposed instead the term "idiopathic environmental intolerance." The definition of this disorder generally involves significant disability or distress as a result of symptoms associated with low level exposure to two or more listed chemical agents affecting two or more organ systems.

There is a **high degree of overlap among these illnesses** (especially between CFS and FM in which most patients seem to meet criteria for both conditions) (Table 20.1). Many experts believe they should be conceptualized as a broad category of "functional somatic syndromes" or "medically unexplained syndromes," as opposed to separate entities. Despite the presence of web sites, advocacy groups, and some legal precedence, research support for these conditions is minimal in the pediatric population. Regardless of this controversy and the difficulty drawing firm conclusions, children with these symptoms are **genuinely distressed and are more disabled** by their symptomatology than many patients with other chronic and life-threatening diseases. Parents frequently wonder if, or sometimes insist that, this is their child's diagnosis. Although clearly common in the PCP's office, epidemiologic studies are minimal and the prevalence rates are unclear. The conditions appear to occur **rarely in prepubertal children, affecting girls much more commonly than boys.**

Table 20.1. Diagnostic criteria for pediatric chronic fatigue syndrome and fibromyalgia

	Chronic Fatigue Syndrome	Fibromyalgia
Primary symptom	Fatigue causing activity limitation	General aching at three or more sites
Duration	6 mo	3 mo
Evidence of other medical condition	Absent	Absent
Pain	Arthralgias, myalgia	Severe pain in 5 of 11 tender point sites
Symptom or minor criteria	8 of 12 of following: Malaise Headache Abdominal pain Depression Lymph node pain Sleep disturbance Myalgia Arthralgia Sore throat Cognitive dysfunction Neurologic symptoms Eye pain or photophobia	3 of 10 of following: Fatigue Chronic headaches Irritable bowel syndrome Chronic anxiety or tension Subjective soft tissue swelling Poor sleep Pain modulation by Physical activities Weather factors Anxiety or stress Numbness

Although most reports note these conditions primarily in higher socioeconomic groups, more recent data have suggested a broader population is affected. The **cause is unknown,** but is best thought of as centrally mediated, complex psychobiologic phenomena that involve the interaction of biologic, psychologic, psychiatric, social, and cultural factors. **No specific laboratory test** is available that confirms any of these diagnoses (including Epstein-Barr virus titers, which have no relationship to the presence of CFS). Laboratory evaluation for standard medical conditions is routinely negative, even while the symptoms persist. Comorbidity with anxiety and depressive disorders is common, although it is not thought that these syndromes are merely part of these psychiatric conditions. Follow-up rarely yields a new medical diagnosis that would explain the presenting symptoms. Few outcome data are available, but what exists suggests that adolescents with CFS have a **milder**

course than adults (most of whom have chronic disability with intermittent exacerbations of symptoms), with gradual improvement in symptoms and functioning occurring after a period of years. During the course of illness, extended school absence or refusal is a frequent and serious complication.

G. Developmental considerations

1. It is developmentally normal for very young children to continue a symptom after a real injury, for a short period of time (e.g., limping after a leg injury), while enjoying the extra attention it brings from parents.

2. Prepubertal children are more likely to experience emotional distress as physical discomfort (e.g., stomachaches) than are older children.

3. Prepubertal children complain of abdominal pain and headaches, whereas pain in the extremities, muscular pain, and neurologic symptoms are more often reported by older children and adolescents.

4. Preschool age children will seek comfort for pain, but may have trouble quantifying the intensity of pain. School-aged children tend to have increased pain thresholds, and are better able to describe the level of intensity of a given pain (e.g., by use of visual analog scales, selecting the face that matches their pain).

5. A link exists between anxiety and sensitivity to pain.

6. Anxiety and depression are more commonly found in the families of children who have multiple somatic complaints.

7. Sexual abuse experiences in childhood have been associated with an increased risk of multiple somatic complaints in children.

8. Adolescents with histories of physical and sexual abuse rate themselves as having more physical complaints than adolescents without these histories.

9. Some evidence indicates that a prior diagnosed medical illness can increase the risk of developing a somatoform disorder.

II. Practical office evaluation. Identification of children and adolescents with somatoform disorders frequently occurs in the primary care setting, because these children are brought "early and often" to the PCP's office (Table 20.2). Usually, physical examination findings are normal or not consistent with the patient's complaints. Laboratory tests should be pursued only until the PCP is comfortable that no traditional medical explanation exists. Recognize that it is virtually impossible to rule out all "organic" causes with 100% certainty and that excessive pursuit of a medical explanation may exacerbate the patient's anxiety, promote further workup and search for "an answer,"

**Table 20.2.   Identification of children
and adolescents with somatoform disorders**

Disorder	Clinical Features	Diagnostic Clues	Differential Diagnosis
Somatization disorder	Many organs symptomatic	Multiple doctors, sometimes surgery	Medical illness Major depression
Conversion disorder	Acute dysfunction Motor, sensory, visceral	Symptom incompatible with physiology	Neurologic condition Psychotic disorder
Pain disorder	Persistent pain Treatment resistant	Excessive disruption of school and peers	Major depression Separation anxiety
Hypochondriasis	Preoccupation with fear of severe illness	Inability to accept medical reassurance	Underlying medical disorder Depression
Body dysmorphic disorder	Preoccupation with imagined defect	Obsession with own "repulsiveness"	Psychotic delusions Anorexia nervosa

expose the child to iatrogenic risk, raise healthcare costs, promote disability behavior, and make resolution of symptoms more difficult.

A.   The following historical data raise the likelihood of a somatoform disorder:

1. Family history of similar somatic symptoms
2. History of physical or sexual abuse
3. History of recent stressor
4. Symptoms worsen when the child is being observed.
5. Symptoms do not wake child up from sleep.
6. Symptoms are constant (i.e., do not wax and wane in intensity or respond to changes in patient or environment).
7. Symptoms do not progress (i.e., over time a medical illness does not "declare" itself).
8. Parents have difficulty accepting reassurance.
9. Patient may have seen multiple doctors, with much disgruntlement about previous doctors.

B.   It is critical when asking about the history to convey a **neutral, attentive, but nonjudgmental attitude**

toward the patient's symptoms. Patients and families are highly sensitive to innuendoes that their symptoms are "all in your head" or not worthy of the doctor's time and attention. This can lead the patient or family to feel increased anxiety and humiliation. When this occurs, a patient and family may go to even greater extremes to show the severity of the symptoms and to advocate for more medical workup. Instead, the physician should take a **positive and reassuring approach** when pursuing the history. In addition to evaluating the physical symptoms, it is important to assess for **anxiety and depressive disorders.** It is helpful to ask:

1. What do you think is the cause of the problem?
2. Is there some particular disease you are worried about (e.g., cancer, multiple sclerosis)? If so, do you know anyone who has this disease?
3. What have you tried to make the symptoms better? Have you sought any other treatment from any other healthcare professionals? Others (i.e., alternative medicine)?
4. Is it possible that these symptoms might be a reaction to stress, like when you watch a scary movie your heart rate goes up? Or when you have a headache after a hard day at work?
5. Does anyone else in the family have similar concerns or symptoms?

C. For both diagnostic and therapeutic purposes, it is also helpful to have the patient and parent keep a **symptom diary.** This is a record of the symptoms over a period of several weeks that tracks the following parameters:
   1. Date
   2. Place on body
   3. Frequency and duration
   4. Severity (rate on scale of 0 to 10, or the use of various visual analogue scales; i.e., thermometer, happy face, other scales)
   5. Quality or description
   6. Mood response
   7. Activities avoided or unable to participate in

III. **Triage assessment and treatment planning**
   A. **General issues.** Transient somatization symptoms are common and frequently do not interfere substantially with a child's life. The PCP can handle these **milder situations** with a combination of education, guidance, and support. Treatment goals in these cases are to give consistent reassurance and to promote the independent functioning of the child or adolescent. In mild cases, symptoms generally resolve within a few weeks, and the child or adolescent's life has not been significantly disrupted. Unexplained bodily symptoms can reoccur in children and adolescents who are susceptible to them.

Treatment of children and adolescents with enduring somatoform disorders, however, is more complex. It requires a multidisciplinary collaboration of PCPs, nurses, pediatricians specializing in chronic pain syndromes, child psychiatrists and psychologists, physical therapists, school personnel, and other clinicians. Successful treatment depends on effective cooperation among the clinicians involved in the care and continued psychoeducation for the patient and family.

Perhaps the single most important element in the effective management of these patients' problems is the designation of **one physician,** generally the PCP, as the **"quarterback"** who **oversees the overall treatment plan** and coordinates care with other clinicians. It is critical that this overseeing physician carefully explain each step of the evaluation and treatment to the patient and family. This designated physician's task is to validate the patient's concerns about receiving an appropriate (i.e., not too little and not too much) workup, and also to help families understand that troubling and "real" symptoms can persist even in the absence of a medical condition to account for them. It is important for the coordinating physician to monitor patients with somatoform disorders closely with frequent follow-up visits and phone calls, so that adequate contact is maintained and appropriate ongoing reassurance given.

A **rehabilitation model of treatment** generally allows for optimal outcomes. Treatment goals include an emphasis on improved general functioning as well as amelioration and management of individual symptoms. Although symptom relief is sought, it is not unusual that symptoms wax and wane over a period of years. These conditions do not fit an acute illness treatment model, in which symptoms are treated and resolve within weeks to months. An auxiliary goal is to prevent morbidity from excessive laboratory testing and surgical procedures, which can cause physical harm and also can reinforce illness behavior and interfere with optimal functioning for the child. Comorbid psychiatric disorders, particularly anxiety and depression, should be treated, as outlined in other chapters. In the most severe cases, adolescents with somatoform disorders can require psychiatric partial hospitalization programs or specialized school programs that have expertise in handling the academic and emotional needs of troubled adolescents. Psychiatric hospitalization is only indicated when an adequate outpatient treatment has failed and the patient remains significantly debilitated by the dis-order (e.g., an adolescent who cannot walk, cannot see, or simply will not leave the house despite outpatient treatment). When hospitalization becomes a consideration, it is best to involve a child and adolescent psychiatrist to negotiate this phase of treatment.

B. **Watching**
 1. **When to watch**
   a. Symptoms have been present a short time (i.e., days to weeks) and are improving without any intervention
   b. The child's normal activities have not been disrupted
   c. Symptom's are not interfering with school, peer relationships, and family life
 2. **What to do when watching**
   a. **Psychoeducation of parents and child**
     (1) **Validate the reality and legitimacy** of the symptoms. It is critical to emphasize to patients and families that the symptoms are "real"; they are not voluntary or "all in the adolescent's head." The mind and the body influence each other in real ways. Legitimizing this verbally and nonverbally is crucial. Examples may help (e.g., a child or adult who becomes frightened or anxious can develop a faster pulse and heart rate).
     (2) **Reassurance.** Families and patients should be reassured that all appropriate medical tests will be conducted, medical causes of pain or discomfort will be fully considered, the condition is not life threatening, and over time the child will improve.
     (3) **Provide encouragement.** Symptoms are usually frightening to the patient and the child or adolescent has a sense of helplessness. An adolescent with a somatoform disorder will be relieved to hear that he or she can get better, although he or she feels unable to control the symptoms.
     (4) **Endorse normal functioning.** Although the child is experiencing symptoms, the parents should positively expect that the child will continue to function (e.g., go to school, socialize, participate in the family).
     (5) **Encourage verbalizing feelings.** Encourage children and their families to speak openly about their feelings and to increase their skills in listening to each other's experiences.
     (6) Address the need for sound **sleep.** Reviewing sleep routines and general sleep hygiene is helpful. If a reliable and predictable routine is not occurring, support the parents in problem-solving and putting this into place.

(7) **Regular moderate exercise** should also be emphasized

(8) **Review diet and nutrition.** No specific guidelines have demonstrated value in somatoform disorders, but occasionally pain syndromes can be partially responsive to dietary changes. In general, aim for good, healthy nutrition and eating habits. Any specific changes or additions to this would depend on the family's observations of what helps. This should not be interpreted as encouragement of a "witch hunt" for nutritional culprits, but rather as part of the effort to enlist the active participation of the patient and family in the management of the symptoms. This active participation (versus passive resignation) is a major ingredient in any successful intervention. Referral to a nutritionist is generally not necessary but can be considered in individual cases.

b. **Advocacy.** In the early stages, no specific advocacy is required, except to encourage the maintenance of usual activities and routines.

c. **Psychotherapy** is generally not recommended at this stage, unless patients and families express a desire for such.

d. **Medication** is generally not indicated.

e. **Laboratory and other evaluations.** A complete physical examination, including neurologic, is critical to develop a differential diagnosis, to reassure the family, and to determine whether any additional laboratory tests are indicated. It is important to pay attention to muscle tightness and spasms, and to identify trigger points that can exacerbate a given pain symptom. Being on the lookout for signs of sexual or physical abuse is also important. In the face of a normal physical examination and low level of clinical suspicion, minimal laboratory tests are indicated (e.g., complete blood count [CBC], erythrocyte sedimentation rate, mono spot urinalysis). No specific laboratory tests confirm a diagnosis of any somatoform disorder, including CFS, FM, and MCS.

f. **Monitoring.** The family should be given a follow-up appointment within 6 weeks (and perhaps earlier) to monitor the progress of the patient. This offering of help regardless of the child's condition, rather than only in cases of continued or worsened symptoms, relieves anxiety and generally serves to decrease symptoms.

C. Intervening further

1. When to intervene further

a. When the child has missed more than 1 week of school

b. When peer relationships and family life are becoming disrupted

c. When the family appears to be stressed by the presence of continued symptoms in the child

2. When intervening further

a. **Psychoeducation**

(1) **Validate reality and legitimacy, provide reassurance, and encouragement as above**

(2) **Development of a treatment team.** Decide at this point the necessity of treatment of individual symptoms with medication, and seek any appropriate referrals (e.g., pediatric subspecialist, physical therapy, occupational therapy or psychological evaluations).

(3) **Recognize comorbidity.** Evaluate for anxiety and depressive syndromes that may coexist with somatoform disorders.

(4) **Review sleeping, eating, and exercise routines** (as above)

(5) **Promote realistic goals.** Although the physical symptoms may continue, it is important to support stepwise increases in independent functioning (i.e., encourage school attendance, sports activities, peer relations, and family life). For a child or adolescent who has significantly withdrawn from many aspects of life, reestablishing participation in school and social activities is a **gradual process taken one step at a time.**

b. **Advocacy.** It is often helpful for the clinician to contact the school directly (with the family's permission), to facilitate the child's reentry to school after missing several weeks, or to help the patient to reestablish sports or other social activities that have lagged. Enlisting the help of school personnel (e.g., counselor, social worker) to be available to and support the child is often critical to success. Addressing the involvement of the school nurse (e.g., limiting contact and encouraging a return to school activities) and the circumstances under which the parents will be contacted (e.g., if the child has a fever or in the nurse's view the symptoms are concerning) is crucial. This plan must be discussed and agreed on by the parents.

c. **Psychotherapy** is often indicated at this stage. It is best to raise this earlier rather than later to optimize the chance of family acceptance of a referral. This foreshadowing also allows for the mental health clinician to become an integrated part of the treatment team. Cognitive-behavioral and family therapy approaches are often helpful at this stage.

d. **Medication** may be a component of treatment at this stage (see *Practical Use of Medications* below).

e. **Laboratory and other evaluations.** A physical examination is generally indicated at each stage of evaluation. If the examination remains normal, no additional laboratory tests should be pursued beyond the initial screening.

f. **Monitoring.** Regular (i.e., at least every 2 weeks initially) follow-up for children and adolescents with somatoform disorders is recommended. Symptoms generally do not disappear quickly and it can take weeks or months for medical clinicians to convince adolescents and their families with somatoform disorders to accept the help of psychologists and psychiatrists.

D. **Referring**

1. **When to refer and transfer primary responsibility**

a. The child or adolescent has missed several consecutive weeks of school

b. Social withdrawal is occurring and peer activities curtailed significantly

c. Family life is significantly disrupted or conflict exists in the family regarding the symptoms in the child

d. PCP reassurance does not help and requests or demands for further and more obscure workup are increasing.

2. **When referring**

a. **Psychoeducation**

(1) **Continued validation, reassurance, and encouragement** as above

(2) **Referral and collaboration with multidisciplinary team.** The PCP can explain to the patient and family the need for clinicians with varying expertise to be involved in the care of the patient. Many families resist the notion that a psychiatrist or psychologist can be of help in what they consider to be a "medical" problem that awaits being identified correctly. It is important for the referral to be posed as a cooperative effort between the various disciplines, rather than a transfer of the patient "out" of the medical realm and "into" the psychiatric realm. It is best to explain to the family that both disciplines will be working together to treat the patient. Continuing to schedule appointments for the patient in the PCP office to monitor physical status serves to reassure the families and patients about this. For optimal effectiveness, the PCP should:

(a) Be sure that role definitions are clear between disciplines: the mental health professional's role is to provide mental health treatment, not recommend laboratory tests and so on; the role of the PCP is to evaluate and monitor the physical status of the child.

(b) The PCP should know the mental health professionals working with the family. Families can and do create doubt about the adequacy of other members of the treatment team. Mutual support is critical in these difficult cases and can only occur with genuine confidence in the other members.

(c) Hold the line on further laboratory tests once a somatoform disorder is confirmed. This can be difficult under the pressure of upset or angry parents but is essential to prevent the entrenchment of illness behavior and chronic disability. At times, this can result in the patient seeking treatment with another physician. When this occurs, it is important that other members of a group practice insist that continued treatment in the practice only occur with the initial PCP, and not with another member.

b. Advocacy. The PCP and child psychiatrist can work collaboratively to **encourage as regular school attendance as possible,** as well as participation in team sports and other social activities for the child. Even when full return to activities is not occurring, it is helpful to recognize and reinforce any positive movement towards further participation. Identifying a **contact person at the school** (e.g., school counselor, social worker) to meet briefly with the patient at times of stress is also helpful.

c. Psychotherapy and physiological interventions. At the time of referral, psychotherapy and physical therapies may be indicated.

(1) Cognitive-behavioral psychotherapy for somatoform disorders involving pain symptoms can be focused on either the modification of pain behavior or of the child's subjective experience of pain.

(2) Pain behavior management involves developing a reasonable incentive for the child to gradually exchange a dysfunctional behavioral response to feeling the pain for a functional behavioral response. For instance, if a child remains in bed instead of getting up and getting ready for school when pain is present, develop a program (i.e., rewards and consequences) to provide an incentive for the child to get out of bed.

(3) Self-regulatory strategies (e.g., progressive muscle relaxation, guided imagery, meditative breathing, self-hypnotic techniques) attempt to alter the perception of pain. They all provide the child or adolescent with a predictable method of taking control and changing the focus of his or her own attention. It is useful to first find out what a child or adolescent has spontaneously developed to help cope with pain and diminish distress. Hypnotic techniques aim to remove attention from the discomfort, and refocus attention on an internal sense of calm. A child or adolescent can learn to imagine a scene or a series of scenes in which he or she feels increasingly more relaxed or calm. A child or adolescent can practice paying attention to other sensations (e.g., the air temperature in the room, sounds, tactile sensations). This can then be embellished through imagery of additional pleasing sensations. These techniques aid the child in dissociating from the pain or discomfort and developing a sense of calm. Electromyographic biofeedback has been used to relieve muscular problems (e.g., muscle spasms) or to improve muscle contractility. Children appear able to rapidly understand the meaning of the visual or auditory feedback given during these techniques and can be taught to use these strategies at home.

(4) **Graded exercise therapy** (i.e., initially 5 days/week of 5 to15 minutes walking, biking, or swimming at 40% peak oxygen consumption, then gradually increased to 30 minutes at 60% peak oxygen consumption) has been established as an effective treatment component in CFS in adults. Although this has not been studied in adolescents or other somatoform disorders, it seems reasonable to use this therapy for pediatric populations as well.

(5) **Massage, acupuncture, and transcutaneous electrical stimulation** (TENS) are among the most commonly used mechanical interventions in pain syndromes. Massage is most commonly used to diminish pain, reduce muscle spasm, diminish swelling, and assist flow and circulation. Acupuncture has been a component of treatment for chronic pain for centuries in traditional Chinese medicine. Clinical research indicates that acupuncture and acupressure do have an effect on the central nervous system. It is believed that acupuncture causes reduction of pain through inducing the release of endogenous opioids as well as through effects on various neurotransmitters. TENS is delivered by a portable battery-powered device that is not painful. This form of treatment is effective in reducing pain by producing high-frequency

stimulation of large afferent fibers and inhibition of small fibers in the same area, thereby diminishing the sensation of pain. TENS is generally administered by physical therapists, who are trained to design and implement rehabilitation programs.

(6) **Psychodynamic psychotherapy,** in group, family, or individual formats can also be useful in the treatment of children and adolescents with somatoform disorders.

(7) **Family therapy** may be necessary to assist the family in relinquishing their preoccupying focus on the symptomatic child. Because of the intensity of the child's illness experience, the symptoms can take on a life of their own in the family. The ability of the child to move past the illness depends in part on the ability of the family to do the same. Many families require assistance in making this transition.

d. **Medications** can be useful in the direct treatment of symptoms of pain in somatoform disorders, as well as for comorbid anxiety or depressive disorders. Use of medication is discussed in the next section.

e. **Laboratory and other evaluations.** Further laboratory tests beyond what are done initially are not useful unless comorbid medical conditions warrant follow-up.

f. **Monitoring.** Close monitoring and follow-up are critical components of successful treatment of somatoform disorders. If a functioning multidisciplinary team has been activated, the PCP need continue follow-up every 1 to 3 months.

IV. **Practical use of medications.**
Medications are frequently helpful for the commonly comorbid conditions (i.e., anxiety and depressive disorders) that occur alongside somatoform disorders. On the other hand, few data exist on medication treatment of pediatric somatoform conditions themselves. Because anxiety and depressive syndromes so frequently accompany somatoform disorders, serotonin reuptake inhibitor (SSRI) antidepressants are often the drugs of choice used in children and adolescents with somatoform disorders. Although the data are limited, specific medications have been reported to be helpful for pain disorders and body dysmorphic disorder. Medications used to treat patients with chronic pain syndromes include analgesics (e.g., acetaminophen) and nonsteroidal anti-inflammatory drugs (e.g., salicylates [aspirin], ibuprofen, and naproxen). Antidepressants, anticonvulsants, and alpha-adrenergic agents have also been used in the treatment of pain syndromes. Specific medications have not been found useful for conversion, hypochondriasis, or somatization disorder. The

use of medication in somatoform disorders is most effective when **integrated into a multimodal treatment plan** that includes psychotherapy, school intervention, psychoeducation, and physical therapies when indicated.

A. **Pain syndromes**

1. **Anticonvulsants** (e.g., carbamazepine, valproic acid, and more recently, gabapentin) have been used in the treatment of pain syndromes, particularly neuropathic pain. **Carbamazepine** (Appendix H) has a chemical structure similar to tricyclic antidepressants, and its ability to diminish pain is believed to occur from its effects on type B γ-aminobutyric acid (GABA) receptors. Carbamazepine, which is initiated in children at 100 mg by mouth twice daily, can be increased every 5 to 7 days in increments of 100 mg. Dose range is often 1000 to 1200 mg/day in divided doses. Effective serum levels are not known, although in clinical practice the usual anticonvulsant range is generally used. The most common side effects are blurred vision, gastrointestinal disturbance, dizziness, and sedation. The most serious potential side effects include aplastic anemia and agranulocytosis. Laboratory monitoring guidelines are reviewed in Appendix H. **Valproic acid** (Appendix Q) is an anticonvulsant that is believed to diminish pain through its potentiation of central nervous system GABA. This drug has US Food and Drug Administration approval for adults in the prophylactic treatment of migraine headaches. Laboratory monitoring guidelines are reviewed in Appendix Q. Oral dosage in children usually begins with 125 mg twice daily and with 250 mg twice daily in adolescents. Dosage is increased in increments of 125 to 250 mg every 5 to 7 days as tolerated. Adequate serum concentrations are thought to be between 50 and 100 µg/ml in children and adolescents. The most common side effects are nausea, diarrhea, and sedation. The most serious side effects of this drug are hepatotoxicity, which in rare cases can be fatal. **Gabapentin** (Appendix I) is an amino acid, used in the treatment of partial complex seizure disorders, but has been hypothesized to be effective in reducing pain based on its similarity in chemical structure to GABA. Gabapentin increases the synthesis of GABA, enhancing its activity, and results in dose-related elevations of GABA in the brain without affecting GABA receptors. The optimal dose of gabapentin in the management of pain syndromes has not been established. Gabapentin, for seizure control, has been used in doses that range from 600 mg/day to

more than 3000 mg/day. The most frequent side effects of gabapentin are sedation, dizziness, and ataxia. Gabapentin is eliminated primarily through the kidneys so that renal function should be monitored before and during usage. No known serious toxicities have resulted when gabapentin was taken in overdose.

2. **Tricyclics** (Appendix P) (e.g., amitriptyline or nortriptyline) in low doses (i.e., 10 to 50 mg) have been studied in adults and used in the treatment of chronic pain syndromes, especially recurrent abdominal pain and headaches. Given the potential cardiotoxic side effects of this class of medications, they are not drugs of choice for these conditions for children. However, they can be useful for adolescents.

3. **Alpha-adrenergic agonists. Clonidine** (Appendix A) has been used for its analgesic properties in cases of neuropathic pain and in patients with central pain syndromes. It has also been used while weaning a child or adolescent with chronic pain from opioids. The dose range is 3 to 10 µg/kg. Oral starting dose for children is 0.05 mg at bedtime, and then increased to 0.05 mg twice and three times daily over the course of 2 weeks as tolerated. The average oral dose of clonidine is 0.1 mg three times daily. The main side effects of clonidine are hypotension and sedation. Clonidine is also available as a transdermal patch that delivers 0.1 mg, 0.2 mg, or 0.3 mg per 24 hours. One patch is effective for approximately 5 days in children.

4. **Acetaminophen** controls pain but does not have anti-inflammatory properties. Analgesic medication is most appropriate for controlling pain associated with tissue damage. Acetaminophen is not recommended as a long-term treatment for children or adolescents with chronic pain syndrome. For children, the recommended dose is approximately 10 mg/kg, which can be used four times per day. Acetaminophen is usually well tolerated in the short-term. Side effects include allergy in the form of skin rash.

5. **Nonsteroidal anti-inflammatory agents** (e.g., ibuprofen and naproxen) can control higher levels of pain than acetaminophen and aspirin. Naproxen is approved for the treatment of juvenile arthritis in children above 2 years of age at a dose of 10 mg/kg/day divided into two doses. A 200-mg dose of ibuprofen is comparable to 650 mg of aspirin, but with longer duration; and 250 mg of naproxen is comparable to 650 mg of aspirin and with longer duration. Primary side

effects of these medications include an inhibition of platelet function and gastritis.

6. **Salicylates** (e.g., aspirin) provide anti-inflammatory as well as analgesic relief. Because of the risk of Reyes syndrome, this is not used as a pain reliever in children and adolescents with somatoform disorders. There may be a place for aspirin in the treatment of rare conditions such as Kawasaki's disease or juvenile rheumatoid arthritis.

B. **Other somatoform conditions**

1. **SSRIs** are the drugs of first choice in the treatment of child or adolescent anxiety and depressive syndromes, commonly comorbid with somatoform disorders. These medications, especially fluoxetine, are now also being used in clinical practice for chronic pain syndromes, body dysmorphic disorder, and CFS. Although no randomized control treatment data provide evidence of efficacy for these disorders, anecdotal reports support their usage. Dosing for these syndromes is similar to that used for depression. Children and adolescents with somatoform disorders may be more sensitive to side effects (e.g., sedation, nausea, headache, other gastrointestinal disturbances) (see Appendix N).

2. **Benzodiazepines** (Appendix E) (e.g., clonazepam) have been used in the short-term treatment of anxiety in children and adolescents. No controlled studies support the use of these medications in children and we would discourage their use in somatoform disorders. They may have a place in the treatment of comorbid anxiety disorders (see Chapter 11).

C. **Insomnia.** Many children and adolescents with somatoform disorders complain of insomnia. In some cases, these symptoms improve during treatment of comorbid anxiety or depression with SSRI antidepressants. Hypnotic medications are generally only recommended for short-term use in the treatment of insomnia. For younger children, antihistamines (e.g., diphenhydramine [Benadryl], at doses of 12.5 to 25 mg at bedtime) are safe short-term treatment for insomnia. For adolescents, hypnotics that do not cause physical dependency (e.g., zolpidem [Ambien] and zaleplon [Sonata]) are generally chosen over benzodiazepines for short-term treatment of insomnia. Dosage for these medications is 5 to 10 mg at bedtime and side effects are minimal.

V. **Summary.** Somatoform disorders are complex constellations of symptoms that are best conceptualized as combined physical and psychological entities. It is not possible to divide them into those that are mainly "physiologic," and those that are "psychological." Successful treatment is accomplished through an integrated approach of collaboration among a variety of professionals including pediatricians, child and adolescent psychiatrists, psychotherapists, physical therapists, educators, and families. Although symptom reduction is an important goal, the main focus of treatment for all of the somatoform disorders is to provide interventions that increase the level of functioning of the child or adolescent socially, academically, and in family life.

SUGGESTED READINGS

Albertini RS, Phillips KA, Guevremont D. Body dysmorphic disorder. *J Am Acad Child Adolesc Psychiatry* 1996;35:1425–1426.

Breau L, McGrath P, Ju L. Review of juvenile primary fibromyalgia and chronic fatigue syndrome. *J Dev Behav Pediatr* 1999;20(4): 278–288.

Bursch B, Walco GA, Zeltzer L. Clinical assessment and management of chronic pain and pain-associated disability syndrome. *J Dev Behav Pediatr* 1998;19:45–53.

Campo JV, Fritsch SL. Somatization in children and adolescents. *J Am Acad Child Adolesc Psychiatry* 1994;33:1223–1235.

Chen E, Joseph M, Zeltzer LK. Behavioral and cognitive interventions in the treatment of pain in children. *Pediatr Clin North Am* 2000; 47(3):513–525.

Friedrich WN, Schafer LC. Somatic symptoms in sexually abused children. *J Pediatr Psychol* 1995;20:661–670.

Fritz GK, Fritsch S, Hagino O. Somatoform disorders in children and adolescents: a review of the past 10 years. *J Am Acad Child Adolesc Psychiatry* 1997;36:1329–1338.

Garralda ME. Practitioner review: assessment and management of somatization in childhood and adolescence: a practical perspective. *J Child Psychol Psychiatry* 1999;40:1159–1167.

Sirven JI, Glosser DS. Psychogenic nonepileptic seizures: theoretical and clinical considerations. *Neuropsychiatry Neuropsychol Behav Neurol* 1998;11:225–235.

Wessely S, Nimnuan C, Sharpe M. Functional somatic syndromes: one or many? *Lancet* 1999;354(9182):936–939.

Zeltzer L, Bursch B, Walco G. Pain responsiveness and chronic pain: a psychobiological perspective. *J Dev Behav Pediatr* 1997;18:402–412.

Web Sites

American Chronic Pain Association. Available at www.theacpa.org. Accessed on 6/29/02.

The National Chronic Pain Outreach Association. Available at http:// neurosurgery.mgh.harvard.edu/ncpainoa.htm. Accessed on 6/29/02.

American Academy of Pain Management. Available at www. aapainmanage.org. Accessed on 6/29/02.

Research has indicated that the reaction of a child to trauma is related to several factors, including:

1. Proximity to the trauma (both physical and emotional proximity) and perceived physical threat
2. Loss of family members and friends
3. Parental reaction to the trauma

Parental reaction to trauma appears to affect children through a variety of mechanisms. **Parental support** has been demonstrated to have a **protective impact** on children, subsequent both to acute trauma and to a child's disclosure of more chronic traumas (e.g., ongoing child sexual abuse). Parents with preexisting and serious psychopathology might be less available to support children. In addition, parents who develop PTSD themselves may be less available for support and repeatedly expose the child to high levels of anxiety related to their own traumatic response. An additional issue that has emerged in the aftermath of both the bombing of the Federal Building in Oklahoma City and the September 11, 2001 attacks on the World Trade Center and Pentagon is the **clear relationship between the amount of exposure to television coverage and children's stress responses,** irrespective of the child's emotional or physical proximity to the trauma. These findings have enormous significance for the prevention of full-blown stress reactions in children.

B. There is a spectrum of stress responses that children and adolescents experience following a significant trauma. Specifically, PTSD, acute stress disorder, and adjustment disorder.

These disorders are presented in decreasing order of severity, with PTSD being the most severe response to a stressor. However, it will become clear that acute stress reactions can also be severe and ultimately evolve into a full-blown PTSD.

1. PTSD is a **complex and chronic disorder** that can follow exposure to a severe stressor. No one really knows why some individuals develop PTSD while others do not. No one knows why some children initially develop many of the symptoms of PTSD following trauma exposure, but their symptoms then spontaneously remit while other children remain very symptomatic.

Studies of adults have indicated that **PTSD symptoms are fueled by both psychological and neurobiological factors.** The latter includes **hyperarousal of the sympathetic nervous system coupled with significant changes in the hypothalamic-pituitary-adrenal axis feedback circuitry resulting in lowered plasma and urinary cortisol levels.** Whether these changes in corticosteroids occur in trauma-naive children following their first

21 ♣ Stress and Trauma:

Its Impact and Treatment in Children and Adolescents

Susan V. McLeer

I. **Background.** Losses, including death, are common childhood experiences. Separation, divorce, illness, or death in a parent or grandparent is an occurrence that primary care physicians (PCP) will face frequently in patients. These events are uniformly stressful for children, prompting normal grief and bereavement processes. Under certain circumstances, these events can become traumatic. Although less frequent, but of higher intensity, are traumas (or stressors) that range from acute exposure to disasters (e.g., crashing of a helicopter into an elementary school yard or the attack on Columbine High School) to the repeated and all too frequent trauma of child maltreatment and exposure to adult domestic violence. In the United States, many children and adolescents have been exposed to traumas of sufficient severity to cause not only significant, but possibly long-standing effects across emotional, behavioral, cognitive, and social domains.

A. **Factors in symptom development.** Recently, professionals have tended to assume that trauma, *de facto,* leads to the development of posttraumatic stress disorder (PTSD). However, it is important to recognize that both cross-sectional and longitudinal studies of children's psychological response to trauma have consistently demonstrated that **only a subgroup of exposed youngsters actually develop PTSD** and many respond with other emotional and behavioral problems that arise subsequent to the trauma. Symptoms of **depression are extremely common as is the development of non-PTSD anxiety disorders.** Some children tend to express their upset through behaviors and become increasingly **impulsive, irritable, and confrontational following trauma. Preexisting disorders** (e.g., attention-deficit/hyperactivity disorder [AD/HD], major depressive disorder, and neurodevelopmental disabilities) can have an **impact on a youngster's response to significant stressors.** In addition, some traumas result in the death of family and friends, adding the component of loss and grief to the child's already complicated experience following exposure. If personal loss is accompanied by the child watching a horrific death at the site of a disaster, then the process of mourning becomes complicated further by the traumatic image of the person's death and requires special handling if future disability and dysfunction are to be avoided.

traumatization is not known. Researchers have hypothesized that a developmental course ensues with effects on hypothalamic glucocorticoid receptor sensitivity that differ significantly in first-exposed children as compared with adults who may have experienced multiple traumas. Definitive studies are pending.

Psychological factors that fuel PTSD symptom maintenance include **classic and operant conditioning** as well as changes in cognition. Classic conditioning occurs as people, places, and situations that are, in reality, not dangerous "feel" dangerous because of their being reminiscent of the actually experienced traumatic event. Operant conditioning occurs when these not dangerous, but "feared" stimuli are avoided. With avoidance, anxiety decreases, the child "feels" temporarily better which reinforces further avoidant behaviors. Avoidant behaviors can then prevent children from experiences that are important for cognitive, emotional, and social development.

   a. **Diagnostic criteria.** As with other psychiatric disorders, the stress-related disorders include both symptom and duration criteria. Both need to be met before a specific diagnosis is made. Nonetheless, it should be clearly noted that even if a child does not meet criteria for a stress-related disorder, that fact alone does not imply that treatment services are unnecessary. Studies have indicated that **although 50%, or even fewer children, meet criteria for PTSD following a severe stressor, most have stress-related symptoms,** some of which can be disabling and have an impact on future social and cognitive development. These issues will be discussed in the section on treatment.

   b. **PTSD diagnostic criteria**

      (1) The **experiencing or witnessing of an event that involved actual or threatened death, serious injury, or threat** to the physical integrity of the child or someone else. In addition, the child's reaction included intense fear, helplessness, horror, or disorganized or agitated behavior.

      (2) The traumatic event is **persistently re-experienced** in one or more of the following ways:

         (a) Recurrent and **intrusive distressing recollections** of thoughts, images or perceptions of the event, including reenactment through repetitive play that is thematically related to the trauma. Parents often see examples of repetitive play after a child has visited the PCP for immunizations. The child goes home and for several days gives "shots" to all the dolls, family pets, and family members. This kind of repetitive play is seen repeatedly in traumatized children, with the theme reflecting the theme of the experienced trauma.

(b) **Nightmares** or otherwise distressing dreams, with or without report of an embedded trauma-related theme

(c) Acting or **feeling as if the traumatic event were recurring**

(d) Intense psychological **distress and physiological reactivity on exposure to cues,** people, places, and things that are reminiscent of the trauma

(3) Persistent **avoidance of stimuli associated with the trauma** and numbing of general responsiveness as indicated by three or more of the following symptoms:

(a) Efforts to **avoid thoughts, feelings, or conversations associated with the trauma**

(b) Efforts to **avoid activities, places, and people** that arouse recollections of the trauma

(c) **Inability to recall an important part of the event**

(d) **Decreased interest** or participation in activities that were important to the child before the event

(e) Feelings of **detachment** or estrangement from others

(f) **Restricted range of affect** (e.g., blunted feelings of affection and love for others)

(g) Sense of **foreshortened future** (e.g., the child does not expect to have a career, marriage, children or a normal life span)

    (4) Persistent **symptoms of autonomic hyperarousal** that have developed subsequent to the trauma, as indicated by two or more of the following symptoms:

        1. Difficulty falling or staying asleep

        2. Irritability or outbursts of anger

        3. Difficulty concentrating

        4. Hypervigilance

        5. Exaggerated startle response

    (5) The required symptoms in each category have **persisted for more than a month.**

    (6) The symptoms cause clinically significant distress or impairment in social, educational, occupational, or other important areas of functioning.

c. **Acute stress disorder diagnostic criteria**

    (1) The **experiencing or witnessing of an event that involved actual or threatened death, serious injury, or threat** to the physical integrity of the child or someone else. In addition, the child's reaction included intense fear, helplessness, horror, or disorganized or agitated behavior.

    (2) Either while experiencing the trauma or afterward, the child or adolescent has three or more of the following **dissociative symptoms:**

        (a) Subjective sense of **numbing, detachment** or absence of emotional responsiveness

        (b) A reduction in awareness of his or her surroundings (e.g., **"being in a daze"**)

        (c) Derealization

        (d) Depersonalization

        (e) Dissociative amnesia (i.e., inability to recall an important aspect of the trauma)

    (3) The traumatic event is **persistently re-experienced** in one or more of the following ways: recurrent images, thoughts, dreams, illusions, flashback episodes, or a sense of reliving the experience; or distress on exposure to reminders of the traumatic event.

   (4) Marked **avoidance of stimuli** that arouse recollection of the trauma

   (5) Marked **symptoms of anxiety or increased autonomic arousal**

   (6) The symptoms cause clinically significant distress or impairment in social, educational, occupational, or other important areas of functioning or impair the child's ability to pursue some necessary task such as getting help or mobilizing family support by telling about what has happened.

   (7) **Onset** of the disturbance must be **within 4 weeks** of the trauma and symptoms **must last for a minimum of 2 days and a maximum of 4 weeks.**

   (8) The disturbance is not caused by the effects of a substance, either prescribed or abused, or by a general medical condition. The disturbance is not better accounted for by the criteria for brief psychotic disorder and is not an exacerbation of a preexisting disorder.

 d. **Adjustment disorder diagnostic criteria**

   (1) The development of emotional or behavioral symptoms in response to an identifiable stressor(s). Symptoms must develop **within a time period of 3 months from stressor onset.**

   (2) Symptoms or behaviors are clinically significant as evidenced by either (a) marked distress that is in excess of what would be expected from the exposure to the stressor or (b) significant impairment in social, educational, or occupational functioning.

   (3) The stress-related disturbance does not meet the criteria for another more specific disorder and is not an exacerbation of a preexisting disorder.

   (4) Symptoms **do not represent that of bereavement.**

   (5) Once the stressor, or its consequences, has terminated, the **symptoms do not persist for more than an additional 6 months.**

C. **Differential diagnosis.** What is apparent in examining the diagnostic criteria for each of these three disorders is that both severity and duration appear to be key factors for differentiating one from the other.

The nature of the trauma or stressor is identical in PTSD and acute stress disorder; however, a lesser degree of severity is indicated for adjustment disorder. Adjustment disorder can be invoked by lower-intensity stressors (e.g., death of a pet, having the family move from one location to the other) or by stressors as severe as those found in PTSD and acute stress disorder.

1. **PTSD** requires that a certain number of symptoms from each symptom subcategory persist together for at least 1 month. If the requisite symptoms are present, but persist for less than 1 month the diagnosis of acute stress disorder should be made. If the duration is greater than 1 month but less than 3 months, the PTSD is considered acute. If the **disorder persists for 3 months or more, it is considered chronic.** Interestingly, studies of both adults and children suggest that major neurophysiologic changes are associated with the development of chronic PTSD. The **appearance of the startle reaction occurs at approximately 3 months following a trauma** and is hypothesized to be a marker of these more chronic internal processes.

2. Symptoms of **acute stress disorder** are basically the same as those in PTSD; however, in acute stress disorder, the avoidant behaviors of PTSD have been subdivided into dissociative symptoms and avoidant behavior, with greater emphasis being placed on an individual having three dissociative symptoms during or after the trauma. If three dissociative symptoms are present, the individual clearly meets the symptom criteria for PTSD avoidance. The same number of re-experiencing symptoms is required for both PTSD and acute stress disorder. However, the number of symptoms of autonomic hyperarousal is not stipulated for acute stress disorder, hence, requiring a lesser degree of severity for diagnosis.

3. With **adjustment disorder,** symptoms noted are not as specific as for those of either PTSD or acute stress disorder. The major requirement is for symptoms to be in excess of the expected reaction to the stressor and includes impairment in social, educational, or occupational functioning. Symptoms of bereavement are excluded. Clearly, an adjustment disorder is of lesser symptom severity than either PTSD or acute stress disorder. However, duration requirements overlap with both of these two disorders, requiring onset within 3 months of the stress and duration being for no more than 3 months. Adjustment disorders are further subclassified, depending on whether associated symptoms feature pre-

dominately anxiety, depression, or behavioral disturbances.

4. **Bereavement** is the normal grieving process that humans experience with the death of loved ones. In the immediate aftermath, normal reactions in younger children include sadness and yearning, increased emotionality, sleep disturbances, clinging, separation fears, and other "regressive" behaviors (i.e., acting like a younger child). Older children and adolescents react with increased or decreased emotionality (including sadness, anger, and irritability or, alternatively, isolation) and sleep disturbances. The acute phase of reactions typically lasts a matter of weeks, although distress often lingers at lower levels for months or longer. Generally, children's functioning remains intact (e.g., goes to school, plays with friends) through normal bereavement. Signs that the bereavement process may have become abnormal include:

   1. Missing more than a week of school
   2. Withdrawing from peer and other activities
   3. Suicidal ideation or acts (although wishes to die and be reunited are not uncommon)
   4. Difficulty separating from parents (especially for sleep) for more than 2 weeks

   More specific signs and symptoms of PTSD, as described above, are not present in uncomplicated bereavement. On the other hand, traumatic deaths (sudden and unexpected, or witnessed deaths, suicides, or deaths involving shameful circumstances) may well lead to complicated bereavement or even PTSD.

5. Other psychiatric disorders can coexist with either PTSD or acute stress disorder. **Comorbid disorders** frequently found **include other anxiety disorders and major depression or dysthymia.** Children with preexisting behavioral disorders (e.g., AD/HD) or conduct disorder have a greater propensity to get into dangerous situations and, hence, have an increased risk for exposure to significant trauma. Finally, within the adolescent age range, those who have sustained significant trauma and have developed **chronic PTSD, can be at increased risk for substance abuse.** Conversely, those who heavily use or abuse substances more frequently place themselves in harm's way and, hence, increase their risk for traumatic exposure.

II. **Practical office evaluation.** The primary care office should develop a screening protocol for office assessment of children exposed to trauma. Such a protocol can be adopted from those already in use with a series of questions regarding:

1. A child's exposure to specific stressors (**trauma detection**)
2. Assessment of posttraumatic **symptoms**
   Standardized rating scales are useful, easy to administer, and quick. Always have the child complete the scale as well as the caregiver. If the child is too young to complete the scale, then a staff person can read the questionnaire to the child and complete the form for the child.
   A. **Trauma detection.** Sometimes parents will contact a PCP because their child has been exposed to a death or another substantial stressor. Often the questions revolve around practical issues such as whether the child should attend the funeral or whether the child should be allowed to sleep with the parents and for how long. However, especially in cases of more severe or stigmatized death or trauma, the child will be brought to the office with behavioral or emotional symptoms. The physician's task then is to determine if trauma exposure has occurred. In such cases, it is essential to take a trauma history.

   Traditionally, general screening questions regarding trauma exposure have been used. However, studies have indicated that **open-ended questions such as, "Has anything really bad or scary ever happened to you," are less productive than specific probes.** This is because children and adolescents, adults for that matter, may not define certain experiences as traumas. Interpersonal traumas both within the family and extra-familial can particularly be omitted when only a general probe is used, without inquiring specifically about child physical and sexual abuse, the witnessing of adult domestic violence or community violence, particularly in inner-city environments. Examples of specific questions might be:
   1. Has anyone ever hit, kicked, punched, or pushed you? Ever been beaten up? Were you injured?
   2. Have you ever seen anyone hit, kick, punch, or push someone else in your family? In your neighborhood?
   3. Have you ever seen anyone get shot? Knifed? Killed? Seriously injured?
   4. Has anyone ever touched you in a way that made you uncomfortable? Ever touched you in a sexual way? If so, who? What did they do?
   5. Has anyone ever touched you in your private parts when you did not want them to? Who? Where did they touch you? How did they touch you? Did they threaten you? Did they tell you not to tell anyone else?
   6. Has anyone important to you ever died? Who? When? How did it happen?
   The language used in the above questions will need to be tailored to the age of the child. Another consideration is whether to ask these questions of the parent

alone, the parent with the child present, or the child alone. Although no absolute answers exist for this, if a generally positive relationship is seen between the parent and child, it is preferable to have the discussion with both present. If the child or adolescent appears to be uncomfortable discussing the issue in front of the parent, it may be best to meet with the child alone at first. This is also true in cases in which the child appears to be in some danger, especially if this is because of maltreatment by one or both the parents. If the PCP has met with the child alone initially and maltreatment is discovered, then the PCP can support and help the child by presenting the issues to the parent together. If the assessment is that the situation is too explosive and dangerous to discuss in the office (i.e., the parent will become violent or out of control), it is best to dispense with a discussion with the parent and instead directly refer the case to Child Protective Services or commensurate authority.

An alternative is for the PCP to use a standardized questionnaire to ask about specific traumas. The two most commonly used questionnaires are noted below. The first takes a little more time to administer, but asks about both severe traumas as well as lesser life stressors that are important in understanding what the child is experiencing. The second questionnaire only asks about severe traumas and may be more appropriate for evaluating a child in whom a high index of suspicion for a trauma-related disorder is suggested.

1. The **Child and Adolescent Psychiatric Assessment (CAPA): Life Events Section** (Costello et al., 1998) is a structured clinical interview that can be systematically administered to both children and their parent/s or caretakers. It has been used in both epidemiologic and clinical settings and takes approximately 10 minutes to administer. The Life Events Section of the CAPA provides a listing of events that the child might have experienced, including extreme or "high-magnitude" stressors (e.g., witnessing a shooting) as well as "low-magnitude" stressors (e.g., parental divorce). The latter is clearly an upsetting experience for a child and increases the youngster's vulnerability, but usually does not qualify as a trauma of sufficient severity to precipitate either an acute stress disorder or PTSD. This interview can be particularly useful for the clinician because both the "high" and "low" magnitude events are assessed.

2. A briefer form for assessment is the **Life Events Checklist** (Nader et al., 1998), which only assesses "high" magnitude traumas. This form is more appropriate for most primary care settings.

B. **Evaluation of symptoms.** Once a trauma meeting the necessary severity criteria is identified, it is necessary to determine the presence and duration of symptoms in each of the symptom subcategories, as related to that specific trauma. If two or more traumas exist, symptoms must be directly elicited in relationship to each of the traumas.

Three structured instruments can be used for assessment of stress symptoms. The first two scales—Clinician-Administered PTSD Scale for Children and Adolescents (CAPS-CA) and Children's PTSD Inventory (CPTSDI)—are particularly useful in a primary care setting because they can be administered rapidly and will provide a complete assessment of PTSD symptoms. The third scale (CAPA PTSD) is far too lengthy for use in a clinical setting. It is best used for clinical research.

1. **The CAPS-CA,** developed by the National Center for PTSD in conjunction with the University of California-Los Angeles Trauma Psychiatry Program (Nader et al., 1998), rates both the frequency and the intensity of PTSD symptoms and includes pictorial scales that are easier for younger children to use. This is a scale that is easily administered in a clinician's office. Psychometric studies have yet to be published regarding this instrument.

2. **The CPTSDI** (Saigh et al., 2000) is also a rapidly administered scale that can be used to assess PTSD in children and adolescents between 7 and 18 years of age. Psychometric studies have indicated extremely high levels of validity and reliability.

3. **The CAPA PTSD Scale** (Costello et al., 1998) is a structured interview that details the timing of events and the onset of symptoms to assess issues of causality. It can take up to 60 to 90 minutes to administer and is better used as a research instrument. Psychometric validation has been obtained only for children between 9 and 17 years of age.

C. **Trauma scales should be completed by both the child and parent(s).** Interviewing solely the parent is problematic because it has been demonstrated repeatedly that children and adolescents are far more reliable reporters for their internalizing symptoms, such as symptoms of anxiety, depression, and dissociative experiences. Parents or caretakers are more reliable reporters for externalizing symptoms (e.g., problematic behaviors).

Teachers can also provide helpful information, although for some traumas (e.g., child maltreatment and adult domestic violence), issues of confidentiality preclude contacting the teachers for information specifically related to the trauma. However, teachers can be approached if questions are posed as relating to a more general assessment of the child. It is clearly important to determine if changes have occurred in a child's academic performance, ability to concentrate, or tendency to "daydream." Changes in behavior, both in and outside the classroom, are critical areas for assessment. Determining if the child is more withdrawn or more irritable with peers at school is also important.

D.   Safety considerations. Depression frequently coexists with stress-related disorders. Increased irritability secondary to autonomic hyperarousal can impair behavioral control and increase impulsivity. For trauma associated with child maltreatment and adult domestic violence, self-esteem can decrease considerably. Peer relationships can be impaired and a child or adolescent may feel increasingly trapped and hopeless. Consequently, suicide assessment is critical. Children should be asked if they sometimes feel so bad that they do not want to go on living, or feel like hurting or killing themselves. If a child indicates that he or she feels or has felt like that, ask how the child thinks that he or she would go about hurting or killing self. Determine if the youngster has a plan and further determine if a gun is available. In addition, it is always essential to check on the use and abuse of substances, because suicidal ideation or feelings, coupled with substance use and abuse, present a lethal combination. Add a gun to the mixture and an extremely high-risk situation has indeed been clearly identified. It is critical also to keep in mind that when a child or adolescent has been exposed to both family and community violence, the risk of retaliation and harm to others also needs assessment.

E.   Who should do the assessment. It is not necessary for a physician to do the screening for whether a child or adolescent has been exposed to a significant trauma. A nurse practitioner, physician's assistant, or a social worker can do the screening and, if positive, can assess the presence and duration of symptoms as well as the impact of symptoms on function.

Even if a child or adolescent does not meet criteria for PTSD, it is important to be aware that **almost all children who are exposed to trauma have some posttraumatic symptoms. Of particular concern are the avoidant behaviors** that develop after trauma. These behaviors can result in a child's avoidance of persons, places, and situations that are important for further cognitive, emotional, and social development; hence, it is important to have a trained person in the office who can determine if significant avoidant behaviors are present. If avoidant behaviors are identified that prevent the child from engaging in situations that are developmentally important, then, irrespective of whether the child meets criteria for one of the three stress-related disorders, the child should be referred for targeted, symptom-specific treatment.

The PCP should be involved in the assessment of suicide risk as well as the determination of the risk to others. The *Child Depression Inventory* and the *Beck Depression Inventory* can be used to quantify symptoms of depression and screen for suicidal risk. Direct questioning then needs to be used to further assess risk.

Assurance of confidentiality should not be given whenever a risk is posed regarding self-injurious behaviors. There is an obligation to warn if an imminent threat is present regarding the safety of others.

III. **Triage assessment and general treatment planning**

A. **General issues.** Children and adolescents with either transient symptoms or with an adjustment disorder oftentimes have spontaneous symptom remittance. Others continue to be symptomatic with declining levels of function. Consequently, it is important to monitor the child's level of function and distress.

Immediately following a traumatic event it is critical to talk with parents about how children react to stress. Encouraging parental support and understanding is oftentimes sufficient to help the child through a difficult and stressful time. The parents may also want to tell the child's teacher that he or she is going through a difficult time so the teacher understands the child better and provides emotional support and guidance. Additionally, it is important to determine how the parents are faring, because the emotional availability of parents is important for the child. Many of the "low" magnitude stressors (e.g., divorce) are so stressful that significant depression or anxiety symptoms can emerge in parents. Providing guidance for the parents to access help and support for themselves may be one of the more effective interventions for the child.

Little is known about the treatment of acute stress disorder in children and adolescents. Studies have indicated that on exposure to a severe stressor, **40% to 85% of children who meet diagnostic criteria for acute stress disorder spontaneously recover.** However, **15% to 60% will develop PTSD.** These children need treatment. Clinical case studies have suggested that early intervention during the period of acute stress disorders can facilitate recovery and decrease the development of chronic PTSD for many children. However, definitive studies have yet to be conducted.

B. **Psychosocial treatments.** It is important to note that neither nondirective play nor talking therapies have demonstrated efficacy in children or adolescents with PTSD. In adults, multiple studies have demonstrated cognitive-behavioral therapies are efficacious in treating this disorder. Studies targeting the treatment efficacy of cognitive-behavioral therapies in children with PTSD are less plentiful, but consistent in indicating that a cognitive-behavioral approach is the current "gold standard" for treatment.

Clinicians who have had specific training in providing this therapeutic modality should provide cognitive-behavioral treatments. Psychologists more frequently have had such training, although some child and adolescent psychiatrists and master's level therapists have also been trained in this modality. Both children and parents or caretakers need to understand as much as possible about the origin of the symptoms and the way symptoms can develop and worsen over time. Consequently, the involvement and education of both child and parent are essential to the therapeutic process. A growing body of evidence indicates that including families in cognitive-behavior therapy approaches significantly enhances efficacy.

Cognitive-behavioral treatments essentially use both **desensitization through imagery and *in vivo* desensitization** to reduce symptoms of acute stress disorder and PTSD. Desensitization through imagery aims to reduce trauma-related anxiety that has become attached to people, situations, and places, which, in reality, are not dangerous, but through association with a trauma the child perceives as dangerous.

The **cognitive component** of treatment targets the development of cognitive assessment skills so that the child or adolescent can **differentiate people, places, and situations that may be potentially dangerous from those that are merely perceived as dangerous.** The cognitive treatment also addresses strategies for accessing support and help in the face of danger.

In providing desensitization through imagery, a risk exists of precipitating more avoidant symptoms in the child. This can occur because in the process of retelling the story of the trauma, strong and painful emotions are elicited. If the child leaves treatment at this point, the process of leaving temporarily decreases the level of the child's anxiety. Lower anxiety feels better and, hence, becomes reinforcement for more avoidance. With an increase in avoidant behaviors, a vicious cycle of avoidance is initiated that ultimately causes the child to become more symptomatic. Parents or caretakers as well as the child need to understand this process to provide the commitment, support, and firm encouragement necessary for treatment. Additionally, monitoring the effectiveness of the treatment requires the use of logs or diaries for tracking symptom frequency and severity. Parents or caretakers can be extremely helpful in encouraging the child to complete these records.

By the time that a child or adolescent is referred for treatment, he or she has undoubtedly already developed many avoidant behaviors associated with the trauma. *In vivo* exposure, the most effective treatment, requires the participation of parents or caretakers.

The best way to understand **in vivo exposure** is to consider the behavioral treatment of an elevator phobia. One can talk for a long time about the advantage of using elevators, but the only effective treatment is actually getting the individual into an elevator and having that person use the elevator **long enough for anxiety levels to be reduced by at least 75%.** If the individual flees the elevator before an adequate reduction in anxiety has occurred, the response of avoiding the elevator will be reinforced and the symptoms worsened. Therefore, it is helpful for parents or caretakers to accompany their children for *in vivo* exposure treatments. Parents or caretakers can be taught to help the child rate anxiety levels and ensure that the child remains in the feared situation long enough for anxiety to be reduced adequately. Having the parents or caretakers fully understand the psychological mechanisms for symptom formation is essential if they are to be "co-therapists" who can facilitate the treatment of the child and prevent a worsening of symptoms. *In vivo* exposure treatment is usually not initiated until the child has experienced considerable success in the desensitization through the imagery process.

Newer longitudinal studies have suggested that irrespective of whether or not a child meets criteria for PTSD, the **avoidant posttraumatic symptoms persist and infrequently resolve spontaneously.** Although replication of these findings is necessary, data suggest that even those who do not meet full criteria for PTSD may need treatment of the avoidant symptoms to ensure that the trauma is not compounded by avoidant behaviors that will keep the child or adolescent away from developmentally important experiences.

C. **Watching**
  1. **When to watch**
     a. Symptoms are mild
     b. Symptoms are recent
     c. Child continues to function adequately, even if mild decrease from baseline
  2. **What to do when watching**
     a. **Psychoeducation**
        (1) Recommend that parents or caretakers **be emotionally available** and not judge, criticize, or try to change the child's feelings.
        (2) **Talking about feelings** is one of the most important tools in coping with

tragedy. Recommend that parents do not avoid talking about the trauma; on the other hand, they should not force the child to talk about the situation either.

(3) Children want to **feel reassured and safe.** Parents or caretakers should address concrete safety issues, but avoid false reassurance. For example, following the bombing of the World Trade Center it was reasonable to reassure a child that his or her home was safe, assuming it was not located in a place that was highly likely to be targeted by terrorists. Do not assure a child that nothing bad would ever happen again.

(4) Reassure parents that crying, fears, worries, and anger can all be stimulated in the face of a disaster or trauma. Allow the child to express feelings. **Acknowledge and validate the child's reactions** to the trauma.

(5) Be aware that in situations where traumas occur close to home (e.g., a shooting in a school yard) that children may speak of **feeling guilty.** Help the child understand that it is normal to wish that one had been able to do something to prevent the disaster, but that disasters do happen and that the child was not expected to "fix everything."

(6) **Younger children's understanding of events is often inaccurate** because of limited experiences, immature ways of thinking, and active fantasy lives. Parents can be helpful by addressing misunderstanding and clarifying the reality of a situation.

(7) Reactions to trauma can be worsened by watching **excessive television coverage,** particularly given how graphic TV coverage may be. Exposure to TV coverage should be limited. It is best for children and adolescents to watch with a supportive adult who talks with the child and helps the child understand and process feelings. Both age and emotional stability should be considered in determining how much, if any, TV exposure is reasonable.

(8) Children need to **be with their parents** or other known and trusted adults who are important to them during times of tragedy and disaster.

(9) The decision about **whether to allow a child to attend a funeral** or wake often comes to the PCP's attention. These are complex decisions that need to balance the child's need to feel included in important family events and emotionally process the loss, with the potential for the event to be overwhelming, confusing, or traumatizing for the child. Questions about what to do often reflect parental disagreement about the issue. The PCP can first clarify whether the parents agree and then define the area of disagreement. The PCP is usually best advised not to "take sides" but rather to help the parents in the office come to an acceptable resolution. In guiding the parents, the following points may be helpful:

(a) In general, funerals are important rituals for children to attend. They provide official closure and offer important opportunities for children to connect with the other survivors as well as emotionally process the loss. As noted, children need to be with parents or other trusted adults during difficult times, and attending the funeral with parents is important in promoting healthy reactions to loss. If parents are too emotionally involved with the grieving process to offer support to children, then another trusted family member or adult can be assigned the task of attending to the child's emotional needs.

(b) Adolescents should be expected to attend the funeral of another family member. If they balk, they should be given an opportunity to discuss their fears and supported, but still with the expectation that they will attend.

(c) School-aged children's stated wishes should be taken into account in coming to a decision. If a child feels strongly that he or she not attend, the parents can explore why and offer reasons for the child to come. If the child persists, it may be best for the child not to attend. In any event, the child should not be forced to go. Conversely, the child may desire to go when the adults do not wish them to do so. In this case, it may help to explore and clarify the concerns of the parent. Reassurance by the PCP, if appropriate, that the child will not be damaged can be helpful. Often the concern of the parents is that they themselves will become more emotionally upset and cry if the child is present and shows upset. In this, reassure the parents that this is a normal part of the grieving process.

(d) Children who are judged to be unable to understand the death or will become emotionally overwhelmed should not be expected to attend. If they wish to come, the parents can rehearse or preview what will happen and what to expect. Very young children (<2 years of age) will have limited understanding of death and should not be forced to attend a funeral. Further, the sight of a dead body, especially of a loved one, may traumatize very young children or cognitively limited children. Parents should consider the impact of open casket viewing on the individual child. Generalized assumptions about children are often misguided and must take in the age and maturity of the child, the relationship to the dead person, how the dead person actually appears, family preferences, and the emotional state of the parents.

    (e) Parents need to be honest with themselves to recognize their own level of distress. If the parents are too distraught to be available to the child, then it may be overwhelming for the younger child and best not to attend a funeral.

    (f) It is often consoling for parents and other adults to have children present at a funeral. This is a normal desire on the part of the adults, and should only be challenged when the child's emotional needs are disregarded.

  (10) **Sleeping difficulties** are not uncommon after stressful or traumatic events. PCPs are frequently asked about the younger child wishing to sleep with the parents in this context, after months or even years of sleeping by themselves. The desire of the younger child to be closer to the parents at this time of stress is normal. Consequently, a few days (longer in cases of severe or ongoing trauma) of wanting to sleep with the parents are normal. When the parents start to feel irritated or that the child may be "milking" the situation, they should make efforts to have the child sleep in its own bed once again. Beyond discussions with the child, parents may wish to provide incentives and rewards for the child to sleep in their own bed (e.g., "if you sleep in your own bed for x nights in a row," the parent will do something special with the child; alternatively, they will provide something that the child has been requesting).

b. **Advocacy.** No specific intervention with schools is necessary at this point.

c. **Psychotherapy** is not necessary during this period of time unless specific comorbid psychiatric conditions exist or the trauma is that of child maltreatment.

d. **Medication.** Not indicated.

e. **Laboratory and other evaluations.** Not indicated.

f. **Monitoring.** Parents should be instructed to call if symptoms worsen or function deteriorates. Child's level of functioning and symptoms should be reassessed 4 weeks after the trauma.

D. Intervening further
  1. When to intervene further
    a. Symptoms are mild to moderate and persistent
    b. Access to definitive psychiatric treatment is delayed
  2. What to do when intervening further
    a. Psychoeducation
      (1) Discuss with parents and children the **specific kinds of symptoms that are apt to develop** following a disaster, including re-experiencing symptoms, avoidant behaviors, and symptoms of autonomic hyperarousal.
      (2) Identify avoidance behaviors. Encourage parents to work with their child to identify people, places, and situations that are not dangerous, but perceived to be dangerous after trauma and, hence, are avoided.
      (3) Explain the risks associated with encouragement or reinforcement of further **avoidance** of nondangerous people, places, and situations associated with the trauma.
      (4) Encourage parents to **support their child to confront feared, but nondangerous, situations rather than avoid them.**
    b. Advocacy
      (1) Parents should meet with the child's teacher and explain what has occurred.
      (2) Functioning in the school setting, including academic and interactions with peers and adults, should be further assessed.
      (3) Child should attend school. If school refusal develops, treat that condition as indicated in Chapter 18.
      (4) Rarely, is it necessary to change school settings. This should be considered only when parents feel that the teacher or school administrator is unduly harsh, lacking in understanding, and unwilling to work with the parents and the child's physician. Undue and excessive peer "scapegoating" may indicate consideration of changing schools. This is particularly

apt to happen if "rumors" regarding child maltreatment, particularly sexual abuse, are circulating among the child's peer group. Group meetings with peers targeting furthering understanding are preferable to removing the child from the school, which should be done only when other interventions are ineffective.

c. **Psychotherapy.** Cognitive behavioral treatments are the psychotherapy of choice. Professionals who are trained and experienced in the use of such treatments should be the providers of this therapy. In most communities, psychologists are more apt to have received such training. The PCP should not undertake cognitive-behavioral treatment of PTSD.

d. **Medication**
    (1) Medications do not provide for definitive treatment of PTSD; however, they do provide for some symptom relief while awaiting definitive treatment.
    (2) Selective serotonin reuptake inhibitors (SSRI) are the drugs of choice. Particularly useful is citalopram or sertraline because of minimal inhibition of the P450 system. The US Food and Drug Administration (FDA) has recently approved sertraline for use in children and adolescents to treat other anxiety-related conditions (OCD). It is expected that paroxetine will receive approval soon for pediatric use. Citalopram has yet to be approved by the FDA, but its "off label" use may be indicated because of its low potential for drug-drug interactions through the P450 system.
    (3) Regarding dosing, start low (2.5 to 5 mg daily of citalopram or equivalent for younger children, and 5 to 10 mg daily for adolescents) and go slow. This minimizes side effects, particularly anxiety or agitation, which can be a problem in children and adolescents with anxiety symptoms.
    (4) Some children with severe anxiety benefit from the short-term use of benzodiazepines (e.g., lorazepam) while waiting for the antianxiety effects of the SSRI to take hold and

for definitive psychosocial treatment to start.

(5) Treatment effects with the SSRI generally take 2 to 3 weeks, and at times 6 weeks, to be noticeable.

e. **Laboratory and other evaluations.** None are necessary.

f. **Monitoring**

(1) Child should be monitored weekly during the treatment phase.

(2) Have parents work with children to maintain a log of re-experiencing symptoms, noting their frequency on a daily basis.

(3) Use one of the PTSD symptom scales at baseline and for follow-up to monitor treatment effect.

(4) Child should be reevaluated immediately if suicidal ideation or behaviors appear.

E. **Referring**

1. **When to refer and transfer primary responsibility**

a. Symptoms are moderate to severe

b. Symptoms are persistent (i.e., >4 weeks)

c. Functional impairment is at least moderate

d. Suicidal or homicidal risk

e. Current active child maltreatment or domestic violence

f. Existence of significant comorbid condition (e.g., AD/HD, mood disorder)

g. Bereavement complicated by traumatic imagery

2. **What to do when referring**

a. **Psychoeducation.** Continued application of the principles noted above.

b. **Advocacy.** As noted above, unless suicidal or homicidal risk requires inpatient hospitalization. In such cases, it is important for parents to discuss with the inpatient psychiatrist the anticipated length of hospitalization and whether educational services will be available in the hospital. If not available, then it is important to work with the child's principal and teacher to ensure that education is provided in the inpatient setting.

c. **Psychotherapy,** provided by a well-trained professional, is critical. Cognitive-behavioral treatment is the "gold standard." Successful treatment should remove the necessity of psychotropic medications.

d. **Medication.** The use of medication needs to be discussed with the treating psychotherapist. If re-experiencing symptoms or symptoms of autonomic hyperarousal are severe, medication can be used as noted in the preceding section. Benzodiazepines are rarely used at this point unless they are necessary for sleep during the time that SSRIs are just being introduced.

  e. **Laboratory and other evaluations.** None required.

  f. **Monitoring.** Follow-up appointments every 4 to 8 weeks are important to encourage treatment compliance and monitor progress.

IV. **Use of medications.** Sometimes, following severe trauma, the child or adolescent experiences such intrusive recollections of events, is bombarded by such terrifying nightmares, and experiences such high levels of autonomic hyperarousal that medication may be indicated. Although medications do not provide for definitive treatment of PTSD, they do provide for some symptom relief while awaiting definitive treatment.

To date, no randomized, placebo-controlled studies have been conducted on the use of psychotropic medications in the treatment of acute stress disorder and PTSD among children and adolescents.

Early studies with adults determined that **tricyclic antidepressants and monoamine oxidase inhibitors were effective in decreasing re-experiencing symptoms as well as symptoms of hyperarousal.** Additionally, these agents have been demonstrated in open clinical trials to be effective in children and adolescents with panic disorders. However, sudden death has been reported among children on tricyclics and side effects from both of these agents are not inconsiderable. Therefore, given the safety concerns and the side effect profiles of tricyclic antidepressants and monoamine oxidase inhibitors, **neither of these agents can be recommended for the treatment of pediatric PTSD at this time.**

The newer **SSRIs** (Appendix N) have been demonstrated to be **effective in adults with PTSD.** However, only one study has been published of an open clinical trial using citalopram in adolescents with PTSD. Only eight subjects were in the study, but all demonstrated symptom reduction in all three-symptom subcategories over the course of 12 weeks. Citalopram was well tolerated and adverse experiences were mild. These findings are consistent with the more carefully controlled studies that have been conducted regarding the impact of SSRI on mood and anxiety disorders in children and adolescents. The combination of increased safety, low side effect profile, and tentative efficacy data suggest that the SSRI are the medication of choice for treating PTSD. No data exist regarding the use of these agents for the treatment of acute stress disorder. Regarding dosing, start low (2.5 to 5 mg daily of citalopram or equivalent for younger children, and 5 to 10 mg daily for adolescents) and go slow. This minimizes side effects, particularly anxiety or agitation, which can be a problem in children and adolescents with anxiety symptoms. Another side effect to be aware of in this population is the development of cognitive alterations (dulling, slowing, or "spaciness") and amotivational syndrome, which can be confused with the numbing symptoms of PTSD. Treatment effects generally take 2 to 3 weeks and, at times, 6 weeks to be noticeable.

Some children with severe anxiety benefit from the **short-term use of benzodiazepines** (e.g., lorazepam) while waiting for the antianxiety effects of the SSRI to take hold and for psychosocial treatment to start.

Other psychopharmacologic agents (e.g., **beta-blockers, alpha-2 agonists, and anticonvulsants**) have been studied even less than the SSRI and **cannot be recommended at this time** for use in the pediatric population.

V. **Summary.** In the United States, many children are exposed to traumas of sufficient severity to result in the development of stress disorders, including adjustment disorder, acute stress disorder, and PTSD. Traumas range from severe catastrophic events (e.g., the bombing of the federal building in Oklahoma City) to the all-too-frequent traumas associated with child maltreatment. Systematic screening for trauma exposure is essential, followed by symptom and disorder assessment, to identify those children in need of specialized treatment services. Cognitive-behavioral treatment is the treatment of choice for stress disorders. Non-directive play or talking therapy is not efficacious. Medication, particularly the SSRIs, may be helpful; however, definitive randomized, placebo controlled studies have not yet been conducted.

SUGGESTED READINGS

American Academy of Child and Adolescent Psychiatry. Practice parameters for the assessment and treatment of children and adolescents with posttraumatic stress disorder. *J Am Acad Child Adolesc Psychiatry* 1998;37(suppl. 10):24S–26S.

Costello EJ, Angold A, March JS, et al. Life events and post-traumatic stress: the development of a new measure for children and adolescents. *Psychol Med* 1998;28:1275–1288.

Donnelly C, Amaya-Jackson L, March J. Psychopharmacology of pediatric post-traumatic stress disorder. *J Child Adolesc Psychopharmacol* 1999;9(3):203–220.

Eth S. PTSD in children and adolescents. *Review of psychiatry series, vol. 20.* Washington, DC: American Psychiatric Publishing, 2000: 1–173.

Nader KO, Newman E, Weathers FW, et al. *Clinician administered PTSD scale for children and adolescents for DSM-IV (CAPS-CA).* Lebanon, NH: The Hitchcock Foundation, 1998.

Perrin S, Smith P, Yule W. Practitioner review: the assessment and treatment of post-traumatic stress disorder in children and adolescents. *J Child Psychol Psychiatry* 2000;41(3):277–289.

Perry B, Azad I. Post-traumatic stress disorders in children and adolescents. *Curr Opin Pediatr* 1999;11(4):310–316.

Saigh PA, Yasik AE, Oberfield RA, et al. The children's PTSD inventory: development and reliability. *J Trauma Stress* 2000;13:369–380.

Web Sites

American Academy of Child and Adolescent Psychiatry has a series of brief, one-page information sheets for parents entitled "Facts For Families." Available at www.aacap.org/publications/factsfam/index. htm. Accessed on 6/29/02.

American Psychological Association web site has a section for parents and teens entitled "The Help Center," which includes detailed information about trauma, loss, and coping. Available at www.helping.apa.org. Accessed on 6/29/02.

Child Bereavement Trust is a United Kingdom charity founded to improve support offered by professionals to grieving families. Includes detailed information about loss and grieving for parents and adolescents, professionals, and schools. Available at www. childbereavement.org.uk. Accessed on 6/29/02.

Grief Net is a support and information site for adults facing grief. Has a section for children, Kids Aid (see below). Available at www. griefnet.org. Accessed on 6/29/02.

International Society for Traumatic Stress Studies is a multidisciplinary organization of researchers and clinicians whose focus is PTSD (both adult and pediatric). The web site has much useful information for professionals, along with an extensive set of links for parents and professionals. Available at www.istss.org. Accessed on 6/29/02.

Journey of Hearts: A Healing Place in Cyberspace is a support and education resource site developed by a physician for adults and children who have experienced a loss. Available at www.kirstimd.com. Accessed on 6/29/02.

Kids Aid is a support resource and education site for children. Supervised by a psychologist, it includes an extensive bibliography for parents and children of all ages facing loss. Available at www. kidsaid.com. Accessed on 6/29/02.

National Institute of Mental Health website has sophisticated information for families and professionals about trauma, PTSD, coping, and helping children. Available at www.nimh.nih.gov/publicat/ violence.cfm. Accessed on 6/29/02.

22 ♣ Substance Abuse

David L. Kaye and Gerald E. Daigler

I. **Background.** The use of alcohol and illicit substances is widespread among both adult and adolescent populations in the United States and other western countries. Epidemiologic studies of **adults** report that more than 25% of males and 10% of females 15 to 24 years of age meet criteria for a *Diagnostic and Statistical Manual of Mental Disorders* (DSM) alcohol or substance abuse or dependence disorder. Adolescence, in its best sense a time of experimentation, provides the backdrop for the initiation of drug and alcohol use. The Monitoring the Future (MTF) survey annually reports on the prevalence of drug and alcohol use by a nationally representative sample of nearly 50,000 students in the 8th, 10th, and 12th grades. Over the past 25 years these reports show that:

1. **Alcohol** has the most widespread use and heavy drinking remains the most frequent problem area, although this has moderated over the past 10 years (still, 33% of 12th graders report they have been drunk at least once in the past month).
2. **Cigarette smoking** has gradually decreased but daily smoking remains at high levels (i.e., 19% of 12th graders).
3. **Illicit drug use** of any kind peaked in the early 1980s, decreased over the next 10 to 15 years, but then began to increase in the mid 1990s (54% of 12th graders have used an illicit substance at least once in their lives).
4. **Marijuana** is the most widely abused illicit substance. Usage peaked in the 1970s, declined in the 1980s, but again has been rising since the 1990s (nearly half of 12th graders have smoked marijuana at least once in their lives).
5. Although the use of a number of drugs has decreased over these years (notably **cocaine and phencyclidine,** which both peaked in the 1980s), some have increased (e.g., **heroin, hallucinogens,** and ecstasy [MDMA]).
6. Increases in the use of **MDMA or "Ecstasy"** (11.7% of 12th graders have tried at least once) and **steroid abuse** (3.7% of 12th graders have misused steroids at least once) have been the most alarming recent trends.
7. **Ethnic and cultural** differences exist and, in general, use of all substances (including alcohol) is highest for whites, followed by Hispanics, and then blacks; Asian–Americans have the lowest rates. Native American youth have some of the highest rates of alcohol and cigarette use.
8. **Younger-aged children** (i.e., 8th graders) are substantially involved with alcohol and drugs.

Recent MTF figures are reported in Table 22.1. It should be noted that this study surveys youth who are presently in school and, therefore, probably represents an underestimate of older adolescent use.

A. **Misuse versus abuse and dependency.** With these statistics as a backdrop, it is difficult to delineate what patterns of use represent clinical disorder and which are part of normal adolescent behavior. A helpful schema is to think of the **stages of substance use,** according to Hogan:

1. **Curiosity.** Use of substance on a few occasions at most

2. **Experimentation.** Used on more than a few occasions for "fun" or in response to peer pressure

3. **Regular use.** Substances used every few weeks or more and begin to interfere with optimal functioning

4. **Abuse.** Extensive use with negative consequences present (see below)

5. **Dependency.** Life organized around substances or physically dependent (see below)

Although all substance use represents risky behavior (note the not infrequent tragedy of high school students killed in alcohol-related motor vehicle accidents or the college freshman who dies from acute alcohol poisoning), curiosity is a normal part of adolescence. Reserve a diagnosis for situations in which use is (a) **extensive, involves recurrent negative consequences at school, home, or in the community** (defined as substance **abuse** in DSM-IV); or (b) **is so consuming that the individual's life is organized around substances, or causes physical dependence** (substance **dependence** in DSM). The primary care physician (PCP) can be immensely helpful to adolescents and their families by listening, discussing, monitoring, and counseling about these matters. The PCP's active involvement has the potential for large-scale prevention of serious substance abuse.

B. **Substance use disorders**

1. Substance abuse and dependence occur frequently in the adolescent population. Most adolescents who have used alcohol or drugs do not meet criteria for a substance use disorder (SUD), and when followed do not develop disorders in adulthood. On the other hand, substance use of any kind is associated with a wide variety of **negative health outcomes:**

    a. The **three leading causes of death** in adolescents (motor vehicle accidents, homicide, and suicide) are all closely associated with substance use. Aside from death, substance use is often implicated in serious incidents that result in severe medical consequences (e.g., traumatic brain injury, major organ damage).

Table 22.1. Prevalence of alcohol and drug usage, 2001

	Grade 8: Ever Used	Grade 12: Ever Used	Grade 12: 30-Day Use	Grade 8: Daily Use	Grade 12: Daily Use
Alcohol (any)	51	80	50	1	3.6
Alcohol ("drunk")	23	64	33	0.2	1.4
Any illicit substance	27	54	26	—	—
Marijuana	20	49	22	1.3	6
Cigarettes	37	62	30	5.5	19
Cocaine	4	9	2	—	—
Amphetamines	10	16	6	—	—
Hallucinogens	4	13	3	—	—
Heroin	1.7	1.8	0.4	—	—
Ecstasy	5	12	3	—	—
Steroids	3	4	1.3	—	—

b. **Illnesses,** including the human immuno-deficiency virus (HIV), sexually transmitted diseases (STD), and hepatitis C are all intimately associated with substance use.

c. **Teen pregnancy** resulting from unprotected sex often occurs when the individuals are drunk or high.

d. **Involvement in criminal activity** occurs frequently while under the influence of alcohol or drugs. Conversely, a large percentage of college-aged victims of crime report having used alcohol or drugs before the crime occurred.

e. **School failure and dropping out** is a common consequence of substance misuse.

2. In addition to these negative outcomes, adolescents who use substances are at risk for developing an SUD. This, in turn, significantly raises the risks of the above consequences. Because of these repercussions the PCP should be alert to the need for primary and secondary prevention efforts.

The following are **red flags** for the development of an SUD that warrant particular attention from the PCP:

a. **Age of first use.** Some evidence indicates that adolescents who experiment before the age of 15 are at particularly high risk of developing a disorder. Cigarette use before 13 is also associated with increased risk.

b. History of **conduct disorder,** especially when combined with continuing symptoms of attention-deficit/hyperactivity disorder (AD/HD)

c. History of childhood **mood or anxiety disorder**

d. **Family history of substance abuse or dependence**

e. **Unsupportive or highly conflicted family relations**

f. History of **child sexual abuse**

g. Poor **school** achievement

h. Deviant **peer** affiliations

3. **Etiology.** SUD is thought to result from multiple factors, with contributions from the **culture** (availability, customs, and prohibitions), the **family** (modeling, abuse, conflict, poor supervision), **genetics** (neurobiologic deficits in executive functioning, self-regulation, and reward centers; dopaminergic, serotonergic, γ-aminobutyric acid, glutamate, and opioid systems), and **psychological factors** (alienation and defiance, sensation seeking, low religiosity).

4. **Comorbid conditions.** Most adolescents with SUD have **comorbid** psychiatric conditions. Frequently observed are **conduct disorders, mood disorders, and anxiety disorders.** The association of AD/HD with substance abuse is primarily mediated by its association with conduct disorder, and school-aged children with both disorders are at especially high risk. Adolescents whose AD/HD symptoms persist are also at risk. Despite media airplay, it is unlikely that the treatment of **AD/HD** (i.e., stimulants) presents any independent risk. In fact, evidence indicates that **treatment decreases the risk** of later SUD. Whereas the "self-medication" theory of SUD (i.e., that patients are using substances to treat themselves for an underlying psychiatric condition) has merit, for treatment purposes it is best to think of substance abuse as a condition unto itself, requiring specific intervention. In other words, do not treat the "underlying condition" and assume that the substance abuse will go away on its own.

5. **Physical withdrawal** (except in cases of intravenous heroin abuse) **is rare** in adolescents. In our experience consulting to a residential program, no cases have required medical detoxification or intervention over a 10-year period.

6. Substance abuse and dependency should be understood as a **chronic condition.** It should not be thought of in an acute illness model (i.e., with expectation of full recovery), but rather in one of **chronic illness** (i.e., with a lifelong vulnerability to relapse and a treatment focus on recovery, rehabilitation, and prevention of recurrences). In short the course of substance abuse, is often one of **remission and relapse.** Successful treatment focuses on the substance abuse or dependency itself before addressing other mental health issues (e.g., depression, abuse, anxiety). Previously, treatment approaches focused on these "underlying" conditions with the assumption that the substance abuse would clear up on its own. This was found to be an erroneous and misleading assumption! Substance abuse treatment must come first!

II. **Office evaluation.** The **key** to the recognition of substance misuse and abuse is the **physician's willingness to ask directly about these behaviors.** Ask specific questions of both the teen and parents to obtain information necessary for diagnosis and treatment planning. Because of the widespread use of alcohol and illicit substances, it is important to inquire with a matter-of-fact and nonjudgmental approach. Asking questions of the parent in the presence of the adolescent conveys the ability for honest and direct discussion of the topic. It also projects to the family that it is not a subject that should be talked about secretly. Following up with the adolescent alone assures the greatest likelihood of uncovering a problem. The PCP should realize that **denial** is a common feature of substance abuse and dependency. Although outright lying occurs in more severe situations, denial and minimization by the adolescent **and** the parents should be expected as par for the course. Being prepared for this can counter the inevitable feelings of frustration that PCPs experience when dealing with these problems. Be prepared to **be persistent** with pursuing this focus once a problem is suspected.

A. **Screening.** Although all adolescents should be screened for substance use and misuse, patterns that should **raise the level of suspicion** include:
   1. Recent or sudden **drop in academic achievement and motivation**
   2. Recent or sudden **decrease in school attendance**
   3. Recent **school disciplinary actions**
   4. **Adolescent onset antisocial behaviors**
   5. **Cigarette smoking before age 13**
   6. Associating with **peers** known to be involved with substance abuse
   7. Substance-related **legal or medical problem**

   Many tools can be used to screen adolescents, such as those available from the American Academy of Pediatrics. The **RAFFTS** (adapted from Liepman questionnaire), a brief and informative tool, is one good example:

   R: Do you drink or take drugs to Relax, feel better about yourself, or fit in?
   A: Do you ever drink or take drugs while you are Alone?
   F: Do any of your closest Friends drink or take drugs?
   F: Does a close Family member have problems with alcohol or drugs?
   T: Have you gotten into Trouble from drinking or taking drugs?
   S: Have you ever missed School to get high or because you were hung over?

   Another tool to open up discussion is to present the stages of substance use (see above) to the adolescent. This information can be made into a visual aid by placing these categories on a piece of paper, using graphics, if desired.

   While a routine office visit may not allow for extensive discussion, if time permits other questions that can be asked include:

For the parent(s)

1. Do you think that drugs or alcohol are part of the problem that (child's name) is having?
2. Have you ever been concerned or suspected that he or she was drinking or doing drugs?
3. Have you ever discovered drugs or drug paraphernalia (e.g., pipes, syringes, bongs) around the home?
4. Have you seen (child's name) come home and appear to be drunk or high?
5. Has (child's name) ever told you that he or she has been drunk or high?
6. Has (child's name) ever gotten into trouble while drunk or high? Fights? Encounters with the police? Auto accidents or tickets? Medical problems?
7. What has he or she used? Alcohol? Cigarettes? Pot? Coke? LSD? Other substances?
8. How often? Every day? Weekly? Once in a while?
9. What did (child's name) say about those things? What was his or her attitude about talking about it?
10. Has he or she ever used the car when seeming to be drunk or high? Have you ever discussed this issue? Has he or she been told clearly that any use of a vehicle when drinking is forbidden? Are you willing to pick him or her up if he or she calls to tell you he or she has been drinking?

For the adolescent

1. Have you ever considered that you have an alcohol or drug problem?
2. How often do you drink? What is your preferred drink? How much? More than a case of beer a night? More than a fifth of vodka (should be tailored to adolescent's preferred drink)? Note that asking questions matter-of-factly in this way increases the likelihood of accurate reporting.
3. What about drugs? What have you tried? Pot? Coke? Ecstasy? LSD? Heroin? How often? How have you taken it? Snorted? Smoked? Ever shot anything?
4. When did you first drink? Do drugs?
5. Do you drink or do drugs by yourself? With others?
6. What effect does alcohol or drugs have on you? Does it help in some way? Do you feel less anxious? Less depressed?
7. Have you ever missed school to get high or because you were hung over?
8. Have you ever gone to a Rave? How many times?
9. Have you ever had a medical problem because of alcohol or drugs? Blackouts? Passing out? Emergency room visits? Accidents? Injuries?
10. Have you ever felt suicidal when you were high?

11. Have you ever gotten into trouble with the police because of alcohol or drugs?
12. Have you ever driven while impaired or intoxicated? What would you do if you needed to drive and had been drinking? Do you arrange for a designated driver with your friends? Can you agree never to drive when you have been drinking or high?
13. Have you ever had a motor vehicle accident while you were drinking or high?
14. Have any friends ever told you they thought you had an alcohol or drug problem? Have you ever argued with peers about this?
15. Have you ever thought you should stop drinking or doing drugs?
16. Can you talk to your parents about this? Have you ever tried? What happened?
17. Have you done anything to try to stop? What? How did that go?
18. How do you feel about stopping now?

B. **Confidentiality** is essential when dealing with the teenaged patient. It provides an opportunity for the provider to convey to the parent as well as the patient that he or she is maturing, becoming more of an adult, and has the right to individual time with his or her own provider. Confidentiality is no guarantee that the teen will disclose, but it is unlikely that there will be disclosure without it. Studies have shown that the teens and parents expect that the PCP will spend time discussing potentially sensitive matters. Knowing that their conversation is private and confidential allows for greater likelihood of an open and honest discussion. On the other hand, teens need to understand that confidentiality may need to be broken, but only for reasons of danger or potential harm to self or others. This **should be explained to the teen before** going forward with an exploration of these issues. The patient who has experienced consequences of his or her drug use, drives while drinking, and so on needs intervention. This is when you need to get help from parents, counselors, and so forth. You may temporarily lose the teen's confidence but may well save his or her life.

C. **Drug testing.** Illicit substances can be detected in the urine, serum, and saliva. Most common is urine drug screening, which can detect most drugs for up to a few days (the primary exception being marijuana, which can be detected for up to 30 days after last usage, and alcohol, which is present for a few hours). Although this can be a useful tool in the ongoing management of a substance abuse problem, it has little place in verifying the existence of a problem or establishing a diagnosis. Parents may present to the PCP asking or even demanding that their child be "tested."

Acceding to these demands is almost always counter-productive. Sometimes the tests are negative, further reinforcing the adolescent's denial and avoidance, and frustrating the helpless parents. Forced drug tests also encourage the adolescent to avoid getting caught by attempting to manipulate the test. This, in turn, furthers the alienation between parent and child, and undermines the doctor–patient relationship. Even when positive, the teen can continue to deny the problem by insisting that he or she was clean and that the drug test was defective or erroneous. Again, this does not help the adolescent face the reality of the problem. Under some circumstances, urine drug testing can serve a useful purpose. This can occur when the topic is discussed with the adolescent, who is **willing** to undergo this testing as a way of repairing a frayed relationship with the parents or as a positive deterrent to continued use. Under these circumstances, urine drug testing can be used collaboratively to help the youth, as opposed to something punitive being done "to" the child.

III. **Triage assessment and treatment planning.** First and foremost, the job of the PCP is to **be on the lookout for these problems and to elicit the relevant data** to establish and track the existence of substance misuse and abuse. **Starting discussions** about use and abuse with pediatric patients when they are **young** is important and increases the likelihood that they will graduate high school without beginning to abuse substances. Those who engage in such discussions are statistically less likely to develop future problems. Remain vigilant to the many ways that these problems can become manifest. Maintain a high level of suspicion that substance abuse is present in any adolescent who shows a significant change in functioning at school, with peers, at home, or in the community. The PCP is best positioned to provide preventive efforts, whereas most situations requiring direct intervention will **require referral to adolescent substance abuse specialists.** Of note, these specialists are typically found in specialized treatment agencies for adolescent substance abuse or "chemical dependency." They usually have their own training requirements and licensing procedures that are outside the scope of most generic mental health clinics and practitioners. Lastly, as noted, it is important to appreciate that substance abuse and dependency require treatment and intervention directed at the substance abuse itself, before addressing other "underlying" issues (e.g., depression, abuse, anxiety).

Many primary care providers do not feel comfortable following patients with suspected substance abuse problems. However, **no patient should leave the office without a verbal promise to refrain from driving or being a passenger in a vehicle** driven by anyone under the influence of alcohol, marijuana, or other drugs.

A. **Watching**
1. **When to watch**
   a. Positive family history of substance abuse
   b. Long-standing school problems
   c. Childhood history of AD/HD, especially if comorbid with conduct disorder
   d. Childhood history of mood or anxiety disorder
   e. History of high family conflict
   f. History of child sexual abuse
2. **When watching**
   a. **Psychoeducation**
      (1) **Begin educating the parents early.** Children and families at risk for one of the above reasons need to be aware of the elevated risk of substance abuse and to be vigilant about signs of developing problems. This process should begin by the end of elementary school, or earlier depending on the relationship with the family. Although parents and children need not be frightened by discussion of this topic, they need to be informed.
      (2) **Avoid shaming or excessive fear.** The best approach is a straightforward, informative, and matter of fact one. Inducing fear or shame generally is ineffective and runs the risk of turning off the child and parents, limiting future ability to be helpful.
      (3) **Three areas of parenting require special attention**
         (a) **Parents' involvement in their children's lives is crucial.** Spending time with their children and adolescents, attending their activities (e.g., school, sports, arts, religious), reviewing homework, and so on are major deterrents to drug and alcohol involvement.
         (b) **Keep open lines of communication.** Children who can talk to their parents, especially about difficult or socially unacceptable matters, have a "lifeline" that is a strong buffer to the currents of peer pressure.
         (c) **The "Four Ws" (see Chapter 3).** Parents should know where their child is, who the child is with, when the child will be there and be home, and

what the child will be doing. Children who are monitored feel cared about and are less likely to engage in destructive patterns of substance use or abuse.

(4) **Focus on the child's elevated risk status.** These "higher risk" children and families need to understand that they are taking a big chance, bigger than their friends, when they get involved with alcohol or drugs. Substance abuse, once initiated, can take on a "life of its own" that can overtake the life of an adolescent, despite the best intentions. In most circumstances, this means that adolescents should **abstain completely** from alcohol while a teenager.

(5) **Coach the parents in monitoring the adolescent for signs of substance misuse and abuse.** In **elementary school** parents can be forewarned that their child is coming into the age of risk for substance abuse. Adolescents who begin smoking cigarettes early or whose closest friends are involved with drugs or alcohol need especially close monitoring. From the **beginning of middle school,** parents need to be on the lookout for relevant signs. For example, they should carefully watch for erratic behavior, lying about whereabouts, physical signs (e.g., alcohol on breath, ataxia, bloodshot eyes), missing alcohol, and presence of drugs or paraphernalia.

(6) **Begin discussions and education with the high risk child or adolescent early.** Although it is important to discuss these issues with the parents, it is equally important to address them with the child or adolescent. By the time the child is in middle school time should be set aside for the child to be seen alone. Use a tool such as the continuum of substance use noted above, to engage in this discussion with a high school-aged youth. It is prudent to avoid a shaming or fear-inducing approach when having this conversation, and

to recognize that multiple discussions will probably be necessary.

(7) **Review the dangers of substance use and misuse** with parents and child or adolescent. This is best done in a matter-of-fact way to highlight the potential for medical and mental health complications, school problems, legal problems, and fatalities (see above). The **dangers of driving** or being in a vehicle when the driver is impaired should be especially emphasized. Discuss rehearsals of what can be done in these situations. If parents seem unable or unwilling to provide support for their adolescent under these circumstances (e.g., telling the child "don't call me if you're drunk and can't get home"), the PCP should strongly consider referral of the patient, family, or both for mental health treatment.

b. **Advocacy** is necessary to address any already identified existing problems (e.g., learning disabilities, AD/HD) (see the relevant chapters for guidance on addressing those problems). Schools generally provide drug awareness or **prevention programs.** The PCP should be aware that some programs (most notably D.A.R.E.) do not have empiric support for effectiveness. Programs that have demonstrated effectiveness (e.g., Life Skills Training, Project STAR, Project ALERT) do not rely primarily on fear, but instead combine education about drug effects and substance abuse with interactive skills training (e.g., resistance and social skills training).

c. **Psychotherapy** is necessary for any already identified mental health problems. Specific substance abuse treatment is not indicated at this point, as the primary thrust of intervention is **prevention.**

d. **Medications** may be indicated for treatment sensitive conditions already identified (e.g., AD/HD, mood or anxiety disorder). They are not indicated to prevent the development of a substance abuse problem.

e. **Laboratory and other evaluations** are not indicated unless specific signs or symptoms of another medical disorder exist. Urine drug screening should not be used as a deterrent to the development of substance abuse. No empirical support is found for this approach and it may well promote an atmosphere of mistrust that further erodes the parent–child relationship, as well as the doctor–patient relationship.

    f. Monitoring of the child or adolescent at risk should occur no less than every 6 months—more frequently if signs of incipient substance misuse appear.

B. Intervening further

  1. When to intervene further

    a. Cigarette smoking before 13 years of age

    b. Active parental substance abuse

    c. Critical incident (i.e., legal, medical, peers, or school) involving drugs or alcohol

    d. Pattern of drinking beyond experimentation

    e. Drug usage beyond curiosity

  2. When intervening further

    a. Psychoeducation

      (1) Reinforce need for parents to:

        (a) Spend time with children

        (b) Maintain open lines of communication

        (c) Know the 4 "Ws"

      (2) Reemphasize the dangers of substance use and abuse, especially driving while using.

      (3) Thoroughly discuss the extent of substance use with the adolescent. It is **optimal** if this is done in the **presence of the parents** so that everyone has the same understanding. If the adolescent refuses or feels unsafe doing so, the PCP will need to urge future discussion and make a follow-up appointment within a month. The PCP may ask under what conditions **in the future** the adolescent would feel the issue could be discussed with the parents (e.g., "if I get drunk one more time"). This future-oriented questioning can increase the likelihood of follow through. Although each PCP will have a different threshold for when they feel that they **must** discuss the concern with the parents, the essential question is whether the youth's safety is at risk. If the PCP feels that significant risk exists, then the adolescent should be informed that the matter will be discussed with the parents because of concern for the adolescent and because it would be **unprofessional** not to do so.

(4) **Review signs of substance use and abuse and strategies for monitoring** (i.e., who will monitor, how, when) with the parents and adolescent. A corollary of this is to discuss with the parents under what conditions the PCP would send the adolescent for a **substance abuse evaluation** (e.g., additional un-explained school absences, continued poor grades, one more instance of parental concern).

(5) **Be alert for enabling behaviors by parents.** Substance abuse and dependency "grow" when important adults minimize, ignore, or actively promote drinking or drug use. Common "enabling" behaviors include parents serving or buying youth alcohol, writing school excuses for alcohol- or drug-related impairment, or performing school or other obligations (e.g., homework, delivering newspapers) for the youth. Once such enabling behaviors are identified, the PCP is in a position to challenge the parents to recognize the consequences of their own behavior.

(6) **Review history systematically for signs of impaired functioning in home, school, community, with peers.** A more benign appearing incident may turn out to be more concerning when all areas of potential impairment are reviewed. This may prompt referral for an assessment by a qualified adolescent substance abuse professional or agency.

(7) **"Gateway" theory** may be helpful to present to the parents and youth. According to this theory, youth begin with cigarettes, move on to alcohol, then marijuana, and finally to other "harder" drugs. Whereas this progression is not invariant or inevitable, interrupting the pattern **early** does prevent more serious problems. Parents should not be frightened by this (e.g., "one puff of cigarettes and he'll be on his way to heroin"), but rather be informed so they will be motivated to address the situation early.

(8) **Remain focused on the substance use or misuse.** Parents or youth may feel that their "real" problem is depression, stress, anxiety, and so on. They may further reason, therefore, that they (or professionals) should focus their attention on this problem and assume that the substance use will

abate on its own. Experience has shown that this is generally **not true!** Although these "underlying" problems may need attention, they should not be addressed *in lieu* of or before the substance use is. The substance use requires its own special attention.

b. **Advocacy**

(1) **Schools should be alerted to the concern,** which the **parents** (i.e, not the PCP) should do. The PCP cannot divulge any information to the schools without the parents' written permission. If the parents would like the PCP to be involved it is still preferable to encourage the parents to take the lead and, if necessary, the PCP can take a supporting role.

(2) **Be alert to signs of enabling by the schools.** This is most common when a student of "special" status (e.g., the star athlete) is exempted from the usual negative consequences for alcohol- or drug-related behaviors. This special treatment is no service to the school or the star athlete. The PCP support may be crucial for the school's ability to hold up uniform standards of accountability.

(3) **A monitoring plan should be worked out between the school and parents.** For example, schools need to inform the parents of unexplained absences or other signs of substance abuse. It is best when the adolescent participates in these discussions and understands that the school and parents will be working together on this.

(4) **Consideration of person in need of supervision (PINS) petition** (see Chapter 9). The PCP should alert the parents to the legal means available to enforce supervision of their child or adolescent. Laws differ from state to state and the program may bear a different name (e.g., "child in need of supervision" [CHINS]). These programs are usually accessed through the Family Court by parent written request and allow for court monitoring of the youth. Treatment and other services can be mandated

for the youth with failure to do so resulting in institutional placement.

c. **Psychotherapy**

(1) As noted, **if substance abuse is suspected,** the adolescent should be referred directly for a **specialist adolescent substance abuse evaluation.** If indicated, the patient will then be referred for **outpatient treatment.** This initial treatment consists of weekly **group and individual sessions** focused on the substance use or misuse. **Family therapy** is also a critical element of this treatment. The goal of this treatment is to prevent the progression of this pattern into frank abuse and dependence.

(2) **If it is unclear** whether the substance abuse is a significant problem but the PCP has concerns, then a referral to a **child mental health professional** may be an initial step. This professional should be able to further screen for substance abuse and can be expected to make a referral to a specialist substance abuse professional if appropriate.

d. **Medications** are not used to prevent the progression of substance abuse in adolescents. They can be helpful for comorbid conditions. The PCP needs to monitor personal comfort in this situation. Many will feel uncomfortable with any substance use in the history and will refer these cases to a child and adolescent psychiatrist or pediatrician with specialized expertise.

e. **Laboratory and other evaluations**

(1) **Voluntary urine drug screening** may be considered in selected cases (see above). It must be done in the spirit of being in the service of the adolescent's health, and not as a powerful way to "police" the child.

(2) **A complete physical examination and screening laboratory tests** may be helpful at this stage to look for evidence of medical complications and also to convey the seriousness of the concern of the PCP.

f. **Monitoring** needs to occur in 1 to 3 months, depending on the level of concern. Continued monitoring at this interval may be necessary for an extended period to effectively prevent the progression to frank substance abuse or dependency.

C.   **Referring**
1.   **When to refer and transfer primary responsibility**
  a.   Regular alcohol use in context of other psychiatric condition (e.g., AD/HD)
  b.   More than one substance-related critical incident
  c.   Any behavior that endangers self or others that is associated with substance use or misuse
  d.   Alcohol abuse or dependency
  e.   Regular substance use
  f.   Substance abuse or dependency
2.   **When referring**
  a.   **Psychoeducation**
    (1)   Reinforce above principles of parenting
    (2)   Recognize and challenge enabling behaviors
    (3)   Review parents' plan for monitoring substance use
    (4)   Reinforce medical and other complications of substance abuse to maintain parents' and adolescent's motivation
    (5)   Remain focused on the substance abuse as **the** problem
    (6)   Explain the "chronic illness" model of substance abuse. Parents and youth need support and education to adjust their expectations and prepare themselves for the "long haul." Parents and teens who are not prepared for the ups and downs of recovery are at higher risk for relapses. Identifying "triggers" that will leave them vulnerable to relapse are integral to this "inoculation" approach.
  b.   **Advocacy**
    (1)   **Schools should be fully aware of the problem at this point.** Parents should be supported in their contacts with the schools. The schools often can provide additional support services to monitor and help prevent relapse.
    (2)   **Make sure the adolescent is receiving appropriate educational support services and programming.** Substance abusing adolescents' educational and vocational needs can get lost in the furor over the

substance abuse. The PCP can be helpful by assuring that these issues have been considered and addressed.

(3) **PINS or similar supervision should be in place.** If not, the PCP can alert the parents to this possibility. In many states the laws allow for supervision of children only to the age of 16. This creates tremendous problems for many families and is currently the target of advocacy groups in many states attempting to raise the age limit to 18.

c. **Psychotherapy**

(1) **Adolescents at this stage should be in intensive outpatient specialist substance abuse treatment.** Following a complete evaluation, the treatment initially consists of **group therapy** targeting the substance abuse. These are typically **multiple times per week** at first, and gradually decreasing to lesser frequency over a period of months. Weekly, concurrent **family therapy** is a central element of effective treatment. Again, over time this can be decreased in frequency as sobriety accrues. **Individual therapy** is also a necessary part of the treatment. Referral to **self-help support groups** (e.g., Alcoholics Anonymous or AA, Narcotics Anonymous, Al-Anon, among others) is also typically part of treatment and has been helpful for many individuals. Separate groups are available for the teen and family members. Although these are often helpful, successful treatment does not **require** involvement with these groups. These groups are often based on the **12-step** approach of AA, which provides a structured roadmap for recovery. Other less widely known support groups generally take a similar approach.

(2) **Adolescents who refuse or do not respond to outpatient treatment require more intensive treatments.** Oftentimes, legal intervention is required to hold these patients in treatment. In most communities, a continuum of more intensive treatment can be found.

Although other services may be available in a given community, this continuum generally includes, from most to least restrictive:

(a) **Inpatient detoxification units** usually provide brief (i.e., a few days) medical detoxification in a general hospital or medical center. No substance abuse treatment is offered beyond this and this treatment is necessary with adolescents only under unusual circumstances (e.g., intravenous heroin dependency).

(b) **Short-term rehabilitation units** are locked or unlocked facilities that may be free standing units in the community, or may be contained within a general hospital or a psychiatric hospital setting. Typically, 2 to 6 weeks in length, they provide initial stabilization in an intensive setting, from which a patient progresses into an intensive outpatient program or a community residence (see below). If this "rehab" program is insufficient, the patient will require a long-term residential program (see below). Group, individual, and family treatments are provided. Psychiatric consultation is generally available.

(c) **Long-term residential programs** are available in many communities. They are usually unlocked facilities that provide treatment for 3 to 12 months. They are often "voluntary" facilities, although many youth are sent there as an alternative to jail. Youth live full time in these programs and are often schooled on grounds. A full complement of group, individual, and family treatment is provided to target the substance abuse. Psychiatric consultation and treatment should also be available. These programs are utilized when less intensive or briefer programs have failed.

    (d) Community residences ("halfway houses") are for patients who have graduated from a residential program but who are unable to return home or live in a less structured setting. These are homes or small institutional settings in the community in which youth generally are expected to attend school or work off grounds, and return at night for ongoing treatment, meals, and sleep. Substance abuse treatment may be provided on grounds, although patients may need to receive this treatment, as well as psychiatric consultation and treatment, at an outpatient clinic in the community.

  d. Medications are commonly used in the adolescent substance abusing population for the frequent comorbid conditions present (see next section).

  e. Laboratory and other evaluations. Youth in active substance abuse treatment require standard pediatric care. In addition, they are at high risk for HIV and other STD and may require testing for such.

  f. Follow-up for patients in intensive outpatient treatment should be every 1 to 3 months to maintain patient **and** family motivation to complete treatment. Patients in more intensive programs typically have pediatric care available to them on grounds. The PCP should see these patients no less than every 4 months once they are able to attend outpatient appointments. This allows the PCP to maintain contact and show interest in the child's progress.

IV. Practical use of medications. Medications **are not a primary treatment for substance abuse** and dependency. Although research proceeds at a fast pace, currently no medications are used in the adolescent population for the targeted treatment of the substance-related problem. On the other hand, **medications are used to treat the conditions commonly comorbid** with substance abuse or dependence and may be critical to the maintenance of sobriety. As noted, the most common treatable problems are mood disorders, anxiety disorders, and AD/HD. Medication treatment of these conditions follows that outlined in the respective chapters on those topics. A particular concern is whether and how to initiate medication treatment with a youth who continues to drink or take drugs. If the PCP has established a substance abuse or dependency diagnosis, then **no medication** should be prescribed until substance abuse treatment has been initiated and the **youth has been clean for at least 1 month (more conservative practitioners would wait for 3 months).** At that point, consider treating a comorbid or preexisting mood or anxiety disorder. This washout period is required to assure that the psychiatric symptoms were not merely caused by the effects of the substances or withdrawal from such. When the youth does not appear to have a diagnosable substance abuse disorder, the treatment approach can be more complex. In most situations, ongoing usage that would be considered curiosity or experimentation would not preclude the treatment of a psychiatric condition. Education and ongoing discussion with the youth **and** family would be needed to address the potential dangers of (a) continued usage and (b) interactions with the medication, and to urge the adolescent to refrain from usage. These situations require close monitoring and continuing substance use most likely requires referral to a child and adolescent psychiatrist.

V.   **Summary.** Adolescent substance misuse and abuse is widespread in the United States and other western countries. It causes tremendous morbidity and mortality, and is implicated in large numbers of fatal motor vehicle accidents. The PCP has access to children and adolescents before these issues come to the fore and become problems. As such, they are able to provide both prevention and intervention for these problems. The most important step for the PCP is to consider this as a standard part of pediatric practice, and to ask questions that elicit the relevant data and promote discussion of the issues before a child reaches adolescence and the age of risk.

SUGGESTED READINGS

American Academy of Child and Adolescent Psychiatry. Practice parameters for the assessment and treatment of children and adolescents with substance abuse disorders. *J Am Acad Child Adolesc Psychiatry* 1997;36(suppl. 10):140S–156S.

American Academy of Pediatrics Committee on Substance Abuse. *Substance abuse:* Elk Grove, IL: American Academy of Pediatrics, 2002.

Colby S, Chung T. Adolescents and alcohol: preventive opportunities for health care providers. *Medicine and Health, Rhode Island.* 1997;80(7):223–226.

Dube C. The physician's role in preventing alcohol and drug abuse. *Medicine and Health, Rhode Island,* 1999;82(3):95–98.

Fuller P, Cavanaugh R. Basic assessment and screening for substance abuse in the pediatrician's office. *Pediatr Clin North Am* 1995;42:295–307.

Gilvarry E. Substance abuse in young people. *J Child Psychol Psychiatry* 2000;41(1):55–80.

Heyman R, Adger H. Office approach to drug abuse prevention. *Pediatr Clin North Am* 1997;44(6):1447–1455.

Hogan M. Diagnosis and treatment of teen drug use. *Med Clin North Am* 2000;84(4):927–966.

Hyman S, Malenka R. Addiction and the brain: the neurobiology of compulsion and its persistence. *Nature Reviews Neuroscience* 2001;2(10):695–703.

Koob G. The neurobiology of addiction: toward the development of new therapies. *Ann NY Acad Sci* 2000;909:170–185.

Liepman M, Keller D, Botelho R. Understanding and preventing substance abuse by adolescents. *Prim Care* 1998;25:137–162.

Pediatric Clinics of North America, April 2002 issue devoted to adolescent substance abuse.

Weinberg N, Rahdert E, Colliver J, et al. Adolescent substance abuse: a review of the past 10 years. *J Am Acad Child Adolesc Psychiatry* 1998;37(3):252–261.

Werner M, Joffe A, Graham A. Screening, early identification, and office-based intervention with children living in substance abusing families. *Pediatrics* 1999;103(suppl. 5):1099–1112.

Woolf A, Shannon M. Clinical toxicology for the pediatrician. *Pediatr Clin North Am* 1995;42(2):317–333.

Web Sites

American Academy of Child and Adolescent Psychiatry web site has a number of one-page handouts on substance abuse for parents in their Facts for Families series. Available at www.aacap.org. Accessed on 6/29/02.

American Academy of Pediatrics web site has information for parents on substance abuse in the section "You and Your Family;" search in Child Care Books for Caring for Your School Aged Child and Caring for Your Adolescent. Also have useful public education brochures for parents and adolescents about specific substances of abuse. Available at www.aap.org/family. Accessed on 6/29/02.

Monitoring the Future is a large annual survey, commissioned by the federal government, to monitor a wide variety of youth trends. Included in the study is much information about current trends in drug and alcohol use by youth. Available at www.monitoringthefuture.org. Accessed on 6/29/02.

National Clearinghouse for Alcohol and Drug Information sponsors a huge web site filled with information primarily for families, children, and youth regarding alcohol and drugs. Available at www.health.org. Accessed on 6/29/02.

National Institutes for Alcohol Abuse and Alcoholism (NIAAA), a branch of the National Institutes of Health, has an extensive web site with much information primarily about research and public policy for professionals, but also some educational information for parents. Available at www.niaaa.nih.gov. Accessed on 6/29/02.

National Institute for Drug Addiction (NIDA), a branch of the National Institutes of Health, has a website with extensive information on both research and public policy for professionals, as well as educational information for parents and youth. Available at www.nida.nih.gov. Accessed on 6/29/02.

23 ♣ Suicidal Behaviors in Children and Adolescents

Helen R. Aronoff and Stephanie H. Fretz

I. **Background.** The primary care physician (PCP) is on the front lines and is often the first physician to see and evaluate children and adolescents at high risk to commit suicide. This provides a critical perch for prevention of a major public health concern. Over the past 50 years, rates of suicide in teens in the United States (and many other western countries) have increased 300%, stabilizing in the past 10 years. Many factors have been hypothesized to account for these findings, including widespread exposure to violence (on the streets and in the media), and the decrease in stability of the family and other social institutions. At a biological level, it has also been noted that below-average levels of serotonin have been associated with aggressive behaviors, including self-injury.

A. Some basic facts about suicide in children and adolescents are:
1. Of adolescents, 25% report serious consideration of suicide.
2. Of adolescents, 5% to 10% attempt suicide at some point; 10% to 15% make a second attempt; and 10% eventually complete suicide.
3. In the United States, suicide is the third leading cause of death in adolescents 15 to 19 years of age, and the fourth leading cause for those 10 to 14 years of age.
4. Suicide causes more deaths in teens than heart disease, human immunodeficiency virus (HIV), cancer, chronic lung disease, and congenital defects **combined.**
5. Girls attempt suicide much more frequently than boys. Boys, however, have a higher incidence of completed suicide.
6. Firearms (especially handguns) by far are the leading cause of deaths from suicide in both adolescent boys and girls; ingestion of pills is the second leading cause of death and the primary method of suicide **attempts** in adolescents.
7. Preadolescent children **can** be suicidal. They will present with dangerous behaviors (e.g., running or riding bikes into traffic, fire-setting, head-banging, and other self-injurious behaviors). These children may also make suicidal statements. The lethality of these children's attempts is usually low, so they are less likely to succeed in killing themselves. This does not mean that they should not be taken seriously or that they cannot get hurt. These children often continue to verbalize and act out on their suicidal ideation

into adolescence, when they are more likely to actually cause serious harm. Therefore, their behaviors must be addressed.

8. White males account for the vast majority of completed suicide in adolescents; Native American males, followed closely by white males, have the highest **rates** of completed suicide; African-American females, the lowest.

9. About 50% of suicide attempts come to clinical attention. The rest go untreated by any physician; less than 50% keep their first mental health appointment following a suicide attempt.

10. Fifty percent of those who completed suicide were seen by a pediatrician in the month preceding the event; few were actively in mental health treatment when suicide occurred.

B. Suicide is not an act that any child would choose to do. Suicidal states come about over a period of time (months to years) and result from a convergence of many factors. The final common pathway is that the child feels miserable, desperate, and hopeless about feeling better in the future. Suicide appears to be the only way out of this painful misery. Most youths feel ashamed of their suicidal feelings or acts, so care should be taken to communicate a nonjudgmental attitude. If youths perceive that they are being judged negatively, criticized, or blamed for suicidal thoughts or actions they will refrain from communicating in the future and will also feel more misunderstood and hopeless. This increases the risk of further suicidal ideation and behavior.

C. **Evaluating the risk.** No diagnostic tests or algorithms exist for the assessment of the child at risk of suicide. However, suicidal behavior does not "just happen" as a "mistake." Understanding the following three areas aids in (a) evaluating the dangerousness of a child and (b) making solid treatment recommendations:

1. Risk factors
2. Lethality
3. Treatment history and response

1. Virtually all children who attempt and complete suicide have one or more of the following **risk factors.** Especially important are the presence of the first two, which are present in most:

a. **Psychiatric illness,** especially mood disorders (e.g., depression, bipolar disorder) and psychosis (much less common, but can be highly dangerous when present)

b. Drug and alcohol misuse or abuse

c. Previous suicide attempt

d. Conduct disorder, or patterns of antisocial and aggressive behavior

e. General pattern of impulsive behaviors

   f. **History of abuse:** sexual, physical, and emotional
   g. Family history of suicide
   h. Hopelessness
   i. **Gay or lesbian orientation,** especially when lacking family support
   j. History of HIV positive
  2. Assessing **lethality,** or the intent to do harm to oneself, requires balancing an assessment of each of the following:
   a. **Expressed intent to die** (before and after an attempt)—what the child says about the intent
   b. **Inferred intent to die**
    (1) Plan and effort to conceal (the more, the higher the lethality)
    (2) Lethality of attempt without intervention
    (3) Actions taken after attempt to obtain help (the less, the higher the lethality)
    (4) Emotional reaction after attempt (the less affect, the higher the lethality)
    (5) Suicide notes written as if the child were dead, but delivering message to the survivors (e.g., "I want Susie to have my CDs," "just know that I loved you")
   c. **Reasons to live** (presence of the following argues somewhat against lethal intent)
    (1) Realistic life goal or future plans (may be short- or long-range)
    (2) Religious belief
    (3) Feeling valued in important relationships (e.g., family, girlfriend, boyfriend, best friend)
    (4) Fear of pain or retribution
  3. In assessing **treatment history and response,** the goal is to find out whether any treatment has occurred: what kind, how much, what was the response, and what is the child and family's current motivation. Children who are suicidal and have had adequate outpatient treatment or who have limited motivation need an increased level of intensity of treatment (i.e., day treatment, crisis program, hospitalization).
 D. Suicidal crises can best be thought of as **"episodes" of suicidality** (i.e., they have a beginning, a middle, and an end). Suicidal episodes occur in vulnerable, at risk, youth when they experience stressful events. Some of the common **precipitants** to a "beginning" of a suicidal crisis are:
  1. Death or loss (e.g., separation of parents)
  2. School disciplinary action

3. Police or legal action
4. Breakup of romantic relationship
5. Humiliating event

E. Be highly vigilant when these events occur in youth at risk. Other **warning signs** include:

1. Sudden change in mood (i.e., the child who has been depressed, suddenly and inexplicably, becomes happy)
2. Giving away possessions
3. Depressed youth who become persistently agitated or symptoms intensify
4. Escalating acting out behaviors
5. Preoccupation with death themes in conversation, artwork, writing assignments
6. Casual, "joking" comments about "not being around," or wanting to be dead or gone

II. Practical office evaluation

A. The first task is to become aware that a child is experiencing distress sufficient to cause suicidal ideation. This requires direct discussion with the child or adolescent; parents **may not be** reliable informants about the presence of suicidal thoughts and feelings. Questionnaires are good ways to open the door for further discussion and exploration. However, general screening questionnaires for the **parents** to fill out (i.e., Child Behavior Checklist, or CBCL) are generally not helpful. Instead, a questionnaire for the youth to fill out that includes questions about depression and suicide (e.g., the *Children's Depression Inventory,* or a questionnaire developed by the PCP to tap into these issues) is recommended. If children answer affirmatively on a questionnaire that they are depressed or suicidal, these areas can then be followed up. Even when a child denies suicidal ideation but acknowledges the presence of one or more risk factors, follow up with face-to-face questions about suicidal thoughts, ideas, and acts. If the youth has experienced suicidal thoughts the PCP needs to find out:

1. **Specific acts considered,** including the lethality, and amount of thought or detail
   a. Have you ever thought of hurting yourself?
   b. When you were having that thought, did you think about **how it would happen?**
   c. Are you **still** thinking about hurting yourself?
   d. Do you have a **plan** and, if so, can you tell me the plan?
   e. What would you **do** if you became suicidal or were thinking about hurting yourself? Would you let someone know **before** you did anything? Talk to someone? Call?
   f. Do you want to be dead?
2. **Frequency.** How frequently have you felt like this? Every day? Once in a while? One time?

3. **Persistence.** How long do these thoughts stay with you? For a few minutes? Few hours? All day?
4. **Intensity.** How hard is it to resist the impulse to do something harmful to yourself?

B. For the child who has acknowledged a suicidal episode, it is helpful to ask specific questions about its time course and unfolding (i.e., go through the events of the day in a systematic manner). For example, in the case of a youth who overdosed (or thought about overdosing):

1. What and when did you actually take (or think about taking) pills?
2. What happened that day that led up to this? How did you feel that morning when you woke up? The night before? Did you know you were going to overdose that day when you woke up? If not, when did you decide you were going to do it? Did something happen during the day that prompted you?
3. When you felt like hurting yourself, did you do anything to try to feel better (e.g., call a friend, relative, parent, teacher) or resist the impulse?
4. How did you decide to take the pills at that particular time?
5. How long had you thought about doing this?
6. Did you think anyone would be there or find you?
7. How did you feel after you took them? Did you do anything to tell others what happened or get help?
8. When did you stop feeling suicidal? Did something happen that made you feel better?

C. The child's **developmental level and cognitive understanding** need to be considered in assessing intent of the child's lethality. The younger child or the child who is developmentally delayed or cognitively impaired may not have a sense of the **finality** of death. Normal children under the developmental age of 7 years generally **do not** understand that death is permanent. These children can attempt self-harm out of anger at a change in routine, for example, neither anticipating nor understanding the resulting injury. It is not uncommon to hear a boy say, "I didn't want to die. I was mad at mom for taking away my Nintendo," as the reason to threaten to hurt himself with the big kitchen knife. Adolescents also may not be able to realistically appraise the danger involved in their actions. For example, they can believe that an acetaminophen overdose would not be dangerous or, conversely, that an overdose of five aspirin was enough to die. To fully understand the child's lethality, these issues need to be taken into account. Questions to ask include:

1. What do or did you think would happen if you did that?

2. Where did you hear about that? Friends? Television? Movies?
3. What happens when you die? Can you come back and see your family?
4. How did you decide to take this particular medications?
5. How did you decide to take the amount you did?
6. Why didn't you take more? Was there more in the bottle?

D. In assessing self-injurious symptoms, consider the behaviors termed **parasuicidal,** most notably, cutting. The physician who treats adolescents will see youngsters who "cut" themselves. They will use various sharp objects, usually razors, knives, glass fragments, or other sharp objects, to cut their arms, legs, and occasionally their abdomens. These adolescents often deny that their self-mutilating is intended to kill themselves, although they may also have other, clearly suicidal thoughts. These behaviors generally are meant to **relieve emotional pain** that they are unable to express in a healthier manner. Patients will describe feelings of anger or pain, during which they will cut, followed by immediate release and "feeling better." Most often, these adolescents are clinically depressed. Often, they are in a peer group in which several members are also cutting. The marks, for the most part, are superficial and will occasionally spell out a word or a name. Nevertheless, some of the marks can be deep enough to form scars and may signify suicidal intent. Some questions to ask to help determine the motivation for this behavior are:

1. Did you want to kill yourself when you cut?
2. Why do you cut?
3. When do you cut?
4. Show me **all** your cuts. Are you cutting anywhere else that I cannot see?
5. Did you do this to kill yourself or because it relieves your hurt feelings?
6. Do you know other kids who cut?
7. What can we do to help you stop this behavior and still deal with your angry and sad feelings?

III. Triage assessment and treatment planning. Assessment and treatment planning of the suicidal child or adolescent is first and foremost an issue of **safety.** Ensuring the child's **survival** is the major clinical consideration. If safety cannot be reasonably assured, then hospitalization is the treatment of choice. Hospitalization should provide temporary respite from overwhelming stress and mood. Of note, however, very young children, even with inadequate parental supervision, often have difficulty with the separation involved in psychiatric hospitalization. Psychiatric hospitals generally do not allow parents to stay overnight with their children. This consideration must factor into the decision as well. If a safe alternative to hospitalization is available in your community (such as a crisis intervention team), consider it for the preadolescent.

A. **Watching**
    1. **When to watch**
        a. Suicidal ideation absent
        b. One risk factor (see pages 419–420) is present, but:
            (1) Child has never attempted to hurt self before
            (2) No history of severe, persistent depression
            (3) No evidence of psychosis or gross loss of contact with reality, hallucinations, delusions, and so on
            (4) No substance abuse (i.e., more than the normal adolescent experimentation with alcohol and marijuana)
            (5) No legal involvement or symptoms of conduct disorder
            (6) No evidence of sexual or physical abuse (child denies, family seems functional and supportive)
        c. No precipitating, current, severe emotional crisis
        d. Relationship between the child and PCP is strong
        e. Family is supportive and concerned
    2. **When watching**
        a. **Psychoeducation** for the child and parents about the risk factors and warning signs of lethality. It is imperative that parents take a concerned and empathic view of the child at risk. These children should not be seen as "bad" for being suicidal, but as someone requiring adult help and intervention. Describing a child's suicidal thoughts or acts as "manipulative" is rarely helpful and generally serves to further isolate the youth and increase his or her desperation and hopelessness. It is also critical to reinforce the need for communication, especially about suicidal thoughts or plans. Although talking about suicidal feelings is scary, it allows parents to (a) remain in contact with their child, (b) decrease the sense of isolation and shame of the child, and (c) take necessary actions on behalf of the child. Parents should be reassured that talking about it will not precipitate a violent act if they take an understanding approach.
        b. **Advocacy** with the schools usually is not necessary at this stage, unless an uniden-

tified learning disability or issue has been recognized by the PCP.

c. **Psychotherapy** is indicated for treatment of the underlying psychiatric condition and prevention of the development of suicidal behaviors .

d. **Medications** may be indicated for identified psychiatric conditions (e.g., depression, anxiety disorder, attention-deficit/ hyperactivity disorder).

e. **Laboratory and other evaluations** are not necessary unless comorbid medical conditions (e.g., diabetes mellitus) exist.

f. **Monitoring.** Follow-up appointment with the PCP in 2 to 4 months to monitor the progress of the patient, whether suicidal thoughts have emerged, and whether more aggressive treatment is indicated. If referral has taken place, then the PCP should inquire to make sure the family has followed through.

B. **Intervening further**
1. **When to intervene further**
   a. Child has one or more risk factors present (see pages 419–420)
   b. Suicidal ideation of low lethality
   c. Suicide gesture of fairly low lethality (such as minor overdose but without expressed intent)
   d. Cutting behavior
   e. Family is supportive and concerned
2. **When intervening further**
   a. **Psychoeducation**
      (1) Review of risk factors and warning signs
      (2) The pediatrician, child, and family also need to develop a **safety plan.** This consists of four components:
         (a) Encouraging concerned **monitoring** of the child by the family. Not all families are able to do this without fueling the situation. If this is the case, the child must be referred to a qualified child mental health professional.
         (b) Assist the child to develop a hierarchy of others to contact (parent, then other parent, then grandmother, and so on) and alternative activities (exercising, writing, and so on) should suicidal impulses arise.

(c) Educating the family about **emergency resources** (e.g., crisis services, psychiatric emergency programs, police). This includes giving them the phone numbers to contact these services.

(d) **Removal of access to lethal means.** The family must be instructed to do whatever is necessary to prevent the child from gaining access to medications and especially to guns. This may mean removing them from the premises. Frequently "locking them up" is insufficient and an invitation for a future problem.

b. **Advocacy** to assure child has access to school personnel (i.e., social worker, psychologist) who can monitor child and be available for support in crisis situations.

c. **Psychotherapy.** Referral to qualified child mental health professional for consultation or collaborative treatment.

d. **Medications.** Any suicidality in the context of an ongoing psychiatric condition is reason to consider medications. This is especially so if patient and family have received more than 3 months of psychotherapy treatment without significant improvement.

e. **Laboratory and other evaluations** are indicated only for concomitant medical conditions. No specific laboratory tests or imaging techniques are useful at this time in the evaluation of the suicidal child or adolescent.

f. **Monitoring.** Follow-up. The PCP should telephone the child and family the day following the contact. This tells children that the physician and, by extension, other adults in their life are concerned. Have the child return to the office in 4 to 6 weeks to monitor suicidality, medications, and assure mental health follow-up. **Patients who have been significantly depressed and continue to demonstrate suicidal thoughts or impulses are at higher risk for suicidal behavior when their depression begins to improve.** Improvement in symptoms of depression can lead family and treatment team members to lower their suspicion and vigilance about suicide at a time when the patient is gaining the energy to act on previous plans. Be aware of this risk and monitor patients with significant depression and suicidal thought very closely during the recovery period.

C. Referring

1. **When to refer and transfer primary responsibility**
   a. Two or more risk factors present
   b. Suicidal ideation is persistent or lethality is moderate or high
   c. Attempt of moderate lethality
   d. Repeated cutting behaviors
   e. Family is unable to positively support the child or the treatment effort

2. **When referring.** When the PCP has decided that the child is not safe at home or in the community, then **the referral must be to an emergency program.** In that case, help the parents call the ambulance, if needed, as well as call the emergency room to provide collateral information to the evaluating psychiatrist. Although hospitalization may be necessary, many communities have available other high-intensity outpatient-based programs for seriously suicidal youth. Most PCPs will not be up to date with program availability and so it is best to refer these children to psychiatric emergency services, which will be able to assess and make the most appropriate referral. Examples of youth needing this level of service include (but are not limited to):

   1. Depressed youth with expressed intent to die and a specific plan
   2. Suicidal youth unwilling or unable to commit themselves to asking for help if they feel the urge to hurt themselves
   3. Depressed youth with a history of substance misuse or abuse who voice suicidal ideation and experience an acute stressor that could precipitate action (see page 421)
   4. Conduct-disordered youth with a history of substance misuse or abuse who experience an acute stressor
   5. Youth who make a suicide attempt and continue to express intent, or show moderate to high inferred intent, or no identifiable reason to live

   If the situation is not so acute as to need emergency measures, the PCP should provide the following care:

   a. **Psychoeducation**
      (1) Reemphasis of the need to secure all lethal means

           (2) Reeducate parents about warning signs of immediate dangerousness (e.g., giving away possessions, agitation, abrupt change in mood or behavior)

  b. **Advocacy** with the schools will probably be handled by the mental health professional involved in the case. Supporting letters or telephone calls from the PCP may be necessary to secure educational modifications and resources for the child or adolescent. In general, suicidal children should be encouraged to attend school. Being unable to do so may suggest that the child is debilitated sufficiently and that hospitalization is indicated.

  c. **Psychotherapy**

      (1) If not already done, all children at this stage should be referred to a qualified child mental health professional for ongoing treatment. If this referral is to a psychologist, an evaluation by a child and adolescent psychiatrist is also indicated to address the need for hospitalization and use of medications.

      (2) Child should be seen in psychotherapy at least once per week during the acute phase of treatment.

      (3) Continuation of mental health treatment for a **minimum of 6 months**.

      (4) Psychodynamic and cognitive-behavioral approaches are used most commonly.

      (5) Families must be involved in the psychotherapy of suicidal children and adolescents, although individual therapy is also critical. Group therapy, if available, may also be helpful.

      (6) For maximal support, the PCP and mental health professional should be in contact and share information freely (with the written consent of the child and family.)

  d. **Medications** are indicated for underlying psychiatric conditions (see below).

  e. **Laboratory and other evaluations** are indicated only for concomitant medical conditions. No specific laboratory tests or imaging techniques are useful at this time in the evaluation of the suicidal child or adolescent.

f. Monitoring.
   (1) Immediate monitoring to assure that the family has made and kept the first appointment, which can be done by telephone
   (2) Ongoing phone monitoring between the PCP and family to assure follow through with treatment
   (3) Return to PCP's office within 1 month
   (4) Once mental health treatment is well under way, follow-up with the PCP can be extended to 6 to 8 weeks, or longer.

IV. Practical use of medications. No medications are specifically used to treat suicidality *per se*. The general principle is to treat any underlying psychiatric conditions. Most commonly, this will be depression. Because of their lethality in overdose, tricyclic antidepressants are best avoided in suicidal youth. In addition to their efficacy, the relative safety of the selective serotonin reuptake inhibitors and newer antidepressants (i.e., venlafaxine, nefazodone, mirtazapine, and bupropion) in overdose make them the treatment of first choice in this population. For additional information on their usage, see Chapter 16. A child and adolescent psychiatrist generally best manages the psychopharmacologic treatment of psychotic, bipolar, or seriously conduct-disordered youth who are suicidal.

V. Summary. The PCP will be called on to evaluate children and adolescents who are exhibiting life-threatening behaviors. This is a grave and serious task, which **can be accomplished.** The PCP who has a good relationship with patients and their families and a solid knowledge of the risk factors for suicide, and who practices the techniques of the lethality assessment set forth in this chapter, can make informed decisions in situations of danger. The most important issue must always be the **safety** of the child or adolescent in distress.

SUGGESTED READINGS

American Academy of Pediatrics, Committee on Adolescence. Suicide and suicide attempts in adolescents and young adults. *Pediatrics* 2000;105:871–874.

American Academy of Child and Adolescent Psychiatry. Practice parameter for the assessment and treatment of children and adolescents with suicidal behavior. *J Am Acad Child Adolesc Psychiatry* 2001; 40(7 suppl): 4S–23S.

Bell C, Clark D. Adolescent suicide. *Pediatr Clin North Am* 1998; 45(2):365–379.

Greenhill L, Waslick B. Management of suicidal behavior in children and adolescents. *Psychiatr Clin North Am* 1997;20(3):641–666.

Jellinek M, Snyder J. Depression and suicide in children and adolescents. *Pediatr Rev* 1998;19(8):255–264.

Shaffer D, Garland A, Gould M, et al. Preventing teenage suicide: a critical review. *J Am Acad Child Adolesc Psychiatry* 1988;27(6):675–687.

Web Sites

American Academy of Pediatrics: Information on Suicide. Available at www.aap.org/visit/suicideinfo.htm. Accessed on 6/29/02.

American Association of Suicidology. Available at www.suicidology.org. Accessed on 6/29/02.

Compassionate Friends (for families who are grieving a child's death). Available at www.compassionatefriends.org. Accessed on 6/29/02.

Suicidology Web (for parents, teens, and professionals). Available at www.suicide-parasuicide.rumos.com. Accessed on 6/29/02.

Survivors of Suicide (for those grieving suicide of a loved one). Available at www.survivorsofsuicide.com. Accessed on 6/29/02.

Appendix Abbreviations

ACE, angiotensin-converting enzyme
AD/HD, attention-deficit/hyperactivity disorder
ALT, alanine transaminase
AST, aspartate transaminase
b.i.d., twice daily
BP, blood pressure
BUN, blood urea nitrogen
caps, capsules
CBC, complete blood count
CNS, central nervous system
ECG, electrocardiogram
EEG, electroencephalogram
EPSE, extra-pyramidal side effects
FDA, Food and Drug Administration
GI, gastrointestinal
H/O, history of
HR, heart rate
h.s., at bedtime
IM, intramuscularly
INH, isoniazid
LFT, liver function tests
MAOI, monoamine oxidase inhibitor
MPH, methylphenidate
MR, mental retardation
MR/DD, mental retardation and development disabilities
NMS, neuroleptic malignant syndrome
NSAID, nonsteroidal antiinflammatory drug
OCD, obsessive-compulsive disorder
OD, overdose
PR, pulse rate
p.r.n., as needed
PTSD, posttraumatic stress disorder
q.d., every day
q4h, every four hours
q.h.s., every night
q.i.d., four times daily
SIADH, syndrome of inappropriate antidiuretic hormone secretion
SL, sublingually
SR, sustained release
SSRI, serotonin reuptake inhibitor
T½, half-life
tabs, tablets
TCA, tricyclic antidepressant
TFTs, thyroid function tests
t.i.d., three times a day
TTS, transdermal transport system
U/A, urinalysis
VPA, valproic acid
XR, extended release

Medication Appendices

Medication Appendices

Specific Medications	Appendix
Alprazolam	Appendix E
Bupropion	Appendix F
Buspirone	Appendix G
Carbamazepine	Appendix H
Chlorpromazine	Appendix C
Citalopram	Appendix N
Clomipramine	Appendix P
Clonazepam	Appendix E
Clonidine	Appendix A
Dextroamphetamine	Appendix O
Diphenhydramine	Appendix B
Divalproex	Appendix Q
Fluoxetine	Appendix N
Fluvoxamine	Appendix N
Gabapentin	Appendix I
Guanfacine	Appendix A
Haloperidol	Appendix C
Hydroxyzine	Appendix B
Imipramine	Appendix P
Lithium	Appendix J
Lorazepam	Appendix E
Methylphenidate	Appendix O
Mirtazapine	Appendix K
Nefazodone	Appendix L
Nortriptyline	Appendix P
Olanzapine	Appendix D
Paroxetine	Appendix N
Pemoline	Appendix O
Pimozide	Appendix C
Propranolol	Appendix M
Quetiapine	Appendix D
Risperidone	Appendix D
Sertraline	Appendix N
Thioridazine	Appendix C
Trifluoperazine	Appendix C
Valproate	Appendix Q
Venlafaxine	Appendix R

Classes of Medications	Appendix
Alpha$_2$-adrenergic agonists	Appendix A
Antihistamines	Appendix B
Antipsychotics	Appendix C
Atypical antipsychotics	Appendix D
Benzodiazepines	Appendix E
SSRIs	Appendix N
Stimulants	Appendix O
Tricyclic antidepressants	Appendix P

Appendices

Appendix A ♣ Alpha₂-Adrenergic Agonists

Preparations	Clonidine: Catapres 0.1, 0.2, 0.3 mg tabs; TTS-1,2,3 (transdermal patch) delivering 0.1, 0.2, 0.3 mg/d for 5–7 days Guanfacine: Tenex 1, 2 mg tabs
Use	Tourette's syndrome AD/HD (second or third line) PTSD Sleep disturbance (may be combined with methylphenidate) Aggression Nicotine or opiate withdrawal
Relative contraindications	Depression Cardiac conduction delays
Common side effects	Sedation (less with guanfacine) Hypotension Lowered pulse and cardiac output Headache GI upset Dry mouth
Warnings	Rebound hypertension with abrupt withdrawal; always **taper when discontinuing** Rare cases of sudden death reported
Significant drug interactions	CNS depressants Anticholinergics Beta-blockers
Physical examination and laboratory	BP, pulse Weight
Metabolism	Hepatic (50%) and renal T½: 4–6 h in children, 8–12 h in adolescents
Dosing	Clonidine: Initial 0.05 mg h.s., then increase by 0.05 mg q3d until clinical effect reached or 0.1 mg t.i.d.–q.i.d. (maximum 0.4 mg/d total) Clonidine transdermal patch: Initial TTS-1 for 5 d; if necessary, increase to TTS-2 for 5 d; if necessary, increase to TTS-3 Guanfacine: Initial 0.5 mg q.d. for 4 d, then increase by 0.5 mg q4d, given in b.i.d.–t.i.d.; usual dose 1.5 mg/d, maximum 4 mg/d

Appendix B ♣ Antihistamines

Preparations	Diphenhydramine (Benadryl): 25, 50 mg tabs; elixir 25 mg/5 mL
	Hydroxyzine (Vistaril): 25, 50, 100 caps; suspension 25 mg/5 mL
Use	Sleep onset insomnia (short-term use only)
	Agitation
	Extrapyramidal symptoms
Relative contraindications	Hypersensitivity
	Asthma
Common side effects	Sedation
	Agitation and paradoxical excitation
	Anticholinergic
	GI upset
Long-term considerations	May reduce seizure threshold
Significant drug interactions	CNS depressants
	Medications with anticholinergic effect
Physical examination and laboratory	None needed
Metabolism	Hepatic
	$T\frac{1}{2}$: 1–4 h (adults)
Dosing	Children 25–50 mg h.s. or q6h p.r.n. agitation
	Adolescents 50–100 mg h.s. or q6h p.r.n. agitation

Appendix C ♣ Antipsychotics (Traditional)

Preparations	Chlorpromazinc (Thorazine): 10, 25, 50, 100, 200 mg tabs; concentrate 10 mg/5 mL; suppository; parenteral
	Haloperidol (Haldol): 0.5, 1, 2, 5, 10, 20 mg tabs; concentrate 2 mg/mL; parenteral
	Pimozide (Orap): 2 mg tabs
	Thioridazine (Mellaril): 10, 25, 50, 100, 150, 200 mg tabs; concentrate 30, 100 mg/5 mL; elixir
	Trifluoperazine (Stelazine): 1, 2, 5, 10 mg tabs; concentrate 10 mg/mL; parenteral
Use	Psychosis (hallucinations, delusions, gross loss of touch with reality)
	Severe aggression (including in MR/DD population)
	Tourette's syndrome
	Cyclic vomiting
Relative contraindications	Hypersensitivity
	CNS depression
	Previous NMS
	Seizure disorders
	Cardiac conduction defects (especially thioridazine, pimozide)
	Blood dyscrasia
Common side effects (Table A.2)	Anticholinergic (low potency)
	EPSE (high potency)
	Sedation (low potency)
	Orthostatic hypotension (low potency)
	Weight gain
	Photosensitivity (low potency worse)
	Gynecomastia
Warnings	Tardive dyskinesia
	NMS
	Lowers seizure threshold
	Retinopathy (Thioridazine)
	Thioridazine now carries FDA black box warning re QT prolongation; use restricted to refractory schizophrenia

Significant drug interactions	CNS depressants
	Anticholinergics (low potency)
	Alpha-blockers (in low potency)
Physical examination and laboratory	Baseline: Weight, BP, pulse
	Signs of movement disorder at baseline, and q3mo
Metabolism	Hepatic P450 IID6
	t½: Generally 24 h
Dosing	Table A.1

Table A.1. Traditional and atypical antipsychotics: dose equivalence and dosing

Medication	Dose Equivalency	Child Dosing: Aggression	Adolescent Dosing: Aggression	Child Dosing: Psychosis	Adolescent Dosing: Psychosis
Older agents					
Chlorpromazine	100	Initial: 10–25 mg; maintenance: 25–50 mg b.i.d.	Initial: 25 mg; maintenance: 25–100 mg b.i.d.	Initial: 25 mg; maintenance: 150–300 mg/d as b.i.d.–t.i.d.	Initial: 25–50 mg; maintenance: 100–600 mg/d as b.i.d.–t.i.d.
Haloperidol	2	Initial: 0.25 mg; maintenance 0.5–2 mg/d as q.d.–b.i.d.	Initial: 0.5 mg; maintenance 1–4 mg/d as q.d.–b.i.d.	Initial: 0.5 mg; maintenance 1–6 mg/d as q.d.–b.i.d.	Initial: 0.5 mg; maintenance 2–10 mg/d as q.d.–b.i.d.
Pimozide	1	Not used for this indication	Not used for this indication	Not used for this indication	Not used for this indication
Thioridazine	95	Same as for chlorpromazine	Same as for chlorpromazine	Same as for chlorpromazine	Initial: 25–50 mg; maintenance 100–300 mg/d as b.i.d.–t.i.d.

continued

Table A.1. *Continued*

Medication	Dose Equivalency	Child Dosing: Aggression	Adolescent Dosing: Aggression	Child Dosing: Psychosis	Adolescent Dosing: Psychosis
Trifluoperazine	5	Initial: 1–2 mg; maintenance 2–10 mg/d as b.i.d.	Initial 2 mg; maintenance 5–10 mg/d as b.i.d.	Initial 2 mg; maintenance 2–15 mg/d as b.i.d.	Initial 2 mg; maintenance 5–25 mg/d as b.i.d.
Atypical agents					
Olanzapine	4	Initial: 2.5 mg; maintenance 2.5–7.5 mg/d as q.d.–b.i.d.	Initial: 2.5–5 mg; maintenance 2.5–10 mg/d as q.d.–b.i.d.	Initial: 2.5–5 mg; maintenance 5–10 mg/d as q.d.–b.i.d.	Initial: 5 mg; maintenance 10–20 mg/d as q.d.–b.i.d.
Quetiapine	80	Initial 12.5 mg; maintenance 25–150 mg/d as b.i.d.–t.i.d.	Initial 25 mg; maintenance 50–200 mg/d as b.i.d.–t.i.d.	Initial 25 mg; maintenance 50–250 mg/d as b.i.d.–t.i.d.	Initial 50–100 mg; maintenance 100–600 mg/d as b.i.d.–t.i.d.
Risperidone	1	Initial: 0.25 mg; maintenance 0.5–2 mg/d as q.d.–b.i.d.	Initial: 0.25–0.5 mg; maintenance 0.5–4 mg/d as q.d.–b.i.d.	Initial 0.5 mg; maintenance 1–4 mg/d as q.d.–b.i.d.	Initial 0.5–1 mg; maintenance 1–6 mg/d as q.d.–b.i.d.
Ziprasidone	20	Not established in children	Not established in children	Not established in children	Not established in children

Table A.2. Antipsychotic (Traditional and Atypical Agents) side effect profile comparison

Medication	Sedative Effect	Hypotensive Effect	Anticholinergic Effect	Extrapyramidal Effect	QT Prolongation	Weight Gain
Older agents						
Chlorpromazine	High	High	Medium	Low–medium	+	++
Haloperidol	Low	Low	Low	High	+/–	+
Pimozide	Low	Low	Low	High	++	+
Thioridazine	High	High	High	Low	++	++
Trifluoperazine	Medium	Low	Low	High	+	+
Atypical agents						
Olanzapine	Medium	Medium	Medium	Low	+/–	+++
Quetiapine	Medium	Medium	Low	Low	+/–	+
Risperidone	Low	Medium	Low	Low	+/–	++
Ziprasidone	Low	Low	Low	Low	+/++	+

Based on table in Arana G, Rosenbaum J. *Handbook of psychiatric drug therapy.* Philadelphia: Lippincott Williams & Wilkins, 2000:10–11.

Appendix D ♣ Atypical Antipsychotics

Preparations	Clozapine (Clozaril): 25, 100 mg tabs
	Olanzapine (Zyprexa): 2.5, 5, 7.5, 10, 15, 20 mg tabs (also 5, 10, 15, 20 mg dissolving Zydis tabs)
	Quetiapine (Seroquel): 25, 100, 200, 300 mg tabs
	Risperidone (Risperdal): 0.25, 0.5, 1, 2, 3, 4 mg; concentrate 1 mg/mL
	Ziprasidone (Geodon): 20, 40, 60, 80 mg caps
Use	Psychosis
	Mania
	Schizophrenia
	Tourette's syndrome
	Severe aggression
	Agitation in delirium
	Pervasive developmental disorder
Contraindications	Allergy
	History of NMS
	Tardive dyskinesia
Common side effects (Table A.1)	Sedation
	Weight gain (can be substantial)
	Elevated prolactin and gynecomastia (most with Risperidone, least Quetiapine)
	Constipation
Warnings	NMS: Risk thought to be less than conventional antipsychotics
	Extrapyramidal side effects (akathisia, Parkinsonian-like symptoms, dystonia): Risk much less than conventional antipsychotics
	Tardive dyskinesia: Risk thought to be much lower than conventional antipsychotics
	Glucose intolerance
	Increased LFTs can occur
	QT prolongation can occur (more likely with ziprasidone, perhaps risperidone)
	Clozaril associated with seizures and agranulocytosis and requires utilization of distribution system available only through Novartis Pharmaceuticals; CBC required q1wk for first 6 mo, then q2wk for duration of treatment

Significant drug interactions	Metabolized by P4502D6; any drug that inhibits (e.g., SSRIs, quinidine) would increase level; carbamazepine may decrease levels Potentiates CNS depressants
Physical examination and laboratory	Baseline: Height, weights, BP, pulse, CBC with differential, LFTs, observe for abnormal movements; ECG for clozaril, ziprasidone, risperidone with repeat after maintenance dose achieved, then q6–12 mo Follow-up: Weight, BP, pulse, LFT, observe for abnormal movements q3–6mo Serum levels: Not clinically useful
Metabolism	Hepatic elimination T½: 24 h
Dosing	Table A.1

Appendix E ♣ Benzodiazepines

Preparations	Alprazolam (Xanax): 0.25, 0.5, 1, 2 mg tabs Clonazepam (Klonopin): 0.5, 1, 2 mg tabs Clorazepate (Tranxene): 3.75, 7.5, 15 mg tabs; 3.75, 7.5 mg caps Lorazepam (Ativan): 0.5, 1, 2 mg tabs; parenteral available Oxazepam (Serax): 10, 15, 30 mg caps
Use	Situational anxiety Seizures Night terrors, somnambulism Panic disorder (second line) Bipolar disorder (clonazepam: second–third line) Generalized anxiety disorder (second line)
Relative contraindications	Pregnancy Substance abuse
Common side effects	Sedation Drowsiness or decreased mental acuity Disinhibition
Warnings	No known irreversible, adverse effects on major organs Withdrawal symptoms seen after long-term use, especially short-acting agents (e.g., alprazolam, lorazepam) **Never stop abruptly; taper by 10% to 25% q7d in patients receiving regular treatment for >2 wk** Use lorazepam or oxazepam in hepatic disease Use with caution in renal disease but alprazolam should be avoided
Significant drug interactions	CNS depressants
Physical examination and laboratory	None required before initiating or during treatment Serum levels not clinically useful
Metabolism	Table A.4
Dosing	Table A.3

Table A.3. Benzodiazepine dosing

Name	Trade Name	Dosage Forms	Alternative Routes	Dosing	Initial Dose	Maintenance Dosage
Alprazolam	Xanax	0.25, 0.5, 1, 2 mg tabs	SL[a]	t.i.d.–q.i.d	Ch: 0.25 mg Adol: 0.25–0.5	Ch: 0.25–2 mg/d Adols: 0.75–4 mg/d
Clonazepam	Klonopin	0.5, 1, 2 mg tabs	None	q.d.–b.i.d.	Ch: 0.125 mg Adol: 0.25	Ch: 0.25–1 mg/d Adols: 0.5–2 mg/d
Diazepam	Valium	2, 5, 10 mg tabs		q.d.–b.i.d.	Ch: 1 mg Adols: 1–2 mg	Ch: 1–10 mg/d Adols: 2–20 mg
Lorazepam	Ativan	0.5, 1, 2 mg tabs	IM, SL[a]	b.i.d.–t.i.d.	Ch: 0.25–0.5 mg Adols: 0.5–1.0 mg	Ch: 0.25–3 mg/d Adols: 0.5–6 mg/d

SL, sublingual; IM, intramuscularly; Ch, children; Adol, adolescents.
[a] SL route may be easier than swallowing for children and provide for more rapid onset.

Table A.4.   Benzodiazepine dosage equivalency and pharmacokinetics

Medication	Dosage Equivalency	Onset of Effect after Oral Dose[a]	Half-life[a]
Alprazolam	0.5 mg	Intermediate	9–20 h
Clonazepam	0.25 mg	Intermediate	20–60 h
Diazepam	5 mg	Rapid	20–70 h (double for metabolites)
Lorazepam	1 mg	Intermediate	8–24 h (no active metabolite)
Oxazepam	15 mg	Intermediate	8 h (no active metabolite)

[a] Not well studied in children; these approximates based on studies in adults.
Based on table in Arana G, Rosenbaum J. *Handbook of psychiatric drug therapy.*
Philadelphia: Lippincott Williams & Wilkins, 2000: 176.

Appendix F ♣ Bupropion

Preparations	Wellbutrin 75, 100 mg tabs; 100 (blue dye), 150 mg (contains red dye) SR tabs
Use	Major depression AD/HD Smoking cessation in adults
Relative contraindications	Seizure disorder History of substance abuse (increased risk of seizures) Bulimia or anorexia nervosa (increased risk of seizures) MAOI exposure within past 2 wk Hypersensitivity (especially the 150 mg SR tab; in this case 100 mg SR can be used)
Common side effects	Nausea Agitation and anxiety Insomnia Decreased appetite No weight gain, cardiac, sexual side effects
Warnings	**Risk of seizures higher than other antidepressants, stimulants** Psychotic symptoms may occur. Can cause manic "switch" in predisposed patients, although less likely than other antidepressants
Significant drug interactions	MAOI
Physical examination and laboratory	Height, weight, BP, pulse baseline and q3–6mo
Metabolism	Hepatic (causes some inhibition of P450 IID6) $T\frac{1}{2}$: 10–21 h in adults, unknown in children; given as b.i.d. (adolescents)–t.i.d. (prepubertal)
Dosing	Children: Initial 75 mg q.d. for 7 days, then increase to 75 mg b.i.d. for 7 days; then 100 mg SR b.i.d. and hold for 4 weeks; if no response, increase to maximum 150 mg SR b.i.d. (dosing for AD/HD generally lower) Adolescents: Initial 100 mg SR q.d. for 7 days, then increase to 100 mg SR b.i.d. for 7 days and hold for 4 weeks; further increases by 100 mg q5–7d with maximum total of 400 mg/d for depression (no single dose greater than 200 mg); total 300 mg/d (or 6 mg/kg/d, whichever is lower) for AD/HD.

Appendix G ♣ Buspirone

Preparations	Buspar 5, 10 mg tabs
Uses	Generalized anxiety disorder (second line) May help with temper or aggression in MR/DD, neurologically impaired population Augmentation in OCD Augmentation in major depressive disorder
Contraindications	Hypersensitivity MAOI exposure
Common side effects	Generally no difference from placebo Restlessness
Warnings	May see substantial latency of response (6–8 wk) No major organ (including cardiac) side effects
Significant drug interactions	None reported Grapefruit juice may increase levels
Physical examination and laboratory	None necessary
Metabolism	Hepatic elimination with multiple active metabolites T½: Variable, 1–10 h; clinical effect in 2–3 wk
Dosing	Initial: 5 mg test dose; then 5 mg t.i.d. and hold in children; in adolescents increase to 10 mg t.i.d. after 3–7 d; increases thereafter based on clinical response Maintenance: Children 5–10 mg t.i.d., maximum 45 mg/d; adolescents 10–15 mg t.i.d., maximum 60 mg/d

Appendix H ♣ Carbamazepine

Preparations	Carbatrol 200, 300 mg XR tabs
	Tegretol 100, 200 mg chewable tabs;
	   200 mg tab; 100, 200, 400 mg XR tabs;
	   suspension (100 mg/5 mL)

Uses	Partial complex seizures Bipolar disorder Aggression (especially with CNS compro- mise, developmental disability, and so on) Trigeminal neuralgia (rare in children)
Relative contraindications	Liver or renal disease Blood dyscrasia Pregnancy
Common side effects	Sedation Nausea, vomiting Cognitive dysfunction (i.e., memory, concen- tration, motor speed) Lightheadedness Weight gain Blurred vision and yellow-blue color defect Leukopenia
Warnings	Agranulocytosis Hepatotoxicity Stevens-Johnson syndrome (risk highest first 8 wk) SIADH Teratogenicity

Significant drug
  interactions
  (induces P450 3A4)
	Lowers levels of: Birth control pills, TCAs,
	   SSRIs, antipsychotics, erythromycin,
	   theophylline, T_4 and T_3, acetaminophen
	Raises levels of valproate
	Levels of carbamazepine raised by anti-
	   psychotics, TCAs, SSRIs, methyl-
	   phenidate, cimetidine, erythromycin,
	   clarithromycin

Physical examination
  and laboratory
	Baseline: Height, weight, CBC with differ-
	   ential, LFTs, BUN, and creatinine
	Follow-up: 5 d after each dose increase
	   check serum level (12 h after last dose);
	   q3–6mos: serum level, CBC with differ-
	   ential, LFT

Metabolism	Hepatic; autoinduction leads to increased dosing requirements after 2–6 wk T½: 12 h

Dosing	Initial: 100 mg b.i.d. in children, 200 mg b.i.d. in adolescents; then increase by 100–200 mg/d q5–7d
	Maintenance: 10–20 mg/kg/d; in children: 300–800 mg/d as t.i.d.; in adolescents: 800–1000 mg/d as b.i.d.–t.i.d.; Serum levels 4–14 µg/mL

Appendix I ♣ Gabapentin

Preparations	Neurontin 100, 300, 400, 800 mg caps
Use	Bipolar II disorder (possible)
	Severe mood instability (possible)
Contraindications	Hypersensitivity
Common side effects	Sedation
	Enuresis
	Headache
	Agitation and hyperactivity
	Dizziness
Warnings	Can cause extrapyramidal side effects
	Aggression
	No cardiac, renal, hepatic toxicity
Significant drug interactions	None clinically significant
Physical examination and laboratory	Routine medical monitoring; nothing specific necessary for this medication
Metabolism	Renal (excreted unchanged)
	T½: 5–7 h in adults; probably shorter in children
Dosing	In adolescents, start at 300 mg h.s.; increase by 300 mg q3–5d
	Therapeutic dosing 300–1800 mg/d as t.i.d. divided dose

Appendix J ♣ Lithium

Preparations	Lithium carbonate: Eskalith 150, 300, 600 mg caps, 450 mg coated tab (SR); Lithobid 300 coated tab (SR) Lithium citrate syrup 300 mg/5 mL
Use	Bipolar disorders Impulsive aggressivity (including developmentally disabled, conduct disorder) Augmentation to antidepressants in adult and adolescent major depression Severe affective instability (proposed use)
Relative contraindications	Renal impairment Seizure disorders Hypothyroid Breastfeeding Pregnancy Cardiovascular disease (sick sinus syndrome) Leukemia Severe acne Disorders of bone formation
Common side effects	Tremor Polyuria and polydipsia Worsening of acne Nausea, abdominal discomfort, and diarrhea Fatigue, lethargy, cognitive dulling Weight gain Leukocytosis Antithyroid effect and hypothyroidism
Warnings	**Narrow margin of safety requires close monitoring; lethal in overdose** **Toxicity:** Increased tremor, nausea, tremor, followed by ataxia, lethargy, delirium, seizures, coma **Dehydration and excessive sweating can precipitate toxicity** Lowers seizure threshold Renal risks with long-term use are slight and generally insignificant in adults but could be different with children Theoretically, could decrease bone density

Significant drug interactions	NSAID (aspirin OK) increase lithium (Li) level Diuretics increase Li level Metronidazole increases Li level Marijuana increases Li level Antipsychotics increase Li level ACE inhibitors increase Li level Tetracycline increases Li level "Taco tantrums" (i.e., high salt meals) and caffeine/xanthines **decrease** Li levels
Physical examination and laboratory	Baseline: Height, weight, CBC, creatinine, BUN, U/A, TFTs, SMA-12, electrolytes, pregnancy test ECG (if H/O cardiac or <16 yr) EEG (if clear neurologic signs exist) Serum levels (10–12 h after last dose) should be in 0.5–1.2 range; 7d after each dose change; and then q3–6mo or if clinical status changes Follow-up: CBC, BUN, creatinine, TFTs in 3 mo, then q3–6mo, after stable
Metabolism	Renal elimination $T\frac{1}{2}$: 18 h adolescents, faster in children (given as b.i.d. dosing; occasionally, t.i.d. needed)
Dosing	Children: Initial 150–300 mg q.d. test dose, then increase after 7 days to 150–300 mg b.i.d.0 Hold dose for 7 days and check level. If level subtherapeutic increase dose by 150–300 mg/d and recheck serum level. Once therapeutic level reached, hold dose for 4 weeks. If no response, increase dose by 150–300 mg/d q7d till therapeutic response, side effects occur, or serum level reaches maximum 1.2 mEq/L Adolescents: Initial 300 mg test dose, then increase dose to 300 mg b.i.d.; check level. If level subtherapeutic, then increase by 300 mg/d q7d. Once therapeutic level reached then hold dose for 4 weeks; if no response, increase dose by 300 mg every 7 days until therapeutic response, side effects occur, or serum level reaches a maximum 1.2 mEq/L Sustained release preparations may allow for q.d. dosing in children and adolescents; generally, each 300 mg increase will increase levels 0.2 mEq/L

Appendix K ♣ Mirtazapine

Preparations	Remeron 15, 30, 45 mg tabs
Uses	Depressive disorders Pain disorders
Relative contraindications	MAOI treatment currently or in past 2 wk Hypersensitivity
Common side effects	Sedation (especially at lower doses) Increased appetite and weight gain (first few months) Dizziness Nausea
Warnings	Agranulocytosis (rare, first few months greatest risk) May increase cholesterol May increase ALT No known cardiac risk
Significant drug interactions	Medications that alter P450 metabolism
Physical examination and laboratory	Baseline and follow-up weight, BP No routine laboratory study necessary Serum levels not useful
Metabolism	Hepatic elimination: 2D6, 1A2 T½: 20–40 h in adults
Dosing	Not established in children or adolescents In adults: Start at 15 mg q.h.s., with increases by 15 mg q5–7d, to maximum of 45 mg q.h.s.

Appendix L ♣ Nefazodone

Preparations	Serzone 50, 100, 150, 200, 250 mg tabs
Use	Depression PTSD (second–third line) Social phobia (second–third line)
Contraindications	MAOIs Hypersensitivity
Common side effects	Nausea Sedation Dizziness Dry mouth No weight gain, cardiac, or sexual adverse effects
Warnings	Black box warning concerning hepatotoxicity and liver failure Inhibits P450 IIIA4, (raises levels of benzodiazepines, pimozide, cisapride, astemizole)
Significant drug interactions	As above in *Warnings*
Physical examination and laboratory	Height, weight Monitor LFT
Metabolism	Hepatic elimination T½: 5 h in adults, unknown in children
Dosing	Not well established in children and adolescents In adults, usual starting dose is 50 mg q.h.s. with increases of 50 mg q3–7d, to 450–600 mg given in b.i.d. dosing

Appendix M ♣ Propranolol

Preparations	Inderal 10, 20, 40, 60, 80 mg tabs; 60, 80, 120, 160 mg SR tabs
Uses	Performance anxiety Aggression and rage (especially in developmentally disabled, MR) Akathisia (secondary to antipsychotics)
Contraindications	Asthma Diabetes mellitus Hyperthyroid Cardiac disease Depression
Common side effects	Depression Fatigue Impotence Bradycardia Bronchoconstriction Insomnia Nightmares Congestive heart failure (pre-existing cardiac)
Warnings	Should be tapered when discontinued
Significant drug interactions	MAOI exposure Thyroxine Theophylline Epinephrine
Physical examination and laboratory	BP, pulse
Metabolism	Hepatic elimination T½: 3–6 h
Dosing	Performance anxiety: 10–40 mg 30–45 minutes before performance Aggression: Children: Initial 10–20 mg b.i.d.–t.i.d., then increase by 10 mg b.i.d.–t.i.d. until response or BP <90/60, pulse <50; maximum 400 mg/d total. Adolescents: Initial 20 mg b.i.d.–t.i.d., then increase by 10–20 mg b.i.d.–t.i.d. until response or BP <90/60 or pulse <50; maximum 400–600 mg/d total Usual range 120–240 mg/d

Appendix N ♣ Selective Serotonin Reuptake Inhibitors

Preparations	Citalopram (Celexa): 20, 40 mg tabs; concentrate (2 mg/mL) Fluoxetine (Prozac): 10, 20, 40 mg caps; 10 mg tab; concentrate (20 mg/5 mL); weekly 90 mg cap Fluvoxamine (Luvox): 25, 50, 100 mg tabs Paroxetine (Paxil): 10, 20, 30, 40 tabs; concentrate (10 mg/5 mL) Sertraline (Zoloft): 50, 100 mg tabs; concentrate (20 mg/mL)
Uses	Major depressive disorder Panic disorder OCD Separation anxiety disorder PTSD Social phobia Generalized anxiety disorder Selective mutism Bulimia nervosa Premenstrual dysphoric disorder Ritualistic/stereotyped behaviors in autism-spectrum disorders
Contraindications	MAOI treatment currently or in past 2 weeks Hepatic failure
Common side effects	**Agitation/restlessness/anxiety** (may be severe) Cognitive dulling, amotivational, "spacey" GI upset Diarrhea Sexual dysfunction Insomnia or fatigue/tiredness Decreased appetite (first few days) Weight gain (especially paroxetine; generally not pronounced) Headaches Rash Sweating
Warnings	No known long-term adverse effects on major organs

	Serotonin syndrome: Symptoms resulting from excess serotonin; usually caused by combining with other serotonergic medications (e.g., dextromethorphan, sumatriptan); usually mild to moderate in severity, but can be severe including seizures, coma, and death.
Significant drug interactions	Mediated through P450 inhibition (Tables A.5, A.6)
Physical examination and laboratory	No specific tests before initiating or during treatment Serum levels not clinically useful
Metabolism	Hepatic elimination T½: (Table A.7)
Dosing	Table A.7

Table A.5. P-450 Interactions

P-450 Isoenzyme	Substrates	Documented Inhibitors	Documented Inducers
CYP 1A2	**Acetaminophen**	Cimetidine	Charcoal broiled beef
	Caffeine	**Ciprofloxacin**	**Cigarette smoke**
	Propranolol	Diltiazem	Cruciferous vegetables
	Tacrine	**Enoxacin**	Omeprazole
	Theophylline	Erythromycin (weak)	Phenobarbital
	Tricyclics	Fluoxetine (weak)	Phenytoin
		Fluvoxamine	
		Grapefruit juice	
		Paroxetine (weak)	
		Sertraline (weak)	
		Tacrine	
		Verapamil	
		Zileuton	
CYP 2C9/10	Amitriptyline	Amiodarone	Phenobarbital
	Diclofenac	**Cimetidine**	
	Ibuprofen	Fluconazole	
	Naproxen	Metronidazole	
	Phenytoin	Miconazole	
	Piroxicam	Ritonavir	
	Tolbutamide	Sulfamethoxazole	
	Torsemide	Trimethoprim	
	Warfarin	Zafirlukast	
	Zafirlukast	Zileuton	

continued

Table A.5. Continued

P-450 Isoenzyme	Substrates	Documented Inhibitors	Documented Inducers
CYP 2C18/19	Diazepam Imipramine Lansoprazole **Omeprazole** Pentamidine Phenytoin Propranolol	Felbamate Fluoxetine **Fluvoxamine** Ketoconazole Omeprazole	Phenytoin
CYP 2D6	**Antipsychotics** Captopril Clozapine **Codeine** **Dextromethorphan** **Hydrocodone** Metoprolol Mexiletine Ondansetron Oxycodone Propranolol Quinidine Ritonavir **SSRIs** **Tricyclics** **Venlafaxine**	Amiodarone Cimetidine **Fluoxetine** Fluvoxamine Haloperidol **Paroxetine** Propafenone Quinidine (very strong) Sertraline Thioridazine Tramadol	None identified

	Substrates	Inhibitors	Inducers
CYP 2E1	**Acetaminophen** **Alcohol** Caffeine Chlorzoxazone INH **Theophylline**	Disulfiram INH	Ethanol INH
CYP 3A4/5	**Acetaminophen** Amiodarone Astemizole **Benzodiazepines** Carbamazepine **Cisapride** **Corticosteroids** Cyclosporine Diltiazem Erythromycin **Ethinyl estradiol** Felodipine Lidocaine Lovastatin Nefazodone Nifedipine Propafenone **Quinidine** Ritonavir Sertraline	Bromocriptine Cimetidine **Clarithromycin** Cyclosporine Danazol Diltiazem **Erythromycin** Ergotamine Ethinyl estradiol Fluconazole **Fluoxetine** Fluvoxamine Gestodene **Grapefruit juice** Indinavir Itraconazole Ketoconazole Miconazole Midazolam Nefazodone	**Carbamazepine** Dexamethasone Phenobarbital Phenytoin Rifampin Troglitazone

continued

Table A.5. *Continued*

P-450 Isoenzyme	Substrates	Documented Inhibitors	Documented Inducers
	Simvastatin	Nicardipine	
	Terfenadine	Nifedipine	
	Tricyclics	Omeprazole	
	Verapamil	Paroxetine (weak)	
	Warfarin	Progesterone	
		Propoxyphene	
		Quinidine	
		Ritonavir	
		Sertraline (weak)	
		Testosterone	
		Troleandomycin	
		Verapamil	
		Zafirlukast	
		Zileuton	

Bolded medications are those commonly used.
Adapted from Johnson MD, Newkirk G, White JR Jr. Clinically signficant drug interactions. *Postgrad Med* 1999;105:193–195, 200, 205–206.

Table A.6. Relative effects of SSRI inhibition on P-450 isoenzymes

CYP-450 Isoenzyme	Citalopram	Fluoxetine	Fluvoxamine	Paroxetine	Sertraline
1A2	Unlikely	Unlikely	++	Unlikely	Unlikely
2C9/10	No data	Contradictory	Contradictory	None	None
2C19	No data	++	+++	No data	None
2D6	+	+++	None	+++	+
3A4/5	Unlikely	+	++	Unlikely	Unlikely

Based on table by Preskon S. Clinically relevant pharmacology of SSRIs. *Clin Pharmacokinet* 1997;32 (suppl. 1):1–21.

Table A.7. SSRI dosing in depression and anxiety

Medication	Trade Name	Half-life and Dosing Interval[a]	Initial Dose	Maintenance Dose[b]	Maximum Dose
Citalopram	Celexa	24 h (no active metabolite); q.d.	Ch: 2.5–5 mg Adols: 5–10 mg	Ch: 10–20 mg Adols: 20–40 mg	Ch: 40 mg Adols: 60 mg
Fluoxetine	Prozac	1–3 d (active metabolism 7–9 d); q.d.	Ch: 2.5–5 mg Adols: 5–10 mg	Ch: 10–20 mg Adols: 20 mg	Ch: 40 mg Adols: 60–80 mg
Fluvoxamine	Luvox	14–18 h (no active metab.); q.d.	Ch: 12.5–25 mg Adols: 25–50 mg	Ch: 50–150 mg Adols: 50–200 mg	Ch: 200 mg Adols: 300 mg
Paroxetine	Paxil	20–25 h (no active metab.); q.d.	Ch: 5–10 mg Adols: 10–20 mg	Ch: 10–20 mg Adols: 20–40 mg	Ch: 40 mg Adols: 60 mg
Sertraline	Zoloft	20–28 h (active metabolite 60–70 h); q.d.	Ch: 12.5–25 mg Adols: 25–50 mg	Ch: 50–100 mg Adols: 50–200 mg	Ch: 150 mg Adols: 250 mg

[a] Based on adult studies.
[b] Once lower range of maintenance dose reached, hold for 4 to 6 weeks to check response before further increases. **OCD and bulimia require doses towards the higher ends.**
Ch, children; Adol, adolescents.

Appendix O ♣ Stimulants

Preparations	Dextroamphetamine: (Dexedrine and generics): 5 mg tabs; 5, 10, 15 mg SR caps; concentrate (5 mg/5 mL)
	Mixed salts of d- and l-amphetamine (Adderall): 5, 10, 20, 30 mg tabs; also 10, 20, 30 mg XR caps
	Methylphenidate (Ritalin and generics): 5, 10, 20 mg tabs; 20 mg SR tabs. Concerta (XR) 18, 36, 54 mg tabs. Metadate CD (30% immediate release, 70% XR) 20 mg caps
	Pemoline (Cylert): 18.75, 37.5, 75 mg tabs
Uses	AD/HD
	Narcolepsy
	Target signs of inattention, impulsivity, hyperactivity in autism
	Potentiates narcotic analgesics
Relative contraindications	H/O drug abuse (including family members who may abuse these medications)
	H/O psychosis
	Cardiac diagnosis or hypertension
Common side effects	Decreased appetite
	Insomnia
	Dysphoria
	Stereotypies
	Weight loss
	Irritability
	Abdominal pain or discomfort
	Rebound phenomena at end of day
Warnings	Growth suppression (rarely, clinical significant)
	May worsen Tourette's syndrome or tics
	Tachycardia or hypertension
	Psychosis with hallucinations (unusual)
	Self-biting, picking
	Pemoline: hepatotoxicity and death
Significant drug interactions	Sympathomimetics
	Recreational stimulants (cocaine, amphetamines)
	May inhibit hepatic metab. (TCAs, anti-convulsants)

Physical examination and laboratory	Height, weight baseline and q6mo
	Observe for tics
	BP, pulse
	Cylert: LFT baseline, q2wk for duration of treatment
Metabolism	Hepatic elimination
	T½: Methylphenidate 4–6 h; dextroamphetamine 8–12 h; pemoline > 12 h
	Duration of action: (Table A.8)
Dosing	Table A.8

Table A.8. Summary of stimulant dosing

Medication	Duration of Action	Initial Dose	Maintenance	Maximum
Dextroamphetamine (Dexedrine)	4–7 h	Preschool: 2.5 mg; older: 5 mg	10–30 mg/d as b.i.d.–t.i.d.	40 mg/d total
D, l-Amphetamine (Adderall)	4–7 h; XR 7–12 h	Preschool: 2.5 mg; older: 5 mg	10–30 mg/d as b.i.d.	40 mg/d
Methylphenidate	3–5 h	Preschool: 2.5 mg; older: 5 mg	10–40 mg/d as b.i.d.–t.i.d.	60 mg/d total
Methylphenidate extended release (Concerta)	>12 h with peaks at 1–2, 6–8 h (must be swallowed whole)	Not recommended <6 yr; older children 18 mg q.d.	18–54 mg q.d.	72 mg q.d.
Methylphenidate extended release (Metadate)	7–10 h; peaks at 1.5, 4.5 h (must be swallowed whole)	Not used in preschoolers; school age: 20 mg q.d.	20–40 mg q.d.	60 mg q.d.
Pemoline (Cylert)	8–12 h	Not used in preschoolers; older children 18.75 mg	37.5–112.5 mg/d as q.d.	150 mg/d

Appendix P ♣ Tricyclic Antidepressants

Preparations	Clomipramine (Anafranil): 25, 50, 75 mg caps
	Imipramine (Tofranil and generics):
	   10, 25, 50 mg tabs; 75, 100, 125,
	   150 mg caps
	Nortriptyline (Pamelor and generics):
	   10, 25, 50, 75 mg tabs; concentrate
	   10 mg/5 mL

Use	Enuresis AD/HD (second line) Separation anxiety disorder Panic disorder PTSD OCD (clomipramine only) Trichotillomania (clomipramine only) Bulimia (second line) Chronic pain
Relative contraindications	Cardiac conduction disorders Family history of sudden death Schizophrenia Currently on MAOI History of seizure
Common side effects	Sedation Anticholinergic (clomipramine most) Tachycardia Hypotension (nortriptyline least) Weight gain
Warnings	**Cardiac conduction defect and deaths reported on desipramine** Seizures Sexual dysfunction Withdrawal (not dangerous, but should be tapered off) Cholinergic with rebound Lethal in OD

Significant drug
interactions
	Oral contraceptive pills increase levels
	Additive with anticholinergics and CNS
	   depressants
	Smoking may decrease levels
	Use with MAOIs is potentially life-
	   threatening

Physical examination and laboratory	Heart rate, BP
	Height, weight
	ECG at baseline and then 3 d after each dose increase over 2.5 mg/kg, then q6–12months; discontinue if: PR >200 msec; QRS >120 Msec; QTc > 460 Msec; resting pulse > 120
	Serum levels can be helpful for imipramine, nortriptyline in depression
Metabolism	Hepatic elimination
	$T\frac{1}{2}$: (Table A.9)
Dosing	Table A.9

Table A.9. Tricyclic dosing

Condition	Medication	Initial	Maintenance	Maximum
AD/HD	Imipramine	Ch: 10 mg Adols: 25 mg	50–150 mg as b.i.d.	3 mg/kg
	Nortriptyline	Ch: 10 mg Adols: 25 mg	50–100 mg as b.i.d.	2 mg/kg
OCD	Clomipramine	Ch: 10 mg Adols: 10–25 mg	Ch: 75–150 mg as b.i.d. Adols: 100–200 mg as q.d.–b.i.d.	5 mg/kg
Enuresis	Imipramine	Ch: 10 mg Adols: 25 mg	Ch: 25–75 mg Adols: 50–100 mg	3 mg/kg

Adols, adolescents; Ch, children.

Appendix Q ♣ Valproate/ Divalproex Sodium

Preparations	Divalproex sodium (Depakote): 125, 250, 500 mg caps; sprinkles 125 mg cap Valproic acid (Depakene or generic): 250 mg caps; suspension 250 mg/5 mL
Use	Bipolar I disorder Impulsive aggressivity (including conduct disorder, MR/DD populations) Intermittent explosive disorder Severe affective lability Migraine headaches
Relative contraindications	Hepatic disease Pregnancy Ovarian disease Allergy Thrombocytopenia
Common side effects	GI distress (nausea, vomiting, abdominal discomfort) Weight gain Fatigue, sedation, cognitive slowing Tremor Hair loss Menstrual irregularities
Warnings	**Hepatotoxicity** (risk in first 4 mo of initiating treatment or increase dose); may be primed by L-carnitine deficiency, which develops in 5% of children after 1 yr on valproate; elevated risk if younger (<10 yr), MR/brain damaged, polypharmacy Agranulocytosis (highest risk in first 5 wk) **Pancreatitis** (may be fatal) Polycystic ovarian disease (may be related to weight gain) Teratogenicity risk in pregnancy (assure folate supplementation)
Significant drug interactions (primarily by alteration of P450 effects)	Antipsychotics, SSRIs, erythromycin, clarithromycin, cimetidine, salicylates methylphenidate increase VPA levels Carbamazepine, phenytoin, rifampin decrease VPA levels VPA decreases levels of birth control pills, benzodiazepines, antipsychotics, TCAs, T4 and T3

Physical examination and laboratory	Baseline: Height, weight, CBC with differential, LFTs, history of menstrual irregularities and hirsutism; in first 4 mo of treatment LFTs should be repeated q1mo
	Follow-up: >10 yr of age: Height, weight, CBC with differential, LFT q3–6mos; ≤10 yr of age q1–2mos; Follow more closely if AST or ALT >100 IU/L; discontinue if AST >200 or ALT >150
Metabolism	Hepatic elimination
	T½: Variable, 8–20 h; clinical effect lasts at least 24 h
Dosing	Initially 125–250 mg q.d. (adolescents 250 mg b.i.d.); after 7 days increase by 125–250 mg; check level; if subtherapeutic increase by 125–250 mg and recheck level in 7 days; once therapeutic level reached hold dose for 4–6 weeks before further increases; maximum 2400 mg/d total; dosing b.i.d.–t.i.d.
	Serum levels after each dose change and then q3–6mos; checked after 7 d on a dose; 12 h after last dose
	Therapeutic levels generally 50–100 µg/mL for seizure disorders, but 50–125 for psychiatric use

Appendix R ♣ Venlafaxine

Preparations	Effexor XR: 37.5, 75, 150 mg caps
	Effexor: 25, 37.5, 50, 75, 100 mg tabs
Use	Major depression
	AD/HD (third line)
	Generalized anxiety disorder (adults, possibly in children)
Contraindications	Hypertension
	Hypersensitivity
	MAOI exposure
Common side effects	Nausea
	Increased appetite (usually mild)
	Activation, agitation
	Anxiety and panic
	Insomnia
	Elevated diastolic BP (dose-related)
	Sweating
Warnings	Elevations in BP 5% to 7%
Significant drug interactions	MAOIs
	Any that alters P450 2D6 metabolism
Physical examination and laboratory	Height, weight and BP at baseline and each follow-up visit
Metabolism	Hepatic (P450 2D6) with active metabolite
	$T\frac{1}{2}$: 5 h for parent, 11 h for metabolite; XR is longer
Dosing	XR preparation preferred as it can be given q.d.–b.i.d.; therapeutic range 75–225 mg/d.
	Children: Initial 37.5 mg XR; increase after 7 days to 75 mg XR; hold dose for 4–6 weeks; if no response increase by 37.5 mg XR to maximum 150 mg XR per day (may be lower for anxiety and AD/HD).
	Adolescents: Dosing as for children; maximum to 225 mg XR per day.

PEDIATRIC PSYCHOPHARMACOLOGY BIBLIOGRAPHY
For Practitioners

Arana G, Rosenbaum J. *Handbook of psychiatric drug therapy.* Philadelphia: Lippincott Williams & Wilkins, 2000. This is an excellent, pocket-sized reference book for the clinician wanting "just the facts" about psychopharmacology. Clinically indispensable. Only drawback is mostly oriented to adult treatment; does include much about children and adolescents.

Biological therapies in psychiatry. Sponsored by University of Arizona College of Medicine. This monthly newsletter, which has been published for nearly 20 years, covers adult and pediatric psychopharmacology issues in a timely and thoughtful manner. Excellent for keeping up with the latest.

Brown University child and adolescent psychopharmacology update. This monthly newsletter devoted to pediatric issues is a recent publication that looks promising.

Child and adolescent psychiatric clinics of North America. The January, April 1995, and January 2000 volumes have excellent and recent research-based reviews covering the major topics in pediatric psychopharmacology.

Green W. *Child and adolescent psychopharmacology.* Philadelphia: Lippincott Williams & Wilkins, 2001.

Kutcher S. *Practical child and adolescent psychopharmacology.* Cambridge, UK: Cambridge Press, 2002. This book is written by the editor of *Child and adolescent psychopharmacology,* another monthly newsletter.

Pediatric annals. The April 2001 issue is devoted to pediatric psychopharmacology.

Pediatr Clin North Am. The October 1998 volume is devoted to pediatric psychopharmacology.

Rosenberg D, Holtum J, Gershon S. *Textbook of pharmacotherapy for child and adolescent psychiatric disorders.* New York: Brunner Mazel, 1994. This is an excellent and useful text but is now getting dated. If a new edition comes out, we would expect it to be well done.

Werry J, Aman M. *Practical guide to psychoactive drugs for children and adolescents.* New York: Plenum Press, 1999. A more conservative and cautious view from a New Zealand child psychiatrist. Well done and highly recommended.

For Parents

Dulcan M, Benton T. *Helping parents, youth and teachers understand medications for behavioral and emotional problems: a resource book of medication information handouts.* Washington, DC: American Psychiatric Press, 1999. As advertised, this is a helpful compendium of patient education handouts for youth, parents, and teachers (separate handouts for each). The handouts are well done, current, and ready to use. Comes with a CD-ROM to easily produce the copies you want.

Wilens T. *Straight talk about psychiatric medications for kids.* New York: Guilford Press, 1998. This is a thoughtful, balanced book for the parent who wants more detail than a handout (e.g., the Dulcan book).

Useful Psychopharmacology Related Web Sites

Developmental-Behavioral Pediatrics Online Community. Available at http://www.dbpeds.org/. Accessed on 6/20/02.

Dr. Bob's Psychopharmacology Tips. Available at www.dr-bob.org/tips. Accessed on 6/20/02.

Internet Mental Health. Available at www.mentalhealth.com. Accessed on 6/20/02.

Mental Health Infosource. Available at www.mhsource.com. Accessed on 6/20/02.

Subject Index

References in *italics* indicate figures; those followed by "t" indicate tables